Dr Alan Stewart qualified as a doctor at Guy's Hospital, London, in 1976 and spent five years specialising in hospital medicine. He became a member of the Royal College of Physicians. He worked at the British Homeopathic Hospital in London and qualified as a Member of the Faculty of Homeopathy. For the last eighteen years he has specialised in nutritional medicine and was a founding member of the British Society for Nutritional Medicine. He is also a medical advisor to the Women's Nutritional Advisory Service and is actively involved in educating other doctors on the subject of nutrition. Dr Stewart co-wrote the best-selling books *Nutritional Medicine*, *No More IBS* and *The Vitality Diet*, he wrote *Tired All the Time* and has contributed to other books, including *No More PMS*, *Beat Sugar Craving*, *Inside Science*, *The Migraine Revolution*, *The Sinclair Diet System* and the academic book *Post-Viral Fatigue Syndrome*. He has written several medical papers and regularly gives lectures to doctors, practitioners and health visitors. He has also written articles in both the medical and popular press on various aspects of health and is now the resident doctor for *Healthy Living*. He has contributed to many radio programmes, including BBC *Today* and has appeared on many TV magazine shows, documentaries, including BBC 2's *Healing Arts*, and health debates. He is a keen organic gardener and is also an excellent cook.

Maryon Stewart studied preventive dentistry and nutrition at the Royal Dental Hospital in London and worked as a counsellor with nutritional doctors in England for four years. At the beginning of 1984 she set up the PMT Advisory Service which has subsequently helped thousands of women worldwide. In 1987 she launched the Women's Nutritional Advisory Service which now provides broader help to women of all ages.

Maryon Stewart is the author of the best-selling books *The Zest for Life Plan*, *The Phyto Factor*, *Cruising through the Menopause*, *No More PMS*, now in its third edition, *Beat Sugar Craving* and *Healthy Parents, Healthy Baby*. She is the co-author of *No More IBS*, *Beat PMS Cookbook* and *Every Woman's Health Guide*. She has worked extensively on radio including having her own weekly radio programme on health and nutrition, has co-written several medical papers and has written for many glossy magazines and for the national daily newspapers. She has appeared on many TV programmes on all five channels, and had a regular page in *House & Garden* and *Healthy Eating*, has been both advisor and contributor to *Good Health*, on the expert panel for *Top Santé* and is on the editorial board for *Well Woman*. She was voted one of the most influential women of Great Britain by *Good Housekeeping*. She frequently lectures to both the public and medical profession. She is married to Dr Alan Stewart; they live in Lewes, Sussex, with their four children.

THE
NATURAL
HEALTH
BIBLE

An A–Z guide to drug-free health

Maryon Stewart and
Dr Alan Stewart

VERMILION
LONDON

To Simeon
– fear not, for the world awaits your special skills
with our love

First published in Great Britain in 2001

1 3 5 7 9 10 8 6 4 2

Text © Maryon and Alan Stewart 2001

Maryon and Alan Stewart have asserted their rights to be identified as the authors of this work under the Copyright, Designs and Patent Act 1988.

First published in 2001 by Vermilion
an imprint of Ebury Press
Random House, 20 Vauxhall Bridge Road, London SW1V 2SA

Random House Australia (Pty) Limited
20 Alfred Street, Milsons Point, Sydney, New South Wales 2061, Australia

Random House New Zealand Limited
18 Poland Road, Glenfield, Auckland 10, New Zealand

Random House South Africa (Pty) Limited
Endulini, 5A Jubilee Road, Parktown 2193, South Africa

The Random House Group Limited Reg. No. 954009

www.randomhouse.co.uk

A CIP catalogue record for this book is available from the British Library

ISBN 0 09 185614 0

Papers used by Vermilion are natural, recyclable products made from wood grown in sustainable forests.

Printed and bound in Great Britain by Mackays of Chatham Plc, Kent

Contents

Part Three – EATING FOR HEALTH

APPENDICES

'I make no apology for saying that the health of the majority of human beings depends more on their nutrition than it does any other single factor. However important and dramatic have been the advances of hygiene, medicine and surgery, it is still true that even more important would be the effects that proper nutrition would have on morbidity and mortality. For this reason, I believe that the ultimate objective of nutritionists must be the nutrition education of the public.'

Professor John Yudkin, 1981

Acknowledgements

Setting out to write a comprehensive self-help guide that would dramatically help to improve the health prospects of both men and women around the world was indeed a daunting task. The first challenge was finding the time to put pen to paper with our busy practices and four demanding children. The second hurdle was gathering all the relevant published medical literature to ensure that the book was scientifically based. Our task was made significantly easier because of the hundreds of medical researchers and pioneers who have gone before us. Studying the wealth of published medical literature, on almost every subject we have written about, was enlightening. So our first thanks must go to the authors of the medical papers and textbooks we have quoted in our reference section. We are deeply grateful for their contribution to the overall picture.

Very special thanks must also go to our wonderful patients who have been happy to share their 'stories' in this book with the aim of helping others who are suffering similarly. Over the last seventeen years they have given us the hands-on clinical experience and insight to write a book that could potentially help millions of people around the world to reclaim their health and increase their lifespan. We decided to change the names of our 'Case Stories', despite the fact that many were happy to be identified.

We are also grateful to the team at the Women's Nutritional Advisory Service for their support, particularly Helen Heap, our nutritionist, who spent many hours clawing through the journals and the internet gathering new research, and Cheryl Griffiths for her cool organisational skills and nifty fingers. We would also like to acknowledge the seasoned skills of Charlotte Howard, our agent; Joanna Carreras, our editor at Vermilion, for her expertise and wisdom, and Lisa Highton, Mary Howell and Philippa Sandall at Headline in Australia for their vision and support.

We would not have been able to complete our task without the backup and support of our wonderful helpers at home, Jackie Hartt and Liz Copping, who coped admirably with the household chores and the needs of the children, and always with a smile, whilst we were deeply distracted.

Last but not least, we must thank the children themselves – Phoebe, Chesney, Hester and Simeon – for being both patient and self-sufficient, whilst at the same time supplying us with encouraging words and hugs when the end seemed like a long way off.

Introduction

For seventeen years we have been banging the drum about the wealth of scientifically proven benefits of non-drug medicine, and whilst it is true that there is a great deal more awareness on the subject, the majority of doctors in the medical profession and the general public remain greatly confused. This confusion is hardly surprising when the bulk of the medical profession remain under-educated on the subject of non-drug medicine, seemingly oblivious to the tens of thousands of medical papers published, whilst they continue to use a predominance of drug-based medicine. The press and information providers on the internet, on the other hand, who do their homework, now virtually bombard the public with often conflicting information, which simply results in overwhelming confusion.

Lack of education relating to health is a subject which deserves its own book; there is so much to be told. Repeated surveys we have conducted over the years have demonstrated that over 90 per cent of general practitioners in the United Kingdom, by their own admission, have little or no knowledge about nutritional approaches to health. The average time assigned to this subject being somewhere between two and four hours out of a whole medical training course; and the picture is not a great deal better in Australia or New Zealand. Yet the nutritional state of the human body, male or female, is as fundamentally important to health as good foundations are to a builder. When doctors fail to provide the vital information needed to overcome health problems, we may be forced to resort to long-term medication, or may be left to our own devices, feeling thoroughly frustrated and miserable.

The abundance of published science and seventeen years of clinical application has taught us, without doubt, that we can be the masters of our own health prospects by becoming educated, taking charge of our own menu, and making adjustments to our lifestyle. As well as overcoming common symptoms that detract greatly from our enjoyment of life, without the use of drugs, we now know that we can even help prevent many of the life threatening illnesses such as osteoporosis, heart disease, cancer, diabetes and mental illness, conditions which creep up on us silently as we age.

It sounds incredibly simple, so where have we gone wrong? We have never had a better opportunity to live a longer, happier or healthier life, but the majority of us are making a hash of it through lack of education. We have taken a wrong turning, bought on by a combination of a lack of education and an overdose of consumer advertising. The easy option is to bury our heads in the sand, hoping that our bodies will thrive no matter how much we abuse and ignore them.

Our real needs

The demands placed on our bodies throughout the many stages of life are great and varied. All too often these demands are not met, resulting in poor health of one form or another. Our bodies are very sensitive 'machines' with very specific requirements for optimum performance. When health trouble is brewing, the body is very good at sending warning messages, but the problem is that the majority of us, through lack of education, fail to interpret the message in time. In fact, most of us know more about home improvement or car maintenance than we do about the needs of our bodies.

We are blissfully unaware that the body requires a constant supply of good nutrients in order to function in an optimum way. Although our brain chemistry, hormone function and immune system will be adversely affected by an inadequate nutrient intake, most of us would not have a clue which foods provide the vital nutrients that may be lacking.

When the important systems in the body, like the brain, nervous system, hormones and immune functions fail to serve us well, we can suffer a wide variety of problems ranging from recurrent infections, fatigue, loss of libido, headaches and other aches and pains, constipation, irritable bowel syndrome, depression, anxiety to a whole host of other conditions.

Making poor choices

In addition, our increased prosperity has led us to overindulge in the wrong sort of foods and drinks that often contain chemicals and toxins that would make Mother Nature shudder, and although we now have an incredible choice of fresh food all the year round, more and more people are relying on convenience food. We have reached a point where the traditional kitchen is in danger of becoming obsolete.

Recent reports suggest that children were better nourished when on rations during and shortly after the Second World War, than they are now. With a diet rich in fatty foods, pizzas, burgers, confectionery and fizzy drinks, our children have a battle to be bright and to achieve academically, and as adults we need to have a cast iron constitution in order to escape unscathed.

Our changing habits

Apart from not eating well as individuals, many of us do not sit together as a family to enjoy a good meal, but instead eat 'TV' dinners, skip meals or snack on the hoof.

In the last fifty years we have gone from eating four properly cooked meals per day with approximately one in-between-meal snack each day, to an average of one proper meal each day that is freshly prepared and freshly shopped for, and as many as four snacks. Our bodies were simply not designed to be treated in this way.

Our lifestyle has also changed radically. Most of us no longer have the assistance of the extended family to fall back on, and women often have to be income providers, going out to work as well as caring for a family. For many there never seem to be enough hours in the day. As a result our personal needs are shelved or put on the back burner. We often choose to drive instead of walk, resulting in inadequate exercise. Life in the fast lane with so little time to exercise, often leaves us tired and washed out. Amazingly, in the age of the 'Personal Trainer', with more gyms and health clubs than ever before, over two-thirds of us take insufficient exercise to keep our hearts healthy and our bone mass strong. The result is a greatly reduced quality of life as well as poor health in both the short- and long-term.

To add insult to injury, our food chain has now been heavily tampered with and often contains chemicals and hormones that severely compromise our immune system and challenge our normal body function.

So whilst it is true that we are living longer than ever before, on average until our mid-eighties, unless we ring the changes, we are likely to spend our latter years suffering with either heart disease, cancer, mental illness or osteoporosis, all of which seems to have reached epidemic proportions.

Reclaiming your health

What a tale of potential doom and disaster. However, on a more optimistic note, with a little knowledge it is possible to reclaim your health. We undertook an audit of 100 patients in 1996 who completed our four-month re-education programme. Amongst many other things, we discovered that there was a 92 per cent reduction in generalised aches and pains, 91 per cent decrease in headaches, and an 88 per cent decline in insomnia. Eighty-seven per cent of food cravings had diminished, depression had disappeared in 82 per cent of cases, and 78 per cent of the subjects no longer experienced fatigue. Plus 82 per cent of those who had previously been overweight had overcome their weight problem *without* dieting. In addition, out of the 71 per cent of the sample who had previously suffered with low libido, 78 per cent had significantly regained their sex drive. Which only goes to show that a little knowledge does put us back in the driving seat.

In the many years of working with patients we have been able to help literally thousands of individuals over their long-term ills, and removed unwanted and unjustified 'labels' that they thought they would have for life. To cite a few examples: We have dealt with a significant number of patients who have been labelled psychologically or even psychiatrically ill, and have left them symptom-free after three or four months. Patients who have had severe migraine for years no longer even have headaches. We have former acne sufferers without spots, and irritable bowel victims who no longer have to pay attention to their digestion. The violent and often suicidal PMS sufferer who described herself as Jekyll and Hyde, feels like her old self again all month. Ongoing problems with thrush and cystitis have abated, and the turbulent symptoms of menopause, and high cholesterol levels or blood pressure, have been replaced in many patients by a new vitality for life.

These are some of the weekly achievements of our work at the Women's Nutritional Advisory Service (WNAS). They are not miracles, just the result of the application of existing medical science. The published medical papers on which we base our recommendations are all to be found in post-graduate medical libraries. They are there for the taking, but very few doctors are familiar with them. You may well consider it a scandal that these papers remain behind closed doors, as their application would very often result in the resolution of most chronic symptoms.

There are many myths about the ageing process. In fact with adequate care and attention along the way, most of us should be able to look forward to a very active and healthy old age with most of our 'bits' intact. However, in current practice this is not always the case. We often hear of women having a hysterectomy prematurely, or having their healthy ovaries removed, or of men having invasive treatment for prostate problems. It is also not unusual to encounter patients who have been on sleeping tablets, or antidepressants, for as long as they can remember, and others who are taking numerous types of medication, many of which are given to counteract the effects of other prescribed drugs.

It would be narrow-minded of us to claim that good nutrition is the only answer to good health. At the WNAS we encourage individuals to re-evaluate their whole lifestyle. Their current complaint is seen as a warning light which starts off the process. Our programmes always incorporate dietary and lifestyle changes, the use of relevant nutritional supplements, an exercise regime and regular relaxation, including visualisation techniques. We often incorporate other complimentary therapies like homeopathy, osteopathy, herbal medicine, massage, acupuncture and self-healing.

Many of our ills are the result of past traumatic emotional experiences which get buried away, either because we can't confront them at the time they occur, or because we are too busy to deal with them. Difficulties with relationships, both in childhood and in adulthood, get locked deep inside, and unless we can somehow come to terms with them rationally, they may damage our health later in life.

However, inadequate nutrient levels often affect brain chemistry, which in turn can affect mental processes. So perhaps trying to solve life's troubles *prior* to getting the body into optimum condition is not a good idea. The majority of our patients have been delighted to discover that problems which had seemed almost insurmountable prior to undertaking our programme, looked more like molehills that were relatively easy to deal with afterwards.

The purpose of this book is to provide you with the education that you have missed out on, and to empower you with the information necessary to make a fully informed decision about your life, your health and your treatment plan. It is important to understand the strengths and weaknesses of what your doctor has on offer, as well as to have an overview of what self-help measures are available to you, including the role other complementary therapies can play for specific conditions.

The first part of this book will give you the missing background information and some food for thought. You then have the A–Z of key conditions, followed by suggested dietary and nutritional plans. The scientifically minded will find the medical references for each condition in References on page 495. There is also a recommended reading list and a useful address directory in the Appendices which begin on page 483.

If, after following our recommendations, you would like to share your experiences with us you will find our address on page 511. For those who feel they could use some expert help, we provide a tailor-made service which you can also read about on page 511. Or alternatively you could visit our website, www.wnas@wnas.org.uk

We all have the power to influence not only our own health, but that of our family and future generations. Armed with new knowledge we are confident that you will find that the quality of health you enjoy is for the most part actually in your own hands. In our view we will be many years into the twenty-first century before we can expect the medical profession to provide us with all the answers, and even that assessment may be optimistic. In the meantime, *The Natural Health Bible* will arm you with all the information you need to help yourself, and those near and dear to you, to better health.

Part One

YOUR DIET AND LIFESTYLE

Chapter 1
What's Wrong with Present-day Diet and Lifestyle?

In the last fifty years diet and lifestyle have altered dramatically. The whole of society has changed, and not necessarily for the better. At one time culinary skills were passed from one generation to another, and the woman's role was very definitely the 'home-maker'. She was not expected to go out to work whilst her family were growing, and more often than not she had her mother and other female relatives living close by as back-up. The motor car was a luxury, so her daily shopping was usually done locally on foot. She would expect to purchase fresh food regularly, which would have contained far more nutrients that produce purchased from the supermarket weekly. As fast food didn't exist, part of her role would be to cook wholesome meals for the family on a daily basis.

Fifty years on the picture is quite different. We have learned the art of the short-cut, very often through necessity. We drive to the supermarket once or twice a week to purchase food. Here we are presented with fast option choices which, when short of time and adequate information, seem both convenient and appealing. Much of the food on offer has been preserved, sprayed with chemicals, injected, or indeed grown in chemically rich soil. Unless we buy organic food we have come to accept that our food will be treated with pesticides and insecticides, and that animals have been pumped full of antibiotics and growth hormones, with environmental pollution being the cherry on the top.

Human bodies were not designed to be treated in such a fashion, nor to cope with modern-day stresses, so it is no wonder that our bodies develop problems. We probably treat our domestic appliances or our motor car with more respect than we do ourselves. Few of us wouldn't dream of denying our car the appropriate fuel or oil, so how is it that we neglect our bodies so? In our experience at the WNAS it is the 'education gap' that is responsible, but when we are confronted with the real facts about diet and lifestyle, we usually take stock. Few of us, once enlightened, revert to old habits as we are so pleased with our renewed health, and surprised at how enjoyable the new diet and lifestyle are. As an added bonus we are then able to pass our new-found knowledge on to other members of the family.

Let us examine more closely how our eating habits have changed. A century ago, meat, animal fat and sugar formed a much smaller proportion of our diets than today. The consumption of cereal fibres has also dropped considerably:

- We have increased our consumption of sugar. The UK has become one of the world's largest chocolate and sweet-eating nations. We currently spend over £4 billion per year on chocolate alone.
- The last one hundred years have seen a twenty-five-fold increase in world sugar production. In reality refined sugar is not something that we actually need, and the human race managed quite happily without it for centuries. Mother Nature, with her usual wisdom, has designed the body to convert complex carbohydrates and proteins into the sugar required. Table sugar, or sucrose, contains no vitamins, minerals, protein, fibre or starches; it may contain tiny traces of calcium and magnesium if we are really lucky, but apart from that it just provides us with 'empty calories'.
- We have to really go out of our way these days to reduce our sugar consumption as 'considerate' food manufacturers often add it to some of the most unlikely foods: *cheese, fruit yoghurt, tomato sauce, baked beans, pickled cucumbers, muesli, beefburgers, Worcestershire sauce, sausages, peas, cornflakes,* and *canned drinks.*
- Excessive consumption of saturated animal fats results in a gradual blocking of the arteries that supply the heart, brain and other major organs. This leads to poor circulation, and then to heart attacks and strokes. It is worth noting that smoking accelerates this process. The increased incidence of breast cancer has much to do with animal fat consumption as well.
- We eat far too much salt – ten to 20 times more than our bodies really require each day – which can contribute to high blood pressure.
- We often drink far too much coffee and tea which can impede the absorption of essential nutrients, and aggravate symptoms of nervous tension, irritability, insomnia and headaches. On average we consume four mugs of tea and two mugs of coffee each day, which deliver approximately 800 mg of caffeine into our system. That doesn't include other sources of caffeine like chocolate, cocoa, cola and other caffeinated drinks. It certainly means that there are many women walking about with symptoms of caffeine excess. Count how many cups or mugs you have had today – you may be surprised.
- We consume volumes of foods with a high level of phosphorus, which impedes the absorption of good nutrients and interferes with calcium

absorption by bone tissue. Examples of these foods are soft drinks (low or normal calorie varieties), processed foods, canned, packaged, pre-packed convenience foods and ready-made sauces.

- Alcohol consumption has almost doubled in the UK since the end of the Second World War. Alcohol also impedes the absorption of good nutrients and in excess can cause all sort of other health problems as you will see on page 8.
- Unbelievable as it may seem, we actually eat less food than we did thirty years ago and more. It seems that we expend less energy than those of a generation or two ago, and this has resulted in a 10–15 per cent reduction in food intake. This also means that intake of essential nutrients has fallen, particularly if eating refined or convenience foods.
- Many of the foods available contain chemical additives in the form of flavour enhancers, colouring and preservatives. While some of these are not harmful, some of them are, and our bodies are certainly not designed to cope with them.
- These days our meat animals are bombarded with antibiotics, to the point where they often become resistant to them. Antibiotics are used as a preventative measure and often used for growth promotion.
- Nitrate fertilisers have been used to obtain fast-growing and abundant crops. It is now recognised that nitrates are harmful and can produce cancer, at least in animals.
- Almost all our fresh fruit, cereals and vegetables are sprayed with pesticides at least once. In addition, milk and meat may retain pesticides from feed given to livestock.

All these processes in the rearing and growing of food mean a reduction in basic nutrition, and the answer must lie in eating organic foods.

Although organic food is harder to obtain (although it is becoming more widely available) and more expensive weight for weight, by consuming it you will be decreasing the number of chemicals you consume, and thus increasing your nutrient intake. According to the Soil Association, organic vegetable foods are more nutrient dense for the equivalent weight. As they have not been tampered with chemically they deliver much more of what nature promised.

The same is true for meat. Additive-free or organic meat has not been subjected to drugs, growth promoters or contaminated foods. This type of meat is now far more widely available than before (even our local high-street butcher supplies it and some local farms, and many supermarkets, keep stocks). If you find clean meat, it can be included in your diet approximately three times per week, unless of course, you are vegetarian. An alternative is to limit your intake to lean meat, eat more fish, or become a vegetarian.

There are numerous dietary guidelines for you to follow, depending on your needs, in Part Three. If you haven't already started reading labels in the supermarket have a go next time you shop there, there are a few surprises in store. Make sure you have plenty of time to spare as, sadly, many of the labels are pretty long.

The truth about social substances

Why is it that the things we enjoy the most seem to be bad for us? When we are in good health the general rule is that 'a little of what you fancy does you good'. However, when a personal health crisis appears, it may be necessary to make some sacrifices. Often the thought of making the changes is worse than taking the plunge. Surprisingly, people find the alternatives relatively acceptable, prefer the health benefits and feel delighted to be free from the 'addiction' or dependency. These may sound strong words, but it is not uncommon to find that the withdrawal of regular, but relatively small, amounts of caffeine – one or two mugs per day, say – can result in withdrawal headaches and other symptoms for a few days. The increased sense of well-being which follows the withdrawal symptoms, is certainly worth waiting for. Let us look at these social 'poisons' and see just where they fall down.

Caffeine

Many of us have become slowly dependent on caffeine over the years, and our children follow in our footsteps. You will find caffeine in coffee and tea, but also in chocolate, chocolate drinks, cocoa, cola-based drinks, Lucozade, Lemsip, some painkillers, and the new breed of drinks like Red Bull, Red Kick and Virgin Energy.

Caffeine is one of the group of substances known as methylxanthines, and acts as both a physical and mental stimulant. Although small amounts of caffeine can be of benefit in waking us up and stimulating our thought processes, it can have many adverse effects when used to excess. Over the years caffeine has been linked to heart disease, high blood pressure and even infertility. We know that caffeine worsens nervous tension, anxiety, insomnia and aggravates breast tenderness in women. It can also make you feel restless, nervous, with a rapid pulse and palpitations. High consumers will probably experience withdrawal symptoms when trying to kick the habit, rather like the symptoms produced by alcohol or nicotine withdrawal. If you depend on the caffeine 'buzz', then the road to good health will undoubtedly involve reducing your intake.

Coffee

Coffee is the most widely used drug of our time. We are consuming more coffee than ever before. Since 1950 the consumption of coffee in the UK, for instance, has increased four-fold. There are many unacknowledged 'addicts' who would find it a challenge to give up, and even foregoing that last cup can produce symptoms of restlesness, nervous tension and headaches.

Ground coffee contains approximately 150 mg of caffeine per mug, and a mug of instant coffee roughly 100 mg. When we are well, moderate doses of up to 300 mg may be acceptable, but large doses can produce symptoms that could be mistaken for anxiety neurosis, including headaches, tremors, nausea and diarrhoea.

Weaning yourself off coffee can sometimes be a traumatic experience, but sadly there is no real shortcut. Cutting down gradually over a few weeks is the best option, and even when parting with those last few cups, set aside a few days so that you can hide away if you feel really uptight or out of sorts.

How to kick the habit

- Reduce your intake gradually over the space of a week or two.
- Limit yourself to no more than two cups of decaffeinated coffee per day.
- Try some of the alternative drinks like Barleycup, dandelion coffee, or Bambu which you can obtain from health-food stores.
- If you enjoy filter coffee, you can still use your filter, but with decaffeinated versions or with roasted dandelion root instead. Simply grind it and put it through a filter, treating it just like ground coffee. It makes a coffee-like strong malted drink.

Tea

The bad news is that tea, the great British beverage, is not much better than coffee. It contains about 70 mg of caffeine per cup and approximately 100 mg per mug. However, it also contains tannin, another nasty, which inhibits the absorption of nutrients – zinc and iron in particular. Excesses of tea can produce the same withdrawal symptoms as coffee, but tea also can cause constipation.

Drinking tea with a meal will reduce the absorption of iron from vegetarian sources by one-third, whereas a glass of fresh orange juice, rich in vitamin C, would increase the iron absorption two-fold. Vegetarians and vegans need their iron, so drinking anything other than small amounts of weak tea, in between meals, may mean they risk becoming iron deficient.

Acceptable alternatives

Herbal teas are a good substitute. Unlike conventional Indian or Chinese leaf tea, most of the herbal varieties are free of caffeine and tannin, and can be both cleansing and relaxing. A good herbal tea look-alike is Rooibosch tea or Rooi as it is sometimes known, which looks just like ordinary tea when made with milk. As an added bonus it contains a muscle relaxant and has been used in trials on babies with colic. Many of our patients prefer it to ordinary tea after a few weeks, but it does take a while to get used to. Apart from that there are many delicious varieties of herbal tea, and these days you can buy single sachets to try, which means you are not left with a box full of teabags you dislike. Our current favourites are Raspberry and Ginseng tea, Fennel, Lemon and Ginger, and Mixed Berry Cup. See also The Caffeine-free Diet, page 440.

Caffeinated fizzy drinks

We used to have only cola-based drinks to contend with, but these days there are a new generation of caffeinated drinks such as those mentioned on page 6 to tempt us. Apart from caffeine there is also sugar, or the chemical substitutes, to consider – approximately eight teaspoons per can of cola, together with other additives. Sadly many young people get hooked on these drinks early on in life as the 'ad men' would have them believe the drinks are 'cool' and will enhance their image.

We are all much better off with the healthy varieties of fizzy drink, which thankfully are given substantial space on our supermarket shelves. Appletise, Ame and Irish Spring are all good examples. Or you can simply dilute some fruit juice with some fizzy bottled water yourself.

If you have been a large consumer of the caffeine variety of fizzy drinks, you will have to follow the weaning instructions for coffee. We have had patients who consume two or more litres of cola per day, and know that the withdrawal symptoms are likely to be quite similar.

Decaffeinated drinks

Decaffeinated drinks usually contain small amounts of caffeine as well as other members of the methylxanthine family, and decaffeinated tea also contains tannin. The regulations for decaffeinated cola are no more than 125 mg per litre.

The decaffeination process uses one of two methods, either water and carbon dioxide, or the Swiss water process which uses hot water, charcoal and the use of chemical solvents. In the latter process small residues of chemicals remain, but they are minimal. So decaffeinated drinks are better but not marvellous. At the WNAS we recommend restricting decaffeinated drinks to no more than two mugs per day.

Alcohol

Whilst small amounts of alcohol on a regular basis do not cause us harm, we know that alcohol knocks most nutrients sideways.

Alcohol is enjoyed by over 90 per cent of adults in the UK and most Western societies. In the last 50 years consumption has approximately doubled in the UK at a time when total calorie intake has been falling, so alcohol now represents a bigger percentage of calorie intake than it did two or more generations earlier.

This subtle rise in alcohol intake has to some degree been endorsed by the medical profession, particularly as studies demonstrate the potential protective effect of wine consumption, especially red wine, upon cardiovascular disease. However, more careful appraisal of the potential adverse effects of alcohol intake means that considerable caution needs to be exercised.

Women who are planning a pregnancy or who are already pregnant will need to take particular care about limiting intake of alcohol. Furthermore, excess alcohol consumption is associated with an increased risk of many disorders and these will be covered in the relevant chapters.

In brief, the major adverse effects of alcohol can be divided into roughly three groups.

Firstly, it has an adverse effect upon the balance of many nutrients including thiamine (vitamin B1) which is necessary for the metabolic breakdown of alcohol, and the minerals calcium, magnesium and zinc.

Secondly, alcohol in excess destroys body tissue over the years, and is associated with an increased risk of many physical illnesses. Among them:

- cardiovascular diseases, high blood pressure, stroke
- digestive disorders, peptic ulcer, gastritis and pancreatitis
- inflammation and ulceration of the lining of the digestive tract
- liver disease
- cancer, especially of the stomach and liver, as well as breast cancer. For example, in women consuming three glasses of wine per day – equivalent to at least four units of alcohol – the increased risk of breast cancer in these regular 'moderate' drinkers is 70 per cent.
- brain degeneration: brain damage and dementia
- miscarriages
- damage to unborn children
- a risk factor for osteoporosis in both men and women.

Finally there is considerable increased risk of psychologically related problems including depression, suicide in both men and women, premenstrual syndrome, loss of libido in both sexes and impotence in men. Furthermore there are substantial knock-on adverse effects for the mental health of those who live with heavy or dependent drinkers. One third of divorce petitions cite alcohol as a contributory factor. A significant number of accidents as well as road traffic deaths are associated with alcohol consumption and thus are potentially avoidable. People under stress do sometimes hit the bottle in order to escape from reality, and as most of the above conditions come on gradually, we often don't perceive the real dangers of alcohol until it is too late.

There are specific guidelines as to what the safe limits for alcohol consumption are for men and women. These vary to some degree but are usually in the region of up to 14 units per week for women and up to 21 units per week for men. A unit equals 8 gms or 10 mls of pure alcohol. A bottle of wine will contain usually between eight to nine units of alcohol (i.e. up to 1.5 units per glass), a pint of beer is approximately 2.5 units of alcohol, as is a double measure of spirits in a pub. It is easy to underestimate alcohol consumption when trying to calculate units.

Many individuals will feel better consuming less than these amounts of alcohol. Higher intakes may be possible for those with a more robust metabolism, who are physically active and if they are known to be relative rapid metabolisers of alcohol. However, if your drinking has been escalating slowly, it is advisable to seek help. It is important to cut your consumption to the recommended limits.

Tobacco

Earlier this century, cigarettes were actually recommended by doctors, but more recent research has shown that they are bad for our general health. In addition, smoking during pregnancy affects the unborn child, and women who smoke more than fifteen cigarettes per day can expect to experience menopause two years earlier than non-smokers.

Smoking also affects bone density. But it's never too late to stop. Even at the time of the menopause stopping smoking can reduce a hip fracture risk by 40 per cent.

Despite government health warnings and health-promotion campaigns, women still go on smoking. Research shows that better educated people have cut back, but younger women, who are perhaps not so well educated, are still puffing away. Being parents of teenagers we know that it is still considered 'cool' to smoke behind the bicycle sheds! To demonstrate the stronghold that smoking has over us: in 1922, women in the UK aged between 20 and 30 were smoking an average of 50 cigarettes each per year; by 1975, this had risen to an average of just over 3,000 cigarettes per woman, per year. By 1998 this had increased to an average of 93 cigarettes per woman, per week, i.e. approaching 4,840 per woman, per year.

Giving up

Giving up smoking has never been easy. The first step is to make the decision to quit, knowing that you may well experience true withdrawal symptoms, just as drug addicts and alcoholics do when they try to stop. Here is a plan to help you:

- Choose a day on which to give up, and write down the date.
- On the day before, smoke as many cigarettes as you can until you feel sick. Make sure you stub them all out in the same dirty ashtray.
- Go to the library and get a book that contains pictures of the consequences of smoking.
- On the morning of your chosen day, pour yourself a glass of freshly squeezed orange juice, and sit and write down all the reasons for your decision to give up smoking.

- Pin your list of reasons up on the wall so that you can read it at weak moments.
- Put your cigarettes away in a drawer, and tell yourself you can have one whenever you want one.
- When you crave a cigarette, tell yourself you can have one but first consider the reasons why you decided to quit. Make a new decision not to light up.
- Go shopping and stock up with some of your favourite wholesome food, including some fruit and some raw vegetables and dips.
- Tell your close friends and family that you are giving up smoking.
- Take a good multi-vitamin and mineral pill each day, in addition to improving your diet.
- Try to avoid situations that are likely to make you feel like lighting up. For example, drink fruit juice instead of alcohol.
- If possible, go away for a few days to help you break your daily routine.
- Chew some sugar-free gum rather than sweets or chocolate.
- Put the handle of your toothbrush in your mouth whenever you miss your hand-to-mouth habit.
- Each time you feel you need a cigarette, stop, relax and breathe deeply, so that you get a good supply of oxygen into your lungs.
- Join a gym, and make sure you exercise regularly.
- Don't spend evenings alone, instead arrange to go to the cinema, bowling or out for a walk.
- If you feel edgy in the evenings, have a few early nights.
- Keep a progress chart, ticking each day that you have remained a non-smoker.
- Save your cigarette money in a jar, and spend it on treats for yourself.
- Practise some formal relaxation like yoga or meditation.
- If you have a partner, ask for a massage when you feel tense or a bit ratty.
- Picture your lungs recovering now that they are smoke free.

It is never too late to give up smoking. Whenever you do decide to take the plunge you will be helping yourself to better health and preserving yourself for your loved ones. If you find it difficult to quit, contact one of the organisations listed in Useful addresses on page 512 and read some of the suggested books found in Recommended reading on page 490.

Other drugs

Natural remedies were passed down from one generation to the next, until the advent of the pharmaceutical industry post-Second World War. Drugs in general have revolutionised medicine and medical practice, and they have both advantages and disadvantages. Whereas in years gone by we could easily have died of pneumonia, for example, modern antibiotics make that unlikely now. On the down side however, many of us have come to rely on pills to help us cope with life, induce sleep, and indeed counteract the side-effects of another drug. So whilst some drugs can be lifesaving, others can equally wreck the quality of our existence, and it is therefore imperative to be discerning.

Street drugs

These have become increasingly popular in the last fifteen or twenty years. They are readily available and can sometimes be a tempting option for those whose lives are not going as planned. Women of child-bearing age should avoid all street drugs as they undoubtedly harm the unborn child, and in some case babies are born addicted. Drug users, even more so than smokers, tend to have a less nutritious diet than non-users, and are not so concerned about preserving their health, as they are in the process of spoiling it anyway.

Marijuana and cannabis are both widely used substances and products of the hemp plant. The pro-marijuana lobby claim that it is as safe as smoking cigarettes or drinking alcohol. Whilst marijuana does seem to have some medicinal uses, we are not advocating regular use, any more than we are recommending alcohol or tobacco.

Prescribed drugs

Nearly one hundred years ago, Sir Robert Hucheson, President of the Royal College of Physicians, was writing books about diet and nutrition as a mode of treatment. It seems hard to believe that nutrition is no longer considered a major part of conservative medicine. One wonders how we became such a drug-oriented society. Following the post-war boom in the pharmaceutical industry, it is hardly surprising, as the industry has been allowed to assume increased power and influence over doctors' education.

In the USA in 1991 nearly £35 billion was spent on medicines by a population of 250 million, and in the UK it was £3.5 billion, or £69 per man, woman and child. Doctors issue some 15 per cent more prescriptions today than they did a decade ago. In England alone, over 425 million prescriptions were written in 1992, nearly ten million for antidepressants, at a cost of £81 million.

Even doctors themselves, worldwide, now express concern about the excessive use of benzodiazepine tranquillisers and sleeping tablets. The current recommendation is that these drugs, which include Valium, Mogadon and Ativan, should be used as a temporary measure for only a few weeks, rather than in the long term. Those who have been taking them for any length of time should, if at all possible, have their dosage and frequency gradually reduced under medical supervision.

When we run into health difficulties, our body depends on us to clean up our act so that the immune system can function properly and do its job. The body has exceptional natural healing powers, but you wouldn't expect a wound to heal with a nail in it, any more than you can expect to be well without treating your body with respect.

Chapter 2
Nutrition is the Key to Health

The major causes of death in developed countries are heart disease and cancer which are influenced to a large degree by the type of diet we have. Up to 50 per cent of people with heart disease or cancer could probably have prevented or delayed the onset of their illness if they had eaten a better diet (or stopped smoking). This is particularly true for those who became ill at a relatively young age, i.e. before sixty-five years. Furthermore, many minor ills are also influenced by diet and these include problems such as migraine headaches, high blood pressure, arthritis, kidney stones, premenstrual syndrome, eczema, fatigue, irritable bowel syndrome, insomnia and anxiety. These are only the tip of the iceberg as you will see and in this book alone we have covered over 120 conditions.

When we are children our parents teach us how to eat, dress, wash and generally look after ourselves and we are taught at school how to read, write and add up. But where and how do we learn about our bodies' requirements? Well, it is not at school, neither is it at evening classes, as they seem to concentrate there on car maintenance and the secrets of computer mechanics. The woman, who is often regarded as the 'nutritional head of the household', and is expected to meet the demands of her family's nutrient needs as well as her own, has little or no training for this job. When we consider this rationally, it seems so outrageous, especially as we trade both our cars and our computers in from time to time, but only have one body to last a lifetime.

Because we are so often told by our doctors that a balanced diet is all that we need to maintain our health, the WNAS conducted a random survey a few years ago to find out what people understood by the term 'a balanced diet'. We also asked which foods contained key vitamins like A, B, C, D and E, and some key minerals like calcium, magnesium, zinc and iron. The negative results of this survey would have been entertaining were it not for the fact that the consequences of an unbalanced diet may severely affect the quality of health. The only information that people seemed to have about their diet was from basic lessons at school, if they could remember them. Apart from knowing facts such as 'oranges contain vitamin C' and that 'liver contains iron', hardly anyone had a clue as to what actually constituted a sound balanced diet, or how much of each nutrient was required each day for their body size, (or anyone else's body size for that matter).

Although magazine articles are one of the key sources of information about diet, confusion abounds as we lurch from one diet scandal to another. First we hear that alcohol is bad for us and that animal fats will cause our cholesterol levels to rise. Then we hear that we should be drinking two or three glasses of wine each day to prevent heart disease, and that fats have little influence on our cholesterol levels. Should we be eating liver regularly, or does it contain too much vitamin A? Will soft cheeses and uncooked eggs give us listeria and salmonella? Is decaffeinated tea and coffee *really* better for us or will the other methylxanthines get us anyway? We could well be forgiven for putting our heads in the sand and hoping for the best. Trying to sort out the dietary myths from the facts is an arduous task for anyone.

Essential nutrients

In order to fully understand the role of vitamins and minerals in health, it is necessary to have some idea about the part that each nutrient has to play. A truly balanced diet must provide an adequate supply of energy and protein, plus essential vitamins, minerals and specialised fats called essential fatty acids (EFAs). The majority of energy comes from fats and carbohydrates in the diet, and a small amount from protein-rich foods.

Proteins, fats, carbohydrates and fibre are all essential for normal body function. Let's look briefly at the function they serve.

Protein

This term is used to describe a series of complex chemicals that are widely found in many nutritious foods. Proteins are made up of amino acids, the essential building blocks of health, as well as many hormones, enzymes and other agents involved in the intricate metabolism of living organisms. If protein intake is not adequate in the diet, then tissue growth and repair cannot take place, and protein-rich tissues breaks down, especially muscle.

Sources of protein

Protein can be found in both animal and vegetarian sources – meat, eggs, dairy products including milk and cheese, peas, beans, lentils, nuts, seeds and, to a very small extent, rice and potatoes. It is wise to have a wide variety of protein sources in your diet, especially if you are a vegetarian.

Fats

Fats provide us with energy. There are a wide variety of different fats, which are all chemically similar, and per gram weight they provide us with over twice the energy content as carbohydrate or sugar.

Animal fats

The majority of animal fats are saturated and serve only as a source of calories. Animal fats are not essential to our diet and have a chemical structure that is saturated with hydrogen. This chemical nature means that they are usually solid at room temperature. A diet rich in these saturated animal fats, and lacking in fibre, vitamins and minerals will often predispose to heart disease.

Vegetable fats

Many, but not all vegetable fats are polyunsaturates and these include the specialised essential fatty acids, or EFAs, which are used in the building structure of our cells, especially those of our skin and nervous system, and are also a source of calories. Chemically these fats or oils are unsaturated and are able to accept more hydrogen molecules. This means that they are usually liquid at room temperature. Olive oil and rapeseed oil are rich in monosaturates which are not essential but they do not add to the risk of heart disease in the way that saturated fats do. Good sources of the essential fatty acids are corn, sunflower and safflower oils which provide the Omega-6 series of EFAs. Oily fish such as mackerel, herring and salmon, together with soy bean and walnut oil and to a small extent rapeseed oil provide the Omega-3 series.

Carbohydrates

Carbohydrate is a collective term for the different sugars and starches in our diet. Starches are composed of many individual sugar molecules, predominantly glucose, and are broken down by our digestive system into simple sugars, some of which are better for us than others. The simple sugars are glucose, fructose and galactose (which is part of the sugar found in milk). Table sugar, which is also called sucrose, is made up of one glucose and one fructose unit joined together. Its commercial production from sugar cane and sugar beet leads to the complete loss of vitamins and minerals found in these parent sources. A similar refining process to prepare white flour from wholemeal leads to a substantial reduction in essential vitamins and minerals. Sugars and starch-rich foods all require vitamin B and magnesium in order to be metabolised. Sucrose and to a lesser extent fructose also predispose to tooth decay.

Sources of refined carbohydrates

Cakes, biscuits, sweets, chocolate, table sugar, white bread, white pasta and many breakfast cereals are all refined products that have been depleted of many essential nutrients. Fortunately white flour and some breakfast cereals are fortified with vitamins and flour has added calcium. This helps to make up for these nutritional losses.

Nutritious carbohydrate sources

These include all cereals, potatoes, rice and root vegetables. Fresh fruits and vegetables also provide a mixture of sugars – mainly fructose and a small amount of starch.

Fibre

Fibre is a type of carbohydrate that comes from cellulose – the cell wall of plants – and remains undigested in our gut. Because of its water-retaining properties, it forms the bulk of our stool. There are many types of fibre with differing properties. Most of us associate fibre-rich foods with those containing bran, for example, but bran may inhibit the absorption of certain essential nutrients including calcium and other minerals. It has little effect on blood cholesterol whereas the fibre in fruit, vegetables and oats helps reduce a high level of cholesterol.

Good sources of fibre

A diet rich in fruit, vegetables, salad and cereals lowers blood cholesterol and the risk of heart disease, as well as providing many essential vitamins and minerals.

Vitamins and minerals

There are some 15 vitamins, 15 minerals, and eight to ten amino acids that have been isolated as being essential for normal body function. These nutrients are synergistic, which means they rely on each other in order to keep the body functioning at an optimum level. If you liken the body to a computer for a moment, the computer can only function when it has the correct data and commands fed into it; otherwise it refuses to work or breaks down altogether. Similarly, our bodies require the correct input of nutrients. When one or more nutrient is in short supply the body cannot function properly, and symptoms, be they physical or mental, occur.

Whilst it is true that severe nutritional deficiencies are rare in countries like the UK, Australia, New Zealand and the USA, poor intake of a number of nutrients are acknowledged in some 20 per cent of women of child-bearing age. Combined nutritional inadequacies are likely to have an adverse affect on hormone function and on health in general during the ageing process.

Nutritional needs through the ages

Our bodies are indeed very complex machines that have very specific requirements in order that they may function efficiently. Women in particular have varying needs, not just through their years of physical growth and development, but through each phase as it presents itself. The nutritional requirements for pregnancy are quite different, for example, from those needed by a woman at the time of the menopause.

The following chart will give you some idea about the changing needs throughout life.

Growth & development	All known nutrients.
Puberty of both boys and girls	All nutrients, and particularly iron, zinc, calcium and magnesium.
Premenstrual syndrome	Particularly magnesium, B vitamins, iron and EFAs.
Preconception	Folate, other B vitamins and EFAs.
Pregnancy	All nutrients, particularly EFAs.
Breast-feeding	EFAs, calcium, magnesium and iron.
Menopause	Calcium, magnesium, vitamin E and EFAs.
Post-meonpause	Calcium, magnesium, EFAs, and vitamin D if deficient.
The elderly of both sexes	Vitamins B, C, D, calcium and iron.

Essential nutrients – are we deficient?

To continue the 'machinery' metaphor, learning what your body needs to function properly is a bit like trying to work a complicated computer without a manual. In fact, if the computer arrived without a manual, you would probably either leave it in the box until the manual arrived or, failing that, send it back to the shop. Becoming familiar with your body's needs demands a little patience and determination, because it is not that simple. It's almost like learning a new language.

Although we all have a body, that is where the similarity ends. Each individual body has slightly different requirements. The type of metabolism we have is inherited. There are the lucky robust minority who appear to be able to eat what they like, to maintain their weight and good health, and who seem to be oblivious to environmental and social stresses and strains. They must come from unusually strong stock. As for the rest of us, we have to come to terms with the fact that subtle differences determine the strengths and weaknesses of our make-up, and that one balanced diet for all is a myth.

To understand your own nutrient needs you need to know a little about each individual nutrient. This is presented in the chart on pages 18–21. Look through it and follow up any health problems you might

The Essential Nutrients, Vitamins, Minerals and Essential Fatty Acids

Nutrient	Food source	What they do
Vitamin A	*Retinol (animal vitamin A)* Liver, all dairy products and margarine *Beta-carotene (vegetable vitamin A)* All yellow, green, and orange fruits and vegetables	Essential for vision, especially in the dark, for growth and resistance to infection
Vitamin B1 (Thiamin)	Meat, fish, nuts, wholegrains and fortified breakfast cereals	Essential in the metabolism of sugar, especially in nerves and muscles
Vitamin B2 (Riboflavin)	Milk, meats, fish and vegetables	Involved in energy release from fats and carbohydrates
Vitamin B3 (Nicotinamide)	All forms of meat and fish, liver, fortified breakfast cereals and bread	Energy release from fats and carbohydrates, health of the skin and nervous system
Vitamin B6	Meat, fish, nuts, bananas, avocados, wholegrains	Essential in the metabolism of protein and the amino acids that control mood and behaviour. Affects hormone metabolism
Vitamin B12	All forms of meat, liver, eggs and milk, yeast extract	Involved in the chemical functioning of the nervous system, and the blood cells
Vitamin C (Ascorbic acid)	Any fresh fruits and vegetables	Involved in healing, repair of tissues and production of some hormones
Vitamin D	Milk, margarine, sardines, cod liver oil, eggs (and sunlight)	For the balance of calcium in bones and teeth, and for muscle strength
Vitamin E	Most nuts, seeds and vegetable oils and dark green leafy vegetables	Protect tissues from wear and tear, keep cholesterol and other fats from deteriorating inside the body
Vitamin K	Green leafy vegetables, and the bacteria in our intestines	Help with blood clotting
Folic acid	All green leafy vegetables, liver and fortified cereals	Help maintain the health of the nervous system and the blood

Who is at risk	Symptoms	Visible Signs
The ill, elderly and poorly fed pre-school children	Poor night vision, recurrent chest infections	None
Alcohol consumers, women on the pill, breast-feeding mothers, high consumers of sugar	Depression, anxiety, poor appetite, nausea, personality change	None usually! Heart, nerve and muscle problems if severe
Those on a poor diet. Deficiency rarely severe	Mild fatigue and possibly burning feet	Peeling of the skin on the lips. Red ring around the iris of the eye
Alcoholics, those on a poor diet, and with poor digestion	Diarrhoea, depression and dermatitis	A sore tongue and red scaly rash in light-exposed areas
Women, especially smokers, 'junk-eaters'	Depression, anxiety, insomnia, loss of responsibility	Dry/greasy facial skin, cracking at corners of mouth
Long-term vegans, those who have lost part of their stomach, and the elderly with digestive problems	Anaemia, loss of balance and a sore tongue	Smooth sore tongue, pale appearance, and unsteadiness
Smokers particularly	Lethargy, depression, hypochondria (imagined illnesses)	Easy bruising, look for small pinpoint bruises under the tongue
Urban-dwelling, dark-skinned immigrants, especially young children and pregnant women, those with little sunlight exposure	Softening of the bones, poor teeth and weakness of the hip muscles	Enlarged skull, bowing of the legs and a waddling gait
Those on a very poor diet, or with serious absorption problems	None. Damage to the nervous system if severe	None
Those with a poor diet or on long-term antibiotics	Prolonged bleeding	None
Those on a poor diet, those taking anti-epileptic medication, coeliacs, and a percentage of the normal population of child-bearing women who are at increased risk of having a child with a neural tube defect	Often none. Possibly depression, fatigue and poor memory	None unless anaemic

Nutrient	Food source	What they do
Iron	Meat, wholegrains, nuts, eggs and fortified breakfast cereals	Essential to make blood-haemoglobin. Many other tissues need iron for energy reactions
Zinc	Meat, wholegrains, nuts, peas, beans, lentils	Essential for normal growth, mental function, hormone production and resistance to infection
Magnesium	Green vegetables, wholegrains, Brazil nuts and almonds, many other non-junk foods	Essential for sugar and energy metabolism, needed for healthy nerves and muscles
Calcium	Milk, cheese, bread, especially white, sardines, other fish with bones, green vegetables and beans	Needed for strong teeth and bones, also for normal nerve and muscle function. Lack leads to osteoporosis – bone thinning
Potassium	All vegetables and fruit	Needed for the health of all cells, especially muscles and the nervous system
Selenium	Most wholesome foods, especially seafoods	Involved in two enzymes that protect inflamed and damaged tissues and help thyroid function
Chromium	All wholesome foods, not sugar and other refined carbohydrates	Helps in the action of insulin. Deficiency causes a diabetic-like state
Essential Fatty Acids Omega-3	Cod liver oil, mackerel, herring	Help control inflammation
Fish and related oils	Salmon, rapeseed and soya bean oil	Reduce calcium losses in urine
Essential Fatty Acids Omega-6, evening primrose and related oils	Sunflower, safflower and corn oils, many nuts (not peanuts) and seeds, green vegetables	Control inflammation, needed for health of nervous system, skin and blood vessels

Who is at risk	Symptoms	Visible Signs
Women who have heavy periods (e.g. coil users), vegetarians, especially if tea or coffee drinkers, women with recurrent thrush	Fatigue, poor energy, depression, poor digestion, sore tongue, cracking at corners of mouth	Pale complexion, brittle nails, cracking at corners of mouth
Vegetarians, especially tea and coffee drinkers, alcohol consumers, long-term users of diuretics (water pills)	Poor mental function, skin problems in general, repeated infections	Eczema, acne, greasy or dry facial skin
Women with PMS (some 50 per cent may be lacking), long-term diuretic users, alcohol consumers	Nausea, apathy, loss of appetite, depression, mood changes, muscle cramps	Usually NONE! so easily missed; muscle spasms sometimes
Low dairy consumers, heavy drinkers, smokers, women with early menopause, lack of exercise increases the rate of bone calcium-loss in later years	Usually none until osteoporotic fracture of hip or spine. Back pain	Loss of height
The elderly, after prolonged vomiting, with use of some diuretics and poor diet	Weakness, low blood pressure and muscle cramps	None
The ill, elderly, those on a very poor diet, possibly those with heart failure or long-standing malabsorption, or alcoholics	None that are specific, just not well	None
The elderly, life-long consumers of junk food!	Those of diabetes or of a low blood sugar with episodic weakness and sugar craving	Perhaps a large waistline or sweet wrappers in their pockets!
Those on a poor diet	None	None
Older people, diabetics, drinkers	None	None
Those on a poor diet, diabetics and drinkers. Also those with severe eczema and premenstrual breast tenderness	None	Possibly dry skin

have by referring to the relevant chapters. If you are looking for a general improvement in your health rather than wishing to address a particular condition you would be advised to follow the recommendations for The Very Nutritious Diet on page 437 in order to get a balance of all the essential nutrients. Shop regularly for fresh food, especially for fruit and vegetables, and if you get the opportunity, grow your own fruit and vegetables or buy additive-free or organic produce.

Judith's story

Judith was a very dedicated 45-year-old social worker. She regularly worked long hours at work and had really neglected her social life.

It was thus easy to put her problems of diarrhoea, fatigue and pre-menstrual problems down to her over-caring and rather nervous disposition. Her self-sacrificing nature meant that she had also sacrificed the quality of her diet. She ate erratically, had a poor intake of fresh foods, and would regularly snack on biscuits. She was reluctant even to mention her problem and it was only because of pressure from a friend that she consulted us at all.

There was nothing remarkable to be found from examination but certainly her diet made it likely that she would have some nutritional deficiencies. Tests did reveal somewhat reduced levels of a number of nutrients including zinc and vitamin B1, but the striking feature was the very low level of vitamin B3. Deficiency of this vitamin in particular can cause diarrhoea and can contribute to depression and possibly menstrual disturbances as well.

She had already begun making changes to her diet to improve its nutrient quality and to avoid foods that might be aggravating her bowel problems by the time these results returned. There was no immediate improvement from changing her diet but within a week of beginning high-strength vitamin B her diarrhoea settled completely, her mood improved, and pre-menstrual symptoms lessened. She took this opportunity, with the support of her friends, to make changes to her lifestyle, reducing her work commitment and developing some social interests. A new hairstyle and some evening classes were two further useful steps forward.

Overall there was a very good reduction in her levels of physical symptoms. Her generous, caring nature continues and doubtless she will have to take care that she does not over commit herself both physically and emotionally.

Physical Signs of Vitamin and Mineral Deficiency

Sign or symptom	Can be caused by deficiencies of
Cracking at the corners of the mouth	Iron, vitamins B12, B6, folic acid
Recurrent mouth ulcers	Iron, vitamins B12, B6, folic acid
Dry, cracked lips	Vitamin B2
Smooth (sore) tongue	Iron, vitamins B2, B12, folic acid
Enlargement, prominence of taste buds at the tips of the tongue (red, sore)	Vitamins B2 or B6
Red, greasy skin on face, especially sides of nose	Vitamins B2, B6, zinc or essential fatty acids
Rough, sometimes red, pimply skin on upper arms and thighs	Vitamin B complex, vitamin E or essential fatty acids
Skin conditions such as eczema, dry, rough, cracked, peeling skin	Zinc, essential fatty acids, vitamins A and E
Psoriasis	Folic acid, zinc, selenium, vitamin A, essential fatty acids
Wrinkles	Antioxidants: vitamins A, C, E, selenium, zinc
Poor hair growth	Iron or zinc
Dandruff	Vitamins C, B6, zinc, essential fatty acids, biotin
Acne	Zinc
Bloodshot, gritty, sensitive eyes	Vitamins A, B2
Night blindness	Vitamin A, zinc
Dry eyes	Vitamin A, essential fatty acids
Cracking at corner of eyes	Vitamins B2 or B6
Brittle nails, flattened upturned nails	Iron, zinc, essential fatty acids
White spots on nails	Zinc
Pale appearance due to anaemia	Iron, vitamin B12, folic acid, essential to consult you doctor

Martine's story

Martine was a 45-year-old mother of three who worked part-time as a secretary. Since her mother's death nine months earlier she had been neglecting herself, eating largely junk food, and had put on two stones in weight. She was unhappy, she had dry spotty skin and her hair was in poor condition. She also had dry rough red pimples on her upper arms and thights, split brittle nails and cracking at the corners of her mouth.

'I hadn't been feeling brilliant for some time, so having to cope with my mother's death on top of that was probably the final straw. My eating got out of control and over a period of nine months my weight gradually went up to nearly 12 stones. My normal weight was around $9^1/2$ stones so I felt very uncomfortable and obviously couldn't fit into any of my clothes, which was very depressing. I also noticed that my breasts became incredibly sore each month before my period.

As well as being overweight, I experienced mood swings and noticed that my skin, hair and nails had deteriorated. My nails were split and brittle, my skin became very dry and spotty, and my hair became very dull and split. I felt like a walking wreck. I tried dieting, but found I couldn't stick to a diet for more than a few days which was very demoralising.

I read that cravings for food may be a physiological problem in a report on some research conducted by the WNAS, in Here's Health *magazine. I contacted them for advice and was given a programme to follow that involved eating good food little and often, exercise and nutritional supplements. I started in December which was difficult because of Christmas. But once the new year came, I found I was able to stick to my programme, in fact I was surprised how much I enjoyed it.*

I lost weight gradually, without counting calories, and my vitality returned. Within four months I had lost a stone in weight, my skin was clear, my nails had grown beautifully and even my hair had got its old shine back. The breast symptoms had cleared up too. I felt like a new woman and totally in control. I've had some ups and downs since, but I feel that I now know what my body needs, so it's much easier for me to get back on the right road again.'

See also: Standard References.

Chapter 3
Taking Care of Body and Soul

Pacing ourselves and investing time in our own wellbeing is not something that comes naturally to most of us. When we are preoccupied with caring and providing for our family, our home, as well as coping with our workload outside the home, it sometimes requires real discipline to allocate regular time for personal enhancement. Often, with the best will in the world, our New Year's Resolutions to exercise regularly and make more time for relaxation go out of the window at the first sign of a hiccup in our routine.

There is plenty of hard evidence to suggest that stress underlies many major health problems, and that regular exercise and relaxation are two sound ways of avoiding these, and of keeping both your mind and body in good shape. Taking time out for yourself is not just a nice idea, it is a necessity, especially if you lead a full and demanding life. As a working mother and a busy doctor with four children, we feel pretty qualified to talk about the lifestyle burdens that others have to contend with.

The stress factor

There is a fine line between stress and distress. Stress is reasonably healthy, as it stretches us to capacity and keeps us on our toes. Dealing with challenges as they present themselves is good for our morale, but when we get to the point of overload we cross the line and our modern-day lifestyle often leaves many of us reeling, feeling overwhelmed and under par. If these symptoms continue for more than a short period of time our health can suffer.

The rational ones amongst us do not usually take on a complete 'case load' all at once; we don't ask to be overwhelmed, it just grows on us gradually. We collect our responsibilities as we go along. Perhaps we have been coasting along quite successfully, then a promotion comes along which demands more from us, and at the same time a close relative gets sick, or our partner is made redundant, we find we are expecting another baby, and so on. Additionally, when asked to commit to a project, some of us have not learned to say 'no'. And so we soldier on, believing that we can manage somehow, until one day our body sends out the warning. Whilst this scenario is occurring we are snacking instead of eating properly, and not doing much in the way of exercise or relaxation, or indeed having much fun. Often we lose ourselves along the way because of the many and varied day-to-day pressures of life.

The first warning for some of us could be a bout of flu, or the onset of headaches. Alternatively our digestive system or our energy levels could be affected. Were we to re-evaluate our runaway lifestyle at this point, and invest time in getting our body back into shape, we might well be able to circumvent the health crisis brewing. Invariably though we get up from our sick bed, and go into the ring for the next round. Many of us feel that we have to soldier on, no matter what. There does not seem to be an obvious alternative. Women are particularly prone to this form of martyrdom.

And so we continue, until our bodies say 'no more'. We have both physical and mental limits, and the body can only tolerate so much abuse. It is a vicious circle. Because we feel so awful, usual tasks become more demanding, and looking after ourselves is the last thing to consider. When something goes wrong with the car, the warning light goes on, and when you use a computer wrongly it makes a noise or flashes a message, but our poor bodies fail to communicate their troubles. Most of us wouldn't recognise the signals anyway, until it was too late.

We may not necessarily have a nervous breakdown, but we may develop a weakness in some area of the body as a result of an immune system dysfunction. Some of us develop migraine headaches, others get recurrent thrush, irritable bowel syndrome, panic attacks, depression, chronic fatigue or a nervous rash. The unlucky minority will simply have a fatal heart attack or develop a serious medical condition.

Whilst all this has been going on, it is likely that many of us will have become regular visitors to our doctor's surgery, and have begun taking the 'appropriate' medication. So we are now treating the symptoms, and at best suppressing them. You might even get labelled as 'neurotic' if you are really persistent. What we actually should be doing at this point is looking seriously for the root cause of the problem and addressing it. Whilst some doctors are enlightened and may question you about your troubles or refer you for counselling, they are used to dishing out 'a pill for an ill'. They do not usually have the time in their short consultation to find out what really underlies your symptoms. (At the WNAS we take a whole hour for the first consultation in our clinics, and we have to be organised about using the time wisely in order to get the measure of the real problem.)

There is plenty of medical evidence to support the fact that persistent stress (distress) can affect us both physically and mentally. Let us look at the following case history to demonstrate the point.

Bernice's story

Bernice was a 34-year-old mother of two who, despite her apparently normal life, was at breaking point through stress.

'My husband, who is a conservative, high-powered, executive said I should have been able to "pull myself together" but I was unable to. He wouldn't discuss my upset over the termination I had had after the birth of our last child, or the problems we were experiencing with our sex life, which was now non-existent. I was so anxious and tearful, I honestly don't know how I got through each day. Everything seemed too much, I couldn't even bring myself to answer the telephone when it rang. The most frightening thing of all, which I didn't bring myself to tell anyone, was that I kept seeing "little people" out the corner of my eyes. I knew they weren't there, but they seemed so real. I really thought I was going insane.

Formerly I was such an organised and rational person. I have a very idealistic brain in my head and usually like things to be just so. I used to entertain a lot and loved doing activities with my two children. I have many friends and lots of close family, but I couldn't cope with seeing them as I felt antisocial. One minute I'd feel violent and aggressive, and then I'd think morbid thoughts about dying. I also had chronic back pain and as well as the sleeping pills I took regularly, most days I took at least eight painkillers, which made me very constipated.

My doctor suggested that I got in touch with the WNAS, and in sheer desperation I did. My diet was overhauled, I was sent off to the cranial osteopath, and took Optivite and Efamol. Once my back was feeling better I started to exercise gently and was able to stop taking all the painkillers and sleeping pills. I found the WNAS programme hard to stick to for the first few weeks but was so determined to give it my best as I honestly felt this was the last resort for me.

It did get easier and within a month I was feeling considerably better. Miraculously the osteopath sorted out my back problem, so that I no longer suffered constant pain. My constipation cleared up and the "little men" disappeared thank goodness. After following the programme for three months my symptoms had vanished, and my husband felt that his wife had returned. I was relieved too. I hate to think what might have happened to me and to my family if I had not been pointed in the right direction when I was at such a low ebb.'

Many of us have the ability to cope with near tragedy or disaster, and it is not until it is over, and the dust has settled, that we feel it is safe to 'fall apart'. With hindsight, the warning signals are all there and we can reverse the situation if we come to our senses soon enough.

Here are some tips to help you next time!

- Make sure you make some sacred time for yourself: time to think, and time to switch off from your responsibilities.
- Tell your family how you feel, and ask for their support whilst you get yourself sorted out.
- If your stress comes from work, discuss with colleagues how you can make changes, or if you are self-employed you will need to re-evaluate.
- Try to get away, even if it's only for a few days. Sometimes we can see things more clearly from a distance.
- Learn not to take on too much. If you feel fully committed learn to say 'no'.
- Prioritise your responsibilities and see if you can off-load or delegate some of the less important tasks.
- Eat regular wholesome meals and have a supply of nutritious snacks. Don't fall into the trap of missing meals and eating junk food or chocolate instead.
- Take time each week to exercise. You should be doing three or four sessions of exercise per week, even if it's just skipping or a work-out to a video at home.
- Make time each day to relax formally. You will need 15 minutes, with no interruptions. Really switching off is an art, and you may need some instruction or to read a book on the subject (see page 29).
- Get your partner or a close friend to give you a massage, preferably using some relaxing aromatherapy oils such as geranium or lavender.
- Watch an entertaining film or make time to read a good book.
- Make sure you laugh occasionally. Laughter is so good for us, and yet when we get absorbed with problems in life we seem to lose our sense of humour.
- If you can't see a solution to your current stresses find someone to talk it through with, or get some professional help (don't forget Useful Addresses on page 512).
- Two great books to help you reclaim your life and sort out where you are going next are written by Dr Lucia Capacchione, an American art therapist and teacher, who, when suffering a life threatening illness in 1973, worked out a self-healing method that brought her back to complete health. The first is entitled *Recovery of your Inner Child*, which allows you to search for the root of your stresses and reverse them through journal writing and drawing. She has devised an amazingly powerful technique which is quite enlightening. The second book is entitled *Visioning*, which provides the techniques to work towards living the life you really desire. This involves making a collage, which is fun and therapeutic in itself. Details of both books can be found on page 494.

The benefits of relaxation

Stress and relaxation are at opposite ends of the spectrum. When you are able to maintain the balance there's a good chance of you remaining healthy. However, when the scales tip and stress outweighs relaxation, symptoms of ill-health often rear their heads. With our fast pace of life and our heavy commitments, taking time out for ourselves is often a luxury we consider we cannot afford. But in reality can we afford *not* to make time to relax and unwind? For we know the powerful affect stress can have on us. It has been shown to suppress ovulation in menstruating women, to greatly contribute to digestive disorders like irritable bowel syndrome, to play a key part in migraine headaches, and to increase the number of hot flushes at menopause.

The ability to 'switch off' and refresh ourselves is the key to sanity, but it may not be as easy as it sounds. When you are preoccupied, wound up and tense, it may be hard to lose sight of the benefits of taking time out. Being able to relax thoroughly is actually an acquired skill – which for some of us takes a little practice – but all that is required is some time, and a comfortable space in which to spend that time. Once you have learned the art of relaxation you can practise it at any time, and best of all it is free. Even setting aside time to *think* is therapeutic. Sometimes we go headlong into adverse situations simply because we didn't make time to plan tactics, something which is as true for family and social situations as it is for problems at work.

We all deal with the stresses and strains of life in different ways. Some of us bottle them up and then fall apart one rainy day. Others soldier on feeling disgruntled and perhaps comfort eat or take to the bottle as a result. Regardless of how stress affects you, it is important to take some quiet time each day, as little as 15 or 20 minutes is all that is needed.

Simple relaxation

You will need a quiet space where you can confidently switch off. If necessary, put the answerphone on, or take the phone off the hook. Let other family members know that you don't want to be disturbed for a while, and put on some comfortable loose clothes. Either lie down on a mat, on a soft carpet or firm bed. Make sure that you are comfortable with the room temperature and lighting. You can play some calming music in the background. Once you feel comfortable, do the following, step-by-step:

1 Place a pillow under your head, and stretch out full length. Relax your arms and your lower jaw.
2 Take a few slow deep breaths before you begin.
3 Then concentrate on relaxing your muscles, starting with the toes on one foot and then the other. Gradually work your way slowly up your body, going through all the muscle groups.

4 As you do so, first tense each group of muscles and then relax them, taking care to breathe deeply as you relax.
5 When you reach your head, and your face feels relaxed, remain in the relaxed position for ten to 15 minutes.
6 Gradually allow yourself to 'come to'.

Other methods of relaxation

There are many other relaxation methods available, some of which you will be familiar with. Yoga and meditation are both widely practised doctrines which allow you to practise mind over matter. Massage is a useful tool and so too are creative visualisation, biofeedback and autogenic training. Many of the martial arts like tai chi are therapeutic too. If you find it difficult to close your mind down, it may be a good idea to choose a system of relaxation to try and then to get a little tuition in its principles. Here's an idea of what's on offer.

Yoga

Yoga has been practised throughout the world for thousands of years. It works on the principle of bringing about a harmonious balance between mind, body and soul. It is particularly effective in helping to relieve stress and stress-related conditions. To get started, it's best to attend a yoga class and then to practise the postures at home on a regular basis. There are many good books on yoga (see Recommended Reading on page 490), and there are also a few yoga videos which you might find helpful. Yoga poses can be very powerful, so it is important to have instruction in the early stages.

Massage

We often subconsciously touch or rub a painful area in an attempt to bring about relief. Massage is a term used to describe the ancient art of healing by touch, which is designed to relieve tension, improve circulation and help the body rid itself of toxins. It can also relieve pain by stimulating the production of brain chemicals called endorphins, the body's own painkillers, and by blocking transmission of pain messages by increasing the sensory input to the brain.

There are now many different massage techniques from which to choose, and lovely relaxing aromatherapy oils to use which aid relaxation. If you haven't had a professional massage before, it is worth asking around to find a local person with a good reputation. It is a real treat. If your budget does not permit regular visits to the masseuse, then ask your partner or a friend to do the honours. You could enrol on a massage course with a partner and then practise on each other. Most local authorities have classes and there are many good books on this subject (see Recommended Reading on page 490).

Self-massage

It is possible to massage many parts of your own body, your face, head, neck, shoulders, lower back, abdomen, arms and legs. You will need some almond oil, to which you add a few drops of an aromatherapy oil of choice. Geranium, lavender, orange and melissa are particularly mild and relaxing. It is best to stick to the mild oils as stonger oils which are absorbed through the skin can cause other problems if used inappropriately.

Rub yourself in a clockwise direction on your abdomen, with stroking motions on your arms and legs, kneading your shoulders, and smoothing your neck. Give your face and your temples a rub gently stretching the skin, and with two fingers each side gently massage your temples in a circle. Lastly, rub your ears between your thumb and forefinger, starting at the top and working your way down to the ear lobe, pulling gently at the same time. It feels wonderful and increases circulation to your face and head, as well as easing stress.

Creative visualisation

This is a favoured method of distraction from the stresses of everyday life. If you can recall pictures of holidays when you wished time would stand still or other wholesome fantasies, you can have them all. Creative visualisation is simply a structured method of daydreaming.

Get yourself comfortable in a quiet space, preferably warm and darkened, and without a telephone extension. Lie down, close your eyes and then just float off. Look at those lovely mind pictures until your heart is content. As time goes by, you will develop the ability to 'stay' in your daydream without your mind wandering. When you come round, you should feel warm, calm and relaxed.

Self-hypnosis

This is a self-induced state that makes the mind susceptible to new ideas. When practised regularly it helps to bring about a feeling of calmness and mental agility. It is a system of implanting positive messages which have a therapeutic value, and is thought to be particularly useful in helping to relieve stress, high blood pressure, migraine and insomnia. Some people find that it also helps them to overcome addictive habits. Half an hour each day can leave you feeling refreshed, relaxed and in a more positive mood.

Meditation

Another way of separating you from your body, meditation has a calming and renewing effect on both mind and body. You will need to learn to meditate at a class, but once you have the skill you can use it at any time, and anywhere.

Autogenic training

This method of relaxation, designed to tap into the body's own in-built powers of self-healing, consists of repeating six different commands slowly, in sequence, until you reach a semi-hypnotic state. The end result is a much more relaxed and positive you – and requires only half an hour or so, three times per week initially, but it does involve taking instruction.

Biofeedback

This relaxation technique requires you to link up to a biofeedback machine, or relaxometer. The deep states of relaxation reached through this method have been shown to influence blood pressure levels and brain-wave patterns.

All of these methods and more can be learned at specialist centres through-out the country. It may well be worth investing some time on a few dark winter evenings to learn to outsmart the stresses and strains of daily life.

The benefits of exercise

If you are exercising at least four times per week to the breathlessness stage, and have done so for years, perhaps you should skip this section, which is aimed at the 'reluctant exerciser'.

Many of us wish that our bodies were self-exercising. Whilst we acknowledge that we feel saintly after an exercise session, the thought of getting up on a dark morning in order to exercise before the day begins, understandably, doesn't seem that appealing. But, like most bonuses in life, physical fitness has to be worked for. Why do you need to be phys-ically fit, we hear you ask, as you are not planning on entering any competitions? And anyway you lead a busy life, surely that's enough?

As our knee bone is connected to our thigh bone and so on, it follows that if we exert ourselves physically, it will have a positive overall effect on both our body and our mind. Exercising to the point of breathlessness stimulates the release of brain chemicals, called endorphins, which not only raise our mood, but also influence our hormones. Rushing around and leading a busy life may just leave us feeling absolutely exhausted, especially chasing after children from morning till night. We have yet to meet anyone who feels 'high' from these activities. Exercise, on the other hand, helps to improve energy levels and to overcome symptoms of depression, anxiety, insomnia, and also increases our sense of self-esteem and wellbeing. In fact exercise has been shown to be more successful in overcoming symptoms of depression and anxiety than psychotherapy. Being in good physical shape is also good for the ego, especially as we age, and shouldn't go unnoticed by our partners.

More good news is that exercise may offset ageing of the central nervous system, as well as being cardio-protective. It also stimulates the heart, which in turn stimulates the flow of blood around the body, which flushes out toxins and keeps our skin glowing. So there are many benefits to be had, and we are not talking Olympics here!

Research shows that we need to exercise four or five times per week at least, to the point of breathlessness. But do not treat getting fit like being in a competition. You need only exercise to increase gradually your fitness level. If you haven't exercised for years, it may take only a few minutes initially before you need the armchair. Each exercise session should be slightly longer than the last one, until you feel 'comfortable' exercising for 40 minutes. It may take a few months to build up to that, and it is worth keeping an exercise diary so that you can monitor your progress. If you are currently under your doctor's supervision, and haven't exercised for a while, it is advisable to get a medical blessing before embarking on your exercise regime.

More good news is that you do not necessarily have to join the gym, or do an hour's aerobics class with a group of stick insects, but you do need to choose the kind of exercise you *like* in order to stick at it. For those who haven't exercised for some time, we usually recommend starting with some brisk walking or gentle skipping, and perhaps a short work-out with an exercise video. We particularly recommend the YMCA exercise videos as they are scientifically based, and begin with ten or 12 minute gentle work-outs. They cater for all fitness levels, so if you have a limited amount of time, putting on the exercise video before anyone else is up in the morning is probably the best solution.

An exercise programme should be for life. It takes months to build stamina and only weeks to lose it if we stop exercising, which is rather infuriating. You are likely to be more successful at sticking to your regime if you make yourself a schedule. It is all too easy to cry off because of other commitments. If you find it hard to stick to your schedule, arrange to meet a friend or colleague for a game of tennis or squash, or make a date to have a gentle jog or swim together. That way it will be harder for you to make some sort of excuse.

What we are aiming for

When you make the decision to exercise regularly, your motivation must be sound in order to maintain the commitment. Whilst most women would not object to having the vital statistics of Pamela Anderson and the men amongst us, Arnold Shwarzeneger, your reason for exercising is health. You want to protect yourself from heart disease and to keep your bones strong, thus preventing the bone-thinning disease, osteoporosis. Any visible physical improvements are a bonus. You want to develop and improve your *Stamina, Strength* and *Suppleness*, the three S's.

Stamina

Stamina refers to the efficiency of the heart and lungs in delivering oxygen to the muscles, and can be measured by the amount of time it takes you to get breathless. We can gradually build our stamina, with regular low-intensity aerobic exercise. Aerobic exercise simply uses large muscle groups like the legs and arms, which then demand more oxygen, making the heart work harder. With regular aerobic exercise the heart and lungs become more efficient, which means they will not have to 'work' so hard in daily life. Increasing your stamina also means that you can achieve more for less effort. You should eventually be aiming for four to five 40-minute sessions of low impact aerobic exercise per week in order to reap all the benefits that exercise has to offer.

Strength

The definition of strength is the maximum force needed by a muscle or group of muscles to overcome a resistance. In other words how much effort it takes to push, pull, lift, climb and carry without injuring your-self. We can increase our strength by as much as 50 per cent without gaining muscle size. Stronger muscles will mean that you can get more out of your day, be it in the garden, in the house, or at leisure. Having strong back and abdominal muscles will also improve your posture and guard you from most lower back pain.

Suppleness

Joint mobility is something you take for granted early in life, but as you get older joints naturally stiffen through lack of use. It really is a case of 'use it or lose it'. Stretching exercises will help to maintain your mobility, and are easy to practise at home whilst listening to music or in front of the television. Stretch your muscles slowly, holding each position until you feel the strain, but not pain.

Where specific exercises are of value to a particular condition, like heart disease, osteoporosis, fatigue, PMS, pregnancy and so on, you will see that we give specific instructions and a target to aim for in the relevant section.

The pay-off

If you have always avoided exercise, you are probably grimacing at the thought of what you know should be ahead. Let us assure you that you will reap the benefits of your labour. We have seen so many patients who have not previously exercised begin their exercise programme reluctantly, and then surprisingly come to love it. They feel it improves their energy levels and vitality, and notice improvements in their skin quite quickly. For every hour you spend exercising you will get the equivalent time back in increased stamina, strength and suppleness. Additionally, it is now well accepted that regular exercise helps to protect us against heart disease, arthritis, protects our bones against the bone thinning disease osteoporosis, and helps us to avoid depression. So exercising is not just a nice idea, both the long- and short-term benefits are well worth the investment of a few hours each week.

Chapter 4
The Strengths of Complementary Therapies

Although making dietary changes, exercising, relaxing and taking nutritional supplements are the prime factors in our health, it is also undoubtedly valuable to explore the world of complementary therapy. Unlike orthodox medicine, holistic medicine looks at the *whole person* – the mind, the body and the spirit, and how they interact.

The years of abusing our bodies eventually takes its toll. Strains that are placed upon the body over time – not eating the right diet, consuming too much alcohol and tobacco, coping with stressful situations and for women being pregnant and breast-feeding, premenstrual syndrome and symptoms of the menopause – may well be more than we can easily tolerate, and the stresses can affect the smooth running of our bodily processes. If your symptoms are severe, it may well be worth investigating what acupuncture, acupressure, cranial osteopathy, herbal medicine, homeopathy or indeed the powers of healing or self-healing have to offer. They are powerful tools that can sometimes help to speed up the recovery process.

Acupuncture

Chinese medical thinking is quite different from that in the West in that it considers symptoms rather than named conditions, and the diagnosis and subsequent treatment address the whole person; the mind, body and lifestyle. Acupuncture can be a useful tool in the treatment of health problems and is appropriate for severe symptoms. You should always consult a properly trained and registered practitioner. Information should be available from your public library, and a register is published by the British Acupuncture Council, listing all members of the five recognised and affiliated professional bodies (see Useful addresses on page 513).

The philosophy

Chinese medicine, of which acupuncture is a part, works on the premise that a universal energy known as *chi*, which has two complementary qualities (*yin* and *yang*), must be in perfect balance in order for good health to exist. The term yin encompasses the feminine principle (cold and the state of rest) whereas yang includes the male principle (heat and activity). These principles are active to appropriate degrees in both men and women, and when the balance is upset, illness is the result.

Chi flows through the twelve meridians or channels of the body, which are each associated with a particular organ, such as the lungs, liver or spleen. Herbal remedies and acupuncture are used to restore the balance of yin and yang, and thus promote healing.

What treatment to expect

As well as taking an in-depth medical history, the practitioner will take your pulse at six different points on each wrist to get the measure of each of the twelve vital organs of the body. Your tongue will also be inspected closely, as its texture reflects the condition of the vital organs.

Acupuncture uses stainless-steel needles, which are inserted into specific points along meridians or lines, in order to affect the energy flowing to an organ. The needles, which remain in place for approximately 20 minutes, don't actually hurt, but they may cause a tingle, mild ache or heat sensation.

Chinese medicine also encompasses the use of herbs rather than drugs, which are aimed at keeping the yin and yang in constant harmony. Many of the herbal remedies used by Chinese doctors are available in pill form and are relatively inexpensive. They should only be used with the guidance of a qualified practitioner, as taking a yang preparation when a yin medicine is required will further exaggerate the imbalance and may well make your problem worse.

Acupressure

The Japanese finger pressure method, otherwise known as shiatsu, is more appropriate to minor or occasional problems than acupuncture. In this system the body is influenced in various ways by the stimulation of key points, found along the course of energy channels circulating near the surface of the skin. These are the same as acupuncture meridians, but the points are stimulated by pressure rather than needles.

In order for shiatsu to be effective it is important to apply the right kind of pressure for an appropriate length of time. Some professional instruction would be useful initially so that you can recognise the correct method. Once you have mastered the art of applying pressure to appropriate points, you can self-administer at home.

Cranial osteopathy

Many of us suffer with subtle back or neck problems that occur as a result of general wear and tear. Long-standing headaches can sometimes be totally cured by some good osteopathic treatment. It is certainly worth consulting a cranial osteopath if you feel the tension building up in your back or neck, or if you suffer from regular headaches.

The philosophy

Cranial osteopathy, or cranio-sacral therapy as it is also known, is a specialised form of osteopathy which is gentle yet potent. The aim is to gently coax the muscles, tendons, joints and connective tissue to establish correct function and release restriction, thus restoring normal circulation, the flow of energy and glandular secretions.

The cranio-sacral mechanism is made up of the cranium (the skull), the sacrum (the bone at the base of the spine), the membranes surrounding the brain, the spinal cord and the fascia, a continuous clingfilm-like sheet that surrounds the muscles, organs, joints and bones. The tension of this fascia is all-important. If you have ever worn an all-in-one pants suit that is too tight or too short, you will have felt somewhat uncomfortable. If the tension in the body's fascia becomes too tight, you can't just take it off, and it is possible that body functions can be affected in the long term.

Cranial osteopathy works on two basic principles: first, that structure can affect function, and second, that impairment in the structure, or reduced mobility, will affect blood flow. Blood flow is of supreme importance in osteopathy, and treatment is aimed at improving local circulation and freeing-up the supply of blood to the nerves.

Everything in the body moves with the cranial rhythm, which is the rhythm of the central nervous system. It's like a breathing rhythm, and is constant, even when we sleep. The movement helps blood flow generally and can help impaired local circulation after trauma.

If there are restrictions to soft tissue (like muscles) to the fascia or to the membranes, then blood, lymph and cerebral spinal fluid is restricted; as a result, nutrition to that area is affected.

What treatment to expect

Cranial osteopaths, like acupuncturists, like to take their time over the initial consultation, in order to take a complete history and to assess the problem fully. The patient/client lies on the osteopath's consulting bed whilst balancing takes place. It is extremely subtle. The treatment feels like mild finger pressure, but the effect is powerful. Often patients fall 'asleep' and experience a very pleasant sense of wellbeing. It is important to rest afterwards, and sometimes things feel worse the next day, but this will pass. One treatment takes several days to work, and so you would not be required to attend more than fortnightly or monthly. Courses are usually short, although the course of treatment may be extended for chronic problems.

Herbal medicine

Curiously, herbal medicine is older and more ubiquitous than any other type of medication on earth. It is as old as food and people, and there is no place which has been inhabited by people and plants that has not had its own herbal medicine. The great majority of plant medicines in use today were discovered by the hunter-gatherers, and so pre-date history itself. There is very good evidence that in all past and present hunter-gatherer societies, the responsibilities for gathering and learning about plant medicine belonged to women. So perhaps we can take some comfort in knowing that afflicted women discovered their own remedies.

As civilisations emerged, men became involved with agriculture and medicine, and tended to form analytical systems. As China, for example, evolved the polar principles of yin and yang, so European medicine relied on the concepts of love and strife: these resolved into four elements which in turn were thought to be represented in the body by the four bodily fluids or humours. Many of these concepts still inform the best herbal medical practice in the West today, along with naturopathic ideas, many learned from native North Americans. Like Chinese medicine, European herbal medicine places great emphasis upon diet and exercise and other environmental factors.

The philosophy

While herbal medicine aims to treat your current condition, it takes into consideration your past history from the time you were born, and the health of your parents at the time of conception. So, even if your symptoms are the same as your neighbour's, your prescriptions are unlikely to be the same. In other words, while we are all subject to the same biophysical laws, each one of us has a unique tissue profile and therefore the treatment (by a once-living plant organism) needs to be unique.

What treatment to expect

The prescription you will receive may consist of a combination of a few or many different herbs. Sometimes you will be given herbs to take at different times of the day; and on occasions, herbs for different times of the month. Herbal medicine has been shown to speed up the healing of broken bones and to aid absorption of minerals from the digestive tract. It can be a very powerful tool. If you would like to consult a trained herbalist, you will find the address of The National Institute of Medical Herbalists on page 517.

Homeopathy

The word homeopathy comes from two Greek words: *homoio* which means 'same' and *pathos* with means 'suffering'. It was developed by Dr Samuel Hahnemann in the eighteenth century, as a system of treating sick people with safe medicine. Whereas orthodox medicine (or allopathic medicine, as it is referred to) aims to treat symptoms with a drug that will produce an opposite effect, homoeopathy treats 'like with like'.

A homeopathic remedy is designed to produce the same symptoms as those you are suffering, and in doing so aims to cancel them out. The dosages used are minute and may contain no substantial amount of the original material. In this latter case, it is thought that the medicine, pill or liquid contains an energy, or 'spirit', of the original medicine. Even these extreme dilutions have been shown to be effective for many conditions, including arthritis and hayfever.

The philosophy

Homeopathy is an approach to treatment which aims to assist nature with her own process of healing rather than by-passing her altogether. Like other holistic treatments, it treats each person as an individual. A trained homeopath takes an exceedingly thorough history before suggesting the most suitable remedy. It is very much a gentle, preventative, method of treatment which works best in conjunction with improved dietary and lifestyle measures.

Followers of homeopathy regularly use remedies to help themselves and their families for anything from coughs and cold to menstrual problems. The British royal family continue to be staunch supporters of homeopathy, and it will undoubtedly remain an option for us all.

What treatment to expect

Once diagnosed you will usually be presented either with little white pills made from lactose, which melt under your tongue, or a tincture, which is a liquid. You will be given instructions about how frequently to use your remedy, and advice about diet and lifestyle. The remedies are widely available, and they are reasonably priced. Sometimes it's trial and error until you find the remedy that suits you, but it may be worth persisting.

If you do decide to consult an holistic practitioner, use a recommended practitioner or find a properly qualified person from the register kept by each association. Sadly, there are many non-qualified people practising, and these should be avoided. The addresses and telephone numbers of the relevant associations can be found in Useful addresses starting on page 512.

Healing

Until more recent times consulting a healer for 'laying on of hands' was considered by the majority to be a pursuit only entertained by 'believers'. Suspicious was the term many polite folk would have used to describe their feelings about the practice. Despite this, if you care to look back in time, priests in ancient Egypt were said to have cured the sick by laying on of hands and there are many examples of similar miraculous cures in the Bible.

Today, at the start of the 21st century, a wide variety of styles of healing have become quite acceptable and it is not uncommon to be able to book an appointment with a healer with a practice in any High Street. We have even reached the point where medical science has begun to acknowledge the possible benefits of healing, and as a result it is sometimes offered in hospitals to complement orthodox treatment.

The philosophy

The term healing encompasses a wide range of belief systems. Healers often describe their work as the 'restoration of health by non-physical means'. Whilst there is no explanation as to how healing is induced, a variety of clinical trials demonstrate its beneficial effects. Many healers believe that therapeutic changes take place in the patient's soul during treatment, prompting biological responses. Some interpret this power as a form of 'energy', some refer to themselves as a 'channel' for healing and others refer to a 'guide', but it effectively adds up to the same thing in that their goal is to assist the body to heal itself. There are numerous brands of healing to chose from these days, which can be a little confusing. However, most healers are ordinary people who recognise their ability to heal others. Some consider that they possess a special ability, whilst others feel that it is a natural talent common to all. Healers usually consider that they are channels for, rather than possessors of, healing energy.

A variety of clinical trials have produced significant results. In 1993, 155 studies were reviewed by a US healer, Dr Daniel Benor. He found that some 60 per cent of the studies had positive results, particularly in cases of high blood pressure, wound healing and anxiety. In 1998 another American trial, this time on 400 heart patients at San Francisco General Hospital, claimed that absent healing seemed to aid patients recovery. Mathew Manning, a well-known UK healer, has extended the life of blood cells and accelerated plant growth in controlled studies. In addition to clinical studies, there have been numerous case reports, from many countries, of individuals who after being given only two months to live with terminal cancer, have been able to confound the scientists by visualising and healing their tumour completely.

Most of the sceptical doctors who refuse to acknowledge any likely benefit to healing, would agree that it can do little harm, and may even be a comfort to patients.

What treatment to expect

There are so many types of healing to chose from, including spiritual healing, faith healing, absent healing and aura healing. Your consultation will take place in different environments, depending on the sort of healer you chose. It will ideally take place in a quiet, tranquil environment, perhaps with relaxing music playing in the background. After being asked for a brief history of your problem, your healer will usually invite you to sit or lie down, whilst he or she sits or stands beside you. Once attuned, the healer's hands will be placed in the area of the site of your problem, and in various other places. Some healers gently touch, whilst others hold their hands in space away from your body. One of the main aims is that healing energy flows though the healer into your body. Some individuals report being able to feel the warmth or chill of the energy, whilst others see colours or light. Some just drift off into a peaceful state and once fully conscious feel refreshed and energised.

Healing is generally a pleasant experience, but it may release deep and forgotten emotions. You will find contact addresses in the Useful addresses section for the National Federation of Spiritual Healers and for Reiki, which is a Japanese form of spiritual healing which has become popular in the last few years.

Self-healing

Those of us who have had success with self-healing will feel certain about the power that lies within to heal their own body. One of those individuals, Dr Lucia Capacchione, is an art therapist and psychologist, from America, who managed to heal herself from a life threatening illness in 1973. She has since gone on to write twelve books on this and related subjects, and regularly gives workshops that instruct individuals how to heal themselves.

Her methods involve keeping a journal and drawing, all with the non-dominant hand. In her experience this helps us to contact our 'inner child', and in doing so, deep-seated underlying causes for our illnesses. She believes that the inner child, which lives within us all, and who loves to play and discover, is often forced underground by the demands of the adult world. When we consistantly ignore our inner child, we fail to nurture our heart and soul, and the body eventually gets sick. Implementing the simple steps laid out in her books which are detailed on page 494, as well following our suggestions of what you can do to overcome each condition covered in this book, may well help to speed your recovery, and give you a new perception about your life.

Part Two

THE A–Z OF PROBLEMS

Abdominal Wind and Bloating

Gas in the bowel is certainly not something to bring up in social conversation, and yet on average we produce 1.5 litres per day, enough to fill a small balloon, which means that in a year we are talking about some 500 litres! Wind is often accompanied by a sluggish and constipated bowel, but fluid retention or lax abdominal muscles can contribute as well. Bloating can occur at any time, and is often worse for women premenstrually. It is best tackled by addressing the underlying problems of bowel sluggishness and anything that can influence wind production.

The subject of abdominal wind has only been taken seriously in the last decade. A variety of gases are produced by billions of mainly friendly bacteria that inhabit the large colon, the transverse section of the large bowel. (Surprisingly, there are more bacteria in the colon than there are cells in our body.) They are found only in tiny amounts in the small bowel where the majority of digestion and absorption of nutrients takes place. They first appear in our caecum, which is the first part of the large bowel, on the right side of the abdomen at about the point where the appendix is (or was, if it has been removed) and are waiting to pounce on the leftovers from the meal you ate several hours before.

These bacteria produce a variety of gases, some of which our own cells are incapable of producing. They include hydrogen, methane and carbon dioxide, all of which have no smell. The gas that smells like bad eggs is hydrogen sulphide, and it is more commonly produced by those living in the West, because of dietary factors.

What are the symptoms?

The trapped gases cause bloating which may be painful or painless, and often results in the sufferer having a lower self-image because frequently clothes don't fit. Some of the wind manages to escape through burping, or to give it its medical term, erucation, or through the back passage when its passing sometimes creates loud noises or an offensive smell. It may be accompanied by social embarrassment, especially if you cannot control its passing and the smell is noticeable by others. Severe sufferers commonly avoid social events because of their symptoms.

Who gets it?

The degree of wind and bloating is related mainly to the type of diet eaten, and how food is digested. Those with a poor digestion, especially with disease of the pancreas, will find that many foods will aggravate this problem. High-fibre foods are particularly to blame. An excess of fats can make it worse, too.

What causes it?

It is not the result of air we swallow, whilst breathing or eating, as most of this is absorbed during the digestive process or brought back as a burp. The amount and type of wind that any one individual produces is influenced by:

- The type of food eaten, especially fibre-rich foods.
- How well the food is digested in the small bowel.
- How quickly food and residues pass through the small bowel to the colon.
- The type of bacteria present in the colon, which may also be influenced by the type of diet we eat, presence or absence of illness, use of anti-biotics and even the type of bacteria in the colons of those with whom you live.

What causes wind production can and does vary from person to person. Something that encourages wind in one person may well have no effect on another. And what causes you wind at one stage may not cause any problems at another time. So it is really a combination of factors and what goes on in the bowel that can influence many aspects of body health.

Excessive production of wind is more likely to occur if:

- You consume foods to which you are intolerant – and in theory this could be any food depending on your individual sensitivities.
- You eat foods that contain sugars that you cannot easily digest, and these are then fermented by the bacteria in the large bowel and coverted to gas. The same can occur in fewer cases following the excess consumption of table sugar (found in most sweets and sweetened foods), fruit sugar or fructose (found in most fruits and vegetables), or the artificial sweetener Sorbitol (found in cool-tasting mints and some sugar-free sweets).
- You eat foods that are known to be hard to digest, especially if they are not well cooked or are eaten in large amounts. The list is potentially very long, and can certainly consist of any of the following:
  - wheat, especially wheat bran and wholemeal products

- ○ coarse oats, barley and rye
- ○ sweetcorn, especially if whole and not chewed well
- ○ brown rice
- ○ potatoes
- ○ dried beans, lentils and sometimes peas
- ○ vegetables of the Brassica family (cabbage, cauliflower, broccoli and Brussels sprouts) and Jerusalem artichokes
- ○ shells of prawns and other crustacea
- ○ mushrooms
- ○ onions, garlic and leeks
- ○ asparagus
- ○ green peppers.
- You have a rapid gut transit time – which can be encouraged by drinking coffee and eating large meals. A low-fat, high-carbohydrate, high-fibre diet might make the situation worse, too. The combination of rapid passage through the small bowel, especially if the meal was hard to digest, will result in the bacteria of the colon getting their full share.
- You have poor digestion. If you have recently lost weight and experience abdominal pain, you should see your doctor without delay.
- You are making an excessive use of laxatives.
- You have been prescribed some relatively new drugs to control diabetes, as these inhibit the digestion of sugar.
- You eat large amounts of caramel, burnt sugar and modified starch. These have all been chemically altered by heat or the cooking process, which makes them harder to digest. Caramel is widely used as a colouring and flavouring agent, so you will need to read labels carefully. There is also a significant amount in beer.

What your doctor can do

The answer is probably very little, other than investigate for severe wind and bloating accompanied by other digestive symptoms. In truth, as our doctors know relatively little about diet, they too are probably suffering in silence. Occasionally preparations based on mint, such as Colpermin and Mintec, or old fashioned charcoal preparations can be helpful. If the wind is accompanied by diarrhoea, weight loss or blood in the stool then obviously medical investigations will be necessary.

What you can do

- Eat slowly, taking care to chew your food well.
- Avoid the foods that you know upset you.
- Ensure that your vegetables are not undercooked.

- If you enjoy eating dried beans, soak them overnight, shake them to remove the husks and cook them thoroughly. Many, including red kidney beans, need to be cooked for at least 10 minutes at a rolling boil, and then simmered for an hour before they are ready to eat. This reduces the potential wind-producing culprits – two tough carbohydrates called stacchyose and raffinose. Black-eyed beans and red kidney beans are usually the biggest wind producers in the bean family.
- Eat smaller portions and take time to relax after a meal to aid digestion.
- Avoid foods rich in sulphur and sulphites as these chemicals encourage the conversion of hydrogen in the colon to hydrogen sulphide – the bad-eggs gas. The main dietary sources of these chemicals are:
  - bread
  - foods preserved with sulphur dioxide, such as dried fruits, and fruit squashes, plus anything else containing a sulphite or metabisulphite compound (where label reading comes in again)
  - wines, beers and cider, which often contain sulphite as a preservative (this doesn't have to be mentioned on the label)
  - eggs and all members of the onion family.
- Avoid caramel, burnt sugar and foods containing them.
- Don't smoke heavily during or after a meal as this can inhibit digestive function and for some could result in increased wind production.
- Eat charcoal biscuits, an old-fashioned remedy that might help.
- Peppermint tea is useful after a meal or when discomfort starts.
- Ginger in the form of tea or crystallised is useful for nausea.
- Have a pot of live yoghurt each day as this is rich in semi-friendly bacteria.
- Take a probiotic supplement such as acidophillus or lactobacillus bifidus. Probiotics contain 'friendly' bacteria which colonise the colon, helping to alleviate abdominal discomfort. They are particularly important if digestive abnormalities have occurred after taking a course of antibiotics. Acidophillus is available in capsules or can be obtained in powder form.
- It might be worth taking a supplement of fructo oligo-saccharides (FOS) which actually feed the existing 'friendly' bacteria to help re-populate the colon. FOS is a short chain polysaccharide that increases the levels of short chain fatty acids (SCFAs) like butyrate. SCFAs actually provide the primary energy substrate for colonic epithelial cell growth and replication. FOS is taken in powder form and must be introduced slowly or it can cause short-term bloating.
- Be patient, it could take up to six weeks to see stable improvement.
- Swallow your embarrassment and consult your doctor if these self-help measures don't work.

Relaxation

Both relaxation and hypnotherapy seem genuinely to improve the way the bowel functions, and are useful tools for diarrhoea sufferers. It seems that they influence the function of the gut muscles, encouraging them to work in an efficient co-ordinated fashion. It is also possible that with the help of regular relaxation and some hypnotherapy a person may gain more control of their bowels as they perhaps become less sensitive to and more tolerant of the disturbance in function.

Regular massage, of at least the abdomen and lower back, with some of the aromatherapy oils mentioned on page 31, is desirable for severe sufferers. Making sure you take time out to relax each day will also bring its benefits.

Complementary therapies

Herbal medicine is likely to offer you a mixture that will calm your bowel and aid digestion, and it is also worth consulting an acupuncturist. Homeopathy may also have a remedy that would bring relief from your symptoms. Any of these systems may help, but it is important to try one at a time, otherwise there will be a very confusing picture.

Sonya's story

Sonya was a 33-year-old woman from Sussex who was married with two children and worked as an administrator. She was admitted to hospital several times as a result of her symptoms, but was offered little effective help from the doctors who examined her.

'Following the birth of my second baby I began suffering with severe bouts of abdominal bloating and pains. One night I had the most terrible attack and thought I was dying. The doctor was called, and by the time he arrived I was hyperventilating. He called an ambulance, and I was taken to casualty, writhing and groaning in pain. The examining doctor was surprised by the amount of pain I was in, and was unable to make a diagnosis. I was kept in overnight for observation and given pain-killers. The following morning I was sent home with a diagnosis of colic, and no follow-up treatment whatsoever. The only suggestion my doctor had was to eat more wholemeal bread and bran, which made my symptoms even worse.

My symptoms affected my whole life. When I had them I found it hard to work and could hardly cope with my family duties. I had no choice but to leave the parenting to my husband. I dreaded family holidays and wondered what the future held for me.

I was recommended to the WNAS clinic. At my first consultation I was asked about many aspects of my history, diet and lifestyle. I was given diet, exercise and supplement programmes to follow, which I duly did.

Within the first month I noticed a spectacular difference, and within four months the symptoms were gone completely! I am three years on now and can honestly say that I feel better than I have for years. I am now able to cope with my job and am a competent wife and mother, and I am immensely grateful. I do wish that the doctors that I had seen over the years had been armed with adequate knowledge about diet, which would have saved me a lot of pain and trauma.'

See also: Irritable bowel syndrome, Premenstrual syndrome, Recommended reading, Useful addresses, References.

Acne

Acne, or to give it its proper name, 'Acne Vulgaris', is perhaps the commonest skin complaint in that most of us have had some experience of it during adolescence. Three types of spots make up acne:

- the redheads or papules
- the yellowheads or pustules
- the blackheads or comedones

These usually appear on a background of inflamed red skin. This is most commonly on the face, back or shoulders. These red-, yellow- and blackheads are manifestations of the inflammation, infection and resolution that occurs in this condition. Initially there is an increased sensitivity to hormones in the skin. Testosterone, which is present in both men and women, stimulates the production of sebum or grease. The ducts that carry this grease to the surface become blocked, get inflamed, then infected, and then either discharge themselves or resolve, leaving a blackhead behind which is the thickened remains of the infected pus of the yellowhead.

Who gets it?

Many do in adolescence. Boys are more affected than girls and some, due to genetic factors, are not affected at all. Many women in their twenties and thirties are also affected as there may be minor hormonal changes or increased hormonal sensitivity that leads to the persistence of acne. Acne can also be caused by a few drugs: steroids, phynytoin and phenothiazines. Exposure to chemicals containing chlorine can also be a rare cause.

What your doctor can do

Therapy is aimed at reducing the bacteria on the skin surface, reducing the production of sebum or altering the hormonal stimulus to acne especially in older women.

- Local applications of antiseptic, especially benzoyl peroxide, help by inhibiting the growth of bacteria and reducing sebum production. A local application of retinoic acid helps to unblock plugged follicles and is used when blackheads dominate.
- Prescribe an antibiotic skin application or antibiotics by mouth. There are a variety of preparations with around a 75 per cent success rate. Sometimes the bacteria become resistant to one antibiotic, and a change is needed. A swab may help decide the best sort.
- Hormone-based treatment using either the oral contraceptive pill or a combination of oestrogen with a small dose of an anti-testosterone preparation, is useful for more resistant cases.
- A powerful drug derived from vitamin A, 13-cis-retinoic acid, is highly effective as it inhibits the excessive production of sebum. It is only used by hospital specialists in those who have failed to respond to other treatments. As its use is associated with foetal abnormalities, women taking it should use contraception.

What you can do

- Keep your skin clean. Clean your skin thoroughly after using make-up.
- Sunbathe. This often helps, though it may increase the number of blackheads.
- Squeeze the blackheads. This is worthwhile provided that they are not pushed inward into the deeper layers of the skin.
- Change your diet. Despite popular belief, no diet is of proven value in acne! For some avoiding chocolate seems to help. It is possible that a low-fat diet (weight-reducing if necessary) with high intake of fruit and vegetables and a reduced intake of wheat might help some sufferers.

Nutritional supplements

The only one of proven benefit is zinc. It is not as effective as antibiotics. A dose of 30 mg per day is needed. Higher doses should only be taken under supervision. Most useful if there is a lot of inflammation or cystic swellings.

Complementary therapies

Consider homeopathy and herbalism.

Miranda's story

Miranda was a very attractive and petite 42-year-old woman from America, who was trained as a nurse. She had married an Englishman and lived half her life in the UK. She came to the clinic as she was feeling generally low, and had a chronic skin problem. The PMS symptoms she had manifested themselves in terrible depression, mood swings and a near suicidal state of mind.

'I was a very health conscious person and considered myself to be relatively educated on the subject of diet. However, when I reached the age of 41 it seems I stopped ovulating and my general health suddenly went down hill. My previously clear facial skin broke out in painful spots and despite seeing many consultant dermatologists in both the UK and the US nothing seemed to really help. I was very depressed and tearful and the best my GP could offer was Prozac, which I took in desperation.

I had suffered from acne from the age of 16 and despite visiting dermatologists, beauty experts and black magic practitioners, and having swallowed every antibiotic known to man, nothing worked on a permanent basis. I was about to start a hospital supervised course of treatment that had possible bad side effects, but again could not be guaranteed to be permanently successful, when I decided to visit the WNAS.

I was taken off wheat, rye, barley and oats for a period of three months and I began to notice the improvement in my skin. I was also not eating red meat or dairy products, but was taking supplements of Optivite, zinc and Efamol. After approximately three months I incorporated rye bread into my diet without problems. After six months my skin was clear. Several months later I tried to reintroduce wheat into my diet with disastrous results. Even small amounts, i.e. in sausages, soup, casseroles, would bring me out in painful cysts. So wheat was completely removed from my diet, along with dairy products. I do eat red meat occasionally without ill effect.

I use soya products instead, which is really no hardship these days. I recently paid another visit to the clinic as my menopause has now begun, and was delighted to discover that soya products are a rich source of naturally occurring oestrogen. It is so wonderful to have clear skin and not feel ashamed to be seen without make-up. Even my mother, who suffered along with me for so many years, recently remarked that visiting the WNAS has transformed my life both physically and mentally.'

ACNE ROSACEA

This is a mainly facial rash that usually develops in middle-aged to elderly people. Like common acne there is a degree of skin redness, with papules (redheads) and occasionally pustules (yellowheads) but never blackheads. Flushing is prominent on the cheeks and nose and is usually made worse by alcohol. Sometimes the eyes become involved with redness of the eyelids and clouding of the vision in severe cases.

What your doctor can do

The main treatment is use of long-term, low-dose antibiotics, usually tetracycline, as given for acne vulgaris. Those suffering with eye symptoms as well will need special attention.

What you can do

- Avoid known aggravating factors; most commonly these are alcohol and anything else that may trigger a flush, like spicy foods and hot drinks. .
- Try a diet low in amine-rich foods as used for migraine (see page 473). In sensitive individuals this type of chemical can affect the blood vessels in the head, triggering migraine, and the possibility exists that they also affect the blood vessels of the face too. This means avoiding cheese, chocolate, tea and coffee, and many other foods.

Complementary therapies
Consider homeopathy and herbalism.

Barbara's story

Barbara was a 33-year-old woman who developed an increasingly severe facial rash. Her undoubted good looks had been spoiled by a red, pimply looking rash that was distributed mainly across her cheeks, down her jaw line and onto her nose. Over a year ago this had been diagnosed as acne rosacea and had not responded to a course of antibiotics from her own doctor.

Close examination showed that there were possibly two types of rash. The typical acne rosacea was mainly on the cheeks but also there were some red itchy bumps along the jaw line. This latter type of rash we have seen in association with a suspected allergy to wheat.

Barbara was asked to follow the diet using the treatment for migraine – avoiding all amine-rich foods as well as wheat, oats, barley and rye which may all contain gluten. She was also asked to take supplements of zinc and vitamin B.

Within three weeks there was an over 50 per cent improvement in the appearance of her rash. Interestingly, the itchy bumps had cleared almost completely and her skin felt much more comfortable.

The rate of her improvement was probably too quick for it to be anything to do with her supplements and it seemed that the avoidance of certain foods was the particularly important factor.

She reintroduced foods that had previously been excluded on a step-by-step basis and was able to identify those that had contributed to her rash in particular. It transpired that alcohol was a particular culprit.

Ageing

We now live for longer and as time passes there will be more retired people and fewer workers in the western world. Health-care services will be stretched and so it makes sense for us to implement self-help measures to preserve our fitness, health and physical appearance.

It is becoming rapidly obvious that the elderly, those of 65 and over, are all individuals, with varying levels of health. We are also beginning to identify factors that determine those who will age quickly. Factors associated with premature death or rapid ageing are:

- cigarette smoking
- excessive alcohol intake
- poor quality diet
- social deprivation e.g. living alone
- low levels of physical activity
- low levels of mental activity
- genetic factors, identified and unidentified

The genetic factor is interesting as we know that there are genetic predispositions to high blood pressure, heart disease and diabetes. Genetic factors may also play a small part in many other diseases. It is clear that there are interactions between a person's genetic predisposition and the effects of their diet, for example salt intake, and whether it raises blood pressure.

Overall intake of nutrients during the course of a lifetime may be an important factor. Interest is centred upon the antioxidants, vitamins, minerals and other non-essential dietary agents that protect tissues against highly reactive chemicals called free radicals. Free radicals are produced during the course of normal metabolic activity in all cells of the body, and can damage tissues, causing chemical change. There are many protective mechanisms which minimise this damage and, as a result, these free radicals only last for minute fractions of a second. Certain nutrients help mop up these potentially damaging free radicals, including:

- vitamin C
- vitamin E
- vitamin A (both beta-carotene and retinol)
- B vitamins
- zinc
- copper
- manganese

If left unchecked free radicals damage the wall of the cell as well as its internal chemistry in a way that is potentially irreversible. The outward signs are deterioration in skin quality, changes in the eye such as cataract formation, some of the changes seen in arthritis, and the gradual development of atherosclerosis. Diets rich in foods containing the nutrients listed above seem to protect against cardiovascular disease and cancer, in particular. The simple message, therefore, is eat lots of fruit and vegetables, and limit your exposure to noxious chemicals, especially cigarette smoke.

Nutritional deficiencies in the elderly

It is in the extremes of life that we are particularly vulnerable to nutritional problems. Newborn infants, especially premature ones, and ill, elderly patients all have special nutritional needs. These are under-recognised and not easily provided for by a normal healthy diet and simple vitamin and mineral supplements.

A detailed nutritional survey of acutely ill, elderly patients conducted over 20 years ago in Yorkshire, England, found that not one patient had a completely normal nutritional profile. Nutrients that were commonly deficient included iron, vitamin B12 and folic acid, any one of which could cause anaemia, and there were also deficiencies of vitamins A, B complex and C, which could influence mood, muscle function and resistance to infection. Other studies have confirmed these findings and uncovered trace nutrient deficiencies including zinc, which helps resistance to infection, selenium, which is involved in antioxidant protection, and chromium, which may influence predisposition to diabetes.

The risk of nutritional deficiencies in this group rises with:

- history of poor diet
- high alcohol intake

- recent weight loss
- medical problems
- use of drugs, especially diuretics, antibiotics if prolonged use is required, steroids and digoxin, a drug used to treat heart disease.

What your doctor can do

- Be alert to the potential problems of nutritional deficiencies in the elderly.
- Look for signs of nutritional deficiency:
  ○ sore, smooth tongue, cracking at the corners of the mouth
  ○ peeling of the lips
  ○ flattened or upturned finger or thumb nails
  ○ excessively dry skin
  ○ easy bruising
  ○ heart failure
  ○ severe muscle cramps
  ○ depression
  ○ loss of appetite.
- Test nutritional status of ill and elderly patients. Simple blood tests for anaemia, measuring serum zinc, serum and red cell magnesium, and tests for the B vitamin deficiencies, especially vitamin B12 and folic acid, should all be on offer at local hospital level. More specialised tests should also be available.
- Advise patients about healthy eating, and in particular those older patients whose foods may need to be in semi-liquid form and easy to digest. High-fibre diets are inappropriate for the majority of ill, elderly patients. There should not be an over-reliance on sugar and refined foods, even those that are easy to consume. Good nutritious foods include all dairy products, eggs, ice cream (preferably organic, and made from wholesome ingredients), vegetables (especially if prepared as soup), meat (especially if minced), mashed potatoes with added milk or cream, stewed fruit, and fortified drinks which are very useful as meal replacements or between meals when additional calories are required.
- Finally, and most importantly, doctors should be prepared to prescribe nutritional supplements. Despite their age, the elderly do very well with the right treatment. Talk to your doctor regarding whether some supplements are available on prescription. As a general rule patients with proven deficiencies or known risk of deficiencies may receive nutritional supplements under ACBS (Advisory Committee on Borderline Substances) Exemption within the United Kingdom.

Problems of the Elderly and the Nutritional Answer

Recurrent upper respiratory tract infections	Zinc and strong multi-vitamins
Congestive heart failure	Strong doses of vitamin B complex
Osteoporosis	Supplements of marine fish oil, evening primrose oil and calcium (Efacal) daily, or calcium, 1 gram daily, and vitamin D, 400 IU daily, for the housebound elderly
Heart rhythm disturbance	Supplements of magnesium, 300 mg daily, and multi-vitamins
Muscle cramps	Supplements of magnesium and multi-vitamins
High blood pressure	Vitamin C, 1 gram daily, to reduce stroke risk, and supplements of magnesium, 300 mg, to lower blood pressure, especially in women
High risk of cardiovascular disease	Vitamin E, 600 IU daily, but not if receiving the anti-coagulant Warfarin
Diabetes	Supplements of chromium, 200 mcg daily if mildly diabetic, subject to approval by their doctor (see page 165, Diabetes)
Loss of memory	Ginkgo biloba if not on anti-coagulant medication

What you can do

This is given on the basis of the elderly person being a near relative to you, the reader of this book.

- Advise your relative's doctor about his or her recent diet.
- Discuss with your relative which types of foods they like to eat, that are nutritious and are easy to prepare.
- Make regular use of meal replacements when convalescing.
- Be prepared to administer supplements in a number of situations even if they are not prescribed by your relative's doctor.

As a general rule, higher doses of supplements may be needed initially, say for two to three months, until nutritional levels are normal, and then pills can be reduced to generally half the amount.

See also: Arthritis and musculoskeletal problems, Ischaemic heart disease, Osteoporosis, Diabetes and Dementia, plus Recommended reading and Standard references.

Allergy and Intolerance

The word 'allergy' simply means altered reaction, and it is used commonly by doctors and the public, but the two terms are often confused. The term 'intolerance' is also used to describe an adverse reaction of a similar sort but with a rather different basis as outlined below.

ALLERGY

The term is now properly confined to adverse reactions involving the immune system. This means that there are changes in the white cells or the antibodies produced by them. These reactions may be to:

- something that is breathed in, an 'inhalant' such as a pollen
- a food, and this can be almost any food
- a food additive, as in the case of colourings
- a drug given by mouth, injection or as a skin preparation
- an insect as with house dust mite allergy or wasp sting allergy
- an animal or their secretions e.g. cat saliva and rodent urine
- chemicals in cosmetics
- dusts e.g. wood or metals
- metals, e.g. jewellery, particularly earrings

The reaction may be immediate as in the case of hay-fever, or delayed as is often the case with allergies to foods.

INTOLERANCE

The term used to describe all other reactions that do not involve immune mechanisms. They are more common than allergies and can vary substantially in type. They involve mainly foods but can also occur with inhaled chemicals such as sulphites, which can trigger asthma. The mechanism of intolerance is fascinating and outside the scope of this book.
  The main types are:

- simple irritants as with asthma and sulphites e.g. in wine
- toxic effects
- effects of chemicals found in some foods, e.g. intolerance of amines in the case of migraine
- metabolic effects of food as in reactive hypoglycaemia
- enzyme deficiencies involved in digestion as in intolerance of milk sugar (lactose) causing diarrhoea
- other enzyme deficiencies especially in the liver, as in the intolerance of fruit sugar

- metabolic effects of food that is spoiled or fermented
- the effects of food on bowel bacteria and flora

All of these are discussed in much more detail in the relevant parts of the book.

What causes them?

Nowadays it would seem that the majority of doctors are prepared to accept that allergies and even intolerances do happen from time to time. What is still not certain, nor indeed widely agreed, is the type of health problems that can be caused and how frequently adverse reactions of one kind or another occur.

Conditions caused by inhalant allergy

- asthma
- rhinitis (seasonal hay fever)
- rhinitis (non-seasonal)
- conjunctivitis – eye irritation

Conditions caused by food allergy

- asthma
- immediate reactions causing mouth, lip or facial swelling (angiodema)
- coeliac disease
- cow's milk protein allergy in children
- colitis in infants and occasionally adults
- Crohn's disease occasionally
- rheumatoid arthritis
- conjunctivitis

Conditions caused by food intolerance

- irritable bowel syndrome
- migraine headaches
- asthma
- rhinitis
- urticaria
- some types of food poisoning
- intolerance of certain carbohydrates, e.g. milk sugar (lactose), ordinary table sugar, fruit sugar
- hyperactive behaviour in children
- possibly mood disturbance in adults

All of these conditions except coeliac disease have a variety of other causes that need to be considered carefully by the doctor. Each topic is dealt with individually throughout the book. The Simple Exclusion Diet and The Strict Exclusion Diet see pages 460 and 466, will be useful.

See also: Asthma, Rhinitis, Coeliac disease, Rheumatoid arthritis, Irritable bowel syndrome, Migraine and Crohn's disease. Plus Recommended reading and References.

Anaemia

Anaemia simply means a lack of blood and there are many causes of this. Iron deficiency, the most usual underlying reason, is one of the most common medical conditions worldwide. Despite the prosperity of western society, it is a problem still often experienced by women of child-bearing age. Additionally, there are a large variety of other blood conditions, some nutritional, some moderately common and many rare, that can also cause anaemia.

Because of it's importance, all hospital laboratories routinely measure the level of haemoglobin, the blood pigment which carries oxygen around the body. There have been many attempts to determine exactly what the normal haemoglobin level is in women, men and children. Definitions vary slightly and in practice the normal range for women is between 11.5 and 16.0 grams per decilitre (1/10 litre). Haemoglobin is carried around inside red cells, which in turn are produced from large 'cell factories' in the bone marrow, concentrated at the ends of the long bones, in the ribs and pelvis. The cells that produce red blood cells are also related to those producing white cells which are involved in resistance to infection, production of antibodies and minute cells called platelets which help in the prevention of bleeding. Occasionally certain blood disorders influence all three types of cell.

Red cells that carry the haemoglobin are actually dying cells. Unlike all other cells of the body they do not contain a nucleus 'brain'; nor do they have the ability to renew themselves, and thus usually have a limited life span of 120 days. During this time they carry oxygen from the lungs through the heart and off to the peripheral tissues such as the brain, muscles and skin where, after depositing the oxygen, they collect carbon dioxide. On the return journey through the lungs they release the carbon dioxide and pick up yet more oxygen. Such is the happy lot of the red cell.

The production of haemoglobin requires a number of factors. Iron is essential as this mineral is found in the structure of haemoglobin itself. Iron is absorbed in the first part of the small intestine, the duodenum. Vitamin B12 and folic acid are needed for the production of chemicals required for the making of the red cell envelope. Adequate protein intake, potassium, vitamin A and other B vitamins are also required but only rarely are deficiencies of these the cause of anaemia.

What are the symptoms?

As anaemia is a condition which comes on gradually, there is time for the body to adapt to it, and a sudden fall in blood pressure or symptoms of shock are rarely seen. The first signs may be:

- mild fatigue and slight paleness
- shortness of breath on effort
- palpitation and worsening of any pre-existing disease of the heart or lungs
- light-headedness, giddiness and buzzing in the ears
- poor appetite and nausea

Very often these are features of nutritional deficiency, especially of iron, as this is the commonest cause of anaemia. This in turn will result in its own symptoms including:

- a sore tongue
- recurrent mouth ulcers
- cracking at the corners of the mouth
- flattening and upturning of the thumb and fingernails
- split and brittle nails
- poor hair growth or hair loss, especially in women
- a blue tinge to the white of the eyes

It is also possible that mild iron deficiency with a low or normal haemoglobin can also cause fatigue, but not all doctors are agreed on this.

What causes it?

The main causes of anaemia are as follows:

- Lack of essential nutrients, especially iron, folic acid and vitamin B12.
- Increased blood loss from heavy periods or bleeding from the bowel. The causes of heavy periods include fibroids, hormonal disturbance and other gynaecological problems. The causes of loss of blood from the bowel include cancer of the colon or stomach, peptic ulcer (especially if aspirin or anti-arthritic drugs are also taken), and also bleeding from a hiatus hernia.
- Poor absorption of essential nutrients can affect the levels of iron, vitamin B12 and folate, either in tandem or with just one of these nutrients being deficient. Disease of the stomach, coeliac disease, pancreatic and small bowel disorders are all possiblities.
- Chronic diseases such as liver and kidney problems, severe arthritis, and chronic infection.

- Genetic disorders, such as thalassaemia which affect the production of haemoglobin. This is very common in Africa, people of Mediterranean origin, and the Far East. Conditions such as thalassaemia and sickle cell disease can, in their mild forms, produce a mild anaemia which may cause relatively little ill health, but in severe forms cause major anaemia in childhood.

Fortunately, even from the result of a simple blood test for anaemia a doctor can very rapidly ascertain the likely cause. This is because many tests on red cells, measures of white cells and platelets, and a test called the ESR that gives a general measure of inflammatory processes throughout the body, is also used.

What your doctor can do

- He can take a variety of tests. The first is a full blood count which measures the haemoglobin and looks at the shape and size of red cells. If the haemoglobin is low then further tests are required. One way is to measure the serum ferritin or some other test of iron adequacy (transferrin saturation), as a low serum ferritin will usually confirm iron deficiency. This is a simple test and is widely available. It is prudent to perform this in most women of child-bearing age presenting with anaemia. Some 13 per cent or more of this category of women had a reduced serum ferritin level in the last government nutritional survey performed in the UK in 1990.

  Often tests measure serum vitamin B12 and red cell folate. These widely available tests, will need to be performed if a certain pattern of anaemia is present on full blood count. Lack of folic acid is likely to occur during pregnancy, as a result of certain blood disorders, malabsorption, or if the diet is very poor. Lack of vitamin B12 may occur after several years in strict vegans whose diet is deficient in this vitamin, in some types of malabsorption, or if the stomach is unable to produce the necessary agents that are required to absorb this vitamin from the diet. This condition is termed pernicious anaemia.

- The doctor may also investigate the cause of the anaemia by assessing the diet, possible blood loss from the gut (stool tests to detect minute quantities of blood may need to be performed but are not always reliable), assessment of symptoms that may suggest malabsorption, e.g. diarrhoea and weight loss, and assessment of menstrual flow. Women are notoriously bad at assessing how heavy their periods are. The presence of flooding severe enough to stain underwear, having to go to bed because of flooding, needing to wear a tampon plus towels are all rough but useful pointers to the menstrual flow being excessive (see page 377).

- In older patients, especially women after the menopause (and in most men), some attempt should be made to assess the possibility of gastrointestinal blood loss. This is particularly important for unexpected iron-deficiency anaemia, and may lead to early detection of colon or gastric cancer. Barium meal, barium X-ray and telescopic investigation of the bowel by a gastroenterologist may all be required.
- Treatment will be in the form of iron supplements, as ferrous sulphate taken by mouth. Occasionally iron will need to be given by injection but this should be extremely rare. Vitamin B12 will need to be given by injection if the deficiency is due to malabsorption, or in tablet form in the case of a vegan with poor oral intake. Supplements of folic acid can be prescribed separately, and doses several times the normal daily intake are recommended if there is any degree of malabsorption. Smaller supplements may need to be given in a variety of blood disorders where there is increased production (and destruction) of red blood cells.
- The treatment of any underlying disorder. This may require a referral to a bowel specialist, dietician or gynaecologist.
- Monitor treatment. If the assessment was correct there should be a rise in haemoglobin level often within two weeks of treatment. Other changes on a blood test should indicate that new red cells are being formed. Blood counts should continue to be monitored until the haemoglobin is normal and it may be prudent for a further check three months later to make sure there has been no subsequent fall.

Despite our knowledge of anaemia, and the ability to investigate patients thoroughly, sometimes the cause is not found. In one recent appraisal of patients with severe iron deficiency anaemia, no cause was found in some 36 per cent of them.

What you can do

- Go and see your doctor if you have any of the symptoms that are potentially attributable to anaemia, and any features that suggest you may be particularly at risk, such as heavy periods or poor diet. A past history of anaemia is an important risk factor too.
- Keep a diet diary for a week and take this along to your appointment. Do this as well if your doctor diagnoses anaemia. It will help aid analysis of your dietary intake of iron, vitamin B12 and folic acid.
- If you have heavy periods keep a record of the number of tampons and towels that you use, and the number of days you bleed in the menstrual cycle. Again this will help your doctor make a decision.
- If you are taking supplements of iron, never take them with tea, coffee, red grape juice or blackcurrant juice. These all contain tannin which

will inhibit the absorption of iron. You normally absorb 10–15 per cent of the amount of iron in your diet, and the same is true of iron supplements, although this rises if we are iron deficient. Taking an iron supplement with tea reduces absorption to a third of these values. Taking it with a supplement of vitamin C (100 mg or more) can double the amount of iron absorbed. A good way of taking your iron pill is with a glass of fruit juice or with a piece of fruit.

- Oxalic acid from rhubarb, spinach and beetroot can inhibit iron absorption, as can phytic acid found in wheat and bran. Limit your consumption of these foods.
- If your iron supplement is causing indigestion, constipation or diarrhoea, a change in the type, reducing the dose, and taking it with food, may all help minimise side-effects. In our experience side-effects are rare if patients take care in this way.
- For most people a simple iron supplement of ferrous sulphate 200 mgs, once or twice daily, will suffice. A variety of more specialised (and more expensive) iron supplements are available on prescription or through health-food stores. The over-the-counter preparations are usually much weaker, and larger doses may need to be taken in order to correct severe iron deficiency. Avoid supplementing with zinc until your iron levels have stabilised because these minerals compete for absorption.
- Do not take time-release iron supplements because the site of absorption is in the initial section of the small intestine.
- If you are deficient in vitamin B12 and need supplements, do not take supplements of folic acid until the vitamin B12 deficiency is corrected. If in doubt about this speak with your doctor. Large supplements of folic acid in a person with untreated vitamin B12 deficiency may lead to increased vitamin B12 problems causing nerve damage.
- Whatever the cause of your anaemia try and eat The Very Nutritious Diet (see page 437) or if vegetarian or vegan see page 455 for your appropriate option. As a general guide, foods that are rich in protein, either of animal or vegetable source, tend to be good sources of iron. Animal sources of iron are better absorbed, and may also enhance the absorption from vegetarian foods. So even allowing small amounts of animal products into a vegetarian diet increases the balance of this mineral.
- Take your iron and other supplements as recommended. You may well need to take the iron supplements for three months after the haemoglobin has risen to normal in order to build up iron stores and to ensure that energy levels rise to their optimum range.

Complementary therapies

There should really be no need of these in the treatment of anaemia.

Belinda's story

Belinda was a 38-year-old South African aid worker who had to spend several months in London as part of her work. On many occasions over the last few years she had been found to be mildly anaemic though this was never fully resolved despite taking iron tablets. Her periods were not particularly heavy. She did complain of mild fatigue, with poor hair growth, abdominal bloating, constipation and some premenstrual symptoms. In the past she had had breast cysts which were still sometimes a problem, and a few years earlier had had several uterine fibroids removed because of severe anaemia.

At the time she was first seen, she was still mildly anaemic, haemoglobin 10.7g (the normal range is 11.5 to 16.5). Other tests revealed that she was indeed iron deficient and there was a very low level for serum zinc. Her weight was steady at 48 kilos. It wasn't clear quite why she had these problems. We prescribed some iron supplements taken with vitamin C or fruit juice, supplements of zinc and multivitamins. This sort of supplement regime could certainly help her fatigue and poor hair growth. There was little clincal improvement in the first two months; she was therefore asked to follow a gluten free diet. This meant avoiding all wheat, oats, barley and rye, which she did most carefully. There was a gradual and gratifying improvement. Abdominal symptoms disappeared, her fatigue lessened, her hair growth improved and best of all her haemoglobin rose significantly well into the normal range at 12.5g. Serum zinc level became normal too. There was a query as to whether she may have been developing coeliac disease, but further tests for this fortunately proved to be negative. She felt better than she had for years. However, every time she tries to introduce wheat into her diet she experiences abdominal symptoms and increased diarrhoea. Hopefully she will grow out of her gluten sensitivity as time passes.

See also: Essential nutrients, Liver disease, Coeliac disease, Pancreatic disease and Irritable bowel syndrome, Recommended reading, References.

Anxiety

Anxiety in its mild form is a natural state associated with stressful situations, and is suffered by everyone at some time. The things people get anxious about include exams, interviews, relationships, finances, acts of violence and rabid dogs. Some degree of anxiety, which subsides after the event, would be considered to be appropriate, given the circumstances.

However, when the anxiety escalates and in some cases brings on panic attacks and palpitations (rapid or irregular heart beats), medical intervention is necessary.

When severe anxiety is present the whole body feels 'wired up'. The person finds it difficult to relax, over-reacts, feels tense, nervous, agitated and finds it difficult to concentrate. Sleep is likely to be disturbed, with periods of insomnia, and early-morning waking. The person may also experience a dry mouth, muscle tremors and diarrhoea, all of which are very distressing.

What are the symptoms?

Heart	palpitations and awareness of missed heartbeats
	discomfort in the chest
Chest	overbreathing
	pain in the chest
Muscular	aches and pains
Nervous System	shakes
	headaches
	dizziness
	tinnitus (ringing in the ears)
	prickling sensations
	poor concentration and memory
Digestive	dry mouth
	difficulty in swallowing
	indigestion
	excessive wind
	diarrhoea
Bladder	frequent need to pass water
Uterus	amenorrhoea – lack of periods
	period pains

There are three main types of anxiety which are quite distinctive:

General anxiety	which is continuous.
Phobic anxiety	which occurs from time to time, when in certain situations or places.
Panic attacks	which occur from time to time, but are not related to a situation or place necessarily; the response is often out of proportion to the situation.

Plus:

Premenstrual anxiety	which is experienced by some women.

GENERAL ANXIETY

The causes of general anxiety are not fully understood, but it is thought that it could be attributable to a combination of any of the following:

- genetic disorders
- insecure relationships in childhood
- stressful events in life
- nutritional deficiencies
- possible food allergies

What your doctor can do

Your doctor can carry out physical investigations to eliminate the possibility that the anxiety is related to a physical disease or problem. An overactive thyroid, hypoglycaemia (low blood sugar) and, rarely, tumours of the adrenal glands can all be accompanied by symptoms of anxiety, as can psychiatric disorders like depression, dementia or schizophrenia.

Once pure anxiety has been diagnosed the treatment your doctor has to offer is mainly psychological:

- Setting your mind at rest is the first step, so that there is a clear understanding that the symptoms are not related to any major illness.
- Stress management advice, to help you to understand and recognise the trigger for your anxiety.
- If you are hyperventilating (overbreathing), you should be given instructions about how to breathe, by re-breathing expired air from a paper bag to restore the normal concentrations of carbon dioxide.
- You may be offered drug treatment like Valium, which produces rapid relief of anxiety, but this should not be prescribed for more than three or four weeks.
- Alternatively, anti-depressants are used to control anxiety, but they are a longer-term treatment and should only be considered as a last resort.

PREMENSTRUAL ANXIETY

The main symptoms of premenstrual anxiety are nervous tension, irritability and mood swings, beginning as early as two weeks before the period and becoming progressively worse as the period approaches.

There are several possible factors, both hormonal and dietary, that might cause it.

- Some doctors think than an excess of the hormone oestrogen or an increased sensitivity to it may trigger changes in brain chemistry, resulting in anxiety. The average diet, high in fat and relatively low in fibre, can increase the levels of this hormone.

- Also, high levels of oestrogen slow down the rate at which the stimulant caffeine is broken down by the liver. This is why some women become more sensitive to tea and coffee when they are pregnant or when taking the oral contraceptive pill.
- A lack of vitamin B and possibly the mineral magnesium can also cause changes in the chemistry of the nervous system, aggravating feelings of anxiety and irritability. Interestingly, it seems that some women and men who are prone to anxiety and panic attacks are more sensitive to caffeine and genuinely have a more sensitive body metabolism, which makes them very susceptible to the effects of a lack of vitamin B or magnesium.
- Kava kava is a herb renowned for its calming and sedative properties and has been used in traditional folklore medicine for centuries in the treatment of anxiety, depression and stress related disorders. The active components of kava are kavalactones, found in the fat soluble resin of the root of the plant. Whilst taking sedatives like Valium can induce unwanted side effects, including addiction, kava does not appear to present any such symptoms. However drowsiness has been reported in some studies. NB Although no side effects have been reported as a result of using standardised kava extract, research does show that it may interfere with levels of the neurotransmitter dopamine and worsen Parkinson's disease. Therefore, until more sound research is published, it should not be taken by anyone with Parkinson's.
- A comparison of caffeine consumption in Chinese nurses and workers in a tea factory revealed a strong association between increased caffeine consumption and the severity of premenstrual symptoms. We conducted our own survey in the United Kingdom with *Fitness* magazine, which was published in 1992. Three hundred and seventy-seven women took part. Caffeine consumption was nearly two and a half times higher in PMS sufferers compared with non-sufferers.
- A final and important factor is hyperventilation. This simply means over-breathing. Often when one becomes anxious it is natural to increase the rate and depth of respiration. This provides more oxygen to the bloodstream but also removes more of the waste gas carbon dioxide. This lack of carbon dioxide causes a change in the body chemistry which can actually aggravate or cause a variety of symptoms, including numbness and tingling in the fingers, hands and around the mouth, muscle cramps, headaches, light-headedness, increased anxiety, physical and mental fatigue, and confusion. The solution is to relax, reduce the rate and depth of breathing, and if symptoms are severe, to breathe in and out of a paper bag for several minutes. When these symptoms chronically occur, formal advice and breathing exercises may need to be given by a physiotherapist or psychologist.

Celia's story

Celia was a 31-year-old mother of two young children who had been suffering for years with mood swings that left her feeling frightened and depressed.

'I'd be chugging along fairly normally, then, suddenly, I would burst into tears over nothing at all. My mood seemed to change from one hour to the next, and the frightening thing was that I had no warning it was about to happen – it was as if I just snapped. I went from feeling perfectly normal, to thoroughly depressed, and my patience threshold was non-existent. The slightest little thing would spark me off and I'd feel like thrashing out. I'd been suffering like this, three weeks out of four, for six years, since the birth of our first son, until I reached crisis point one morning whilst hanging out the washing. All I did was drop a sock on the floor, but I burst into tears. It felt like the end of the world and I was sure I was going mad.

In desperation I opened up to my husband, who was always supportive. We decided that perhaps I needed to get a part-time job, as I hadn't been out of the house whilst the boys were small. Now they were at school it seemed like a good idea, but I didn't manage to get a job and nothing changed.

I went to visit my doctor and explained about my wild moods and tearfulness. He was very sympathetic, but said he only had anti-depressants to offer me. I hate taking pills, but I was so desperate, I promised to try them for three months. I didn't feel I had any choice as by this time I had reached the point where when I woke up each morning I knew I couldn't face the day.

The anti-depressants drained me and left me feeling completely zombified. My quality of life was non-existent and I didn't even feel that I was fit to drive the children around. I tried to stop taking them, but my symptoms returned with a vengeance.

Finally, I thought that my only hope would be to see a psychiatrist, which I did. He asked me all about my sex life, and my marriage. And, as I talked to him it dawned on me that he wasn't going to be able to help me at all. The only thing wrong with my sex life and my marriage was that I was feeling ill. Sex hadn't been that great whilst my moods had been so up and down, but I knew it was not the cause of my bad moods. And so I renewed the prescription for the anti-depressants, and carried on taking them, feeling like a washed-out zombie for the following year. If it hadn't been for my husband and the boys I really think I'd have been suicidal. I can't believe that my husband didn't pack his bags and leave, I must have been so awful to live with.

My husband tried to cheer me up and found a dream house for us to move to, hoping it would pull me out of my problems. I thought long and hard about it, and told him I was going to throw the pills away, and somehow help myself. I booked some counselling sessions which helped a bit. But what really changed my life was an article I read in Family Circle *magazine about a woman describing her mood swings. I read the article over and over again. I just couldn't believe it. She was describing precisely what I had been going through, and had cured her problem, not with pills, but by changing her diet!*

I wrote to the organisation mentioned in the article, the WNAS, and I bought their book. They sent me a questionnaire asking me about my diet, lifestyle and moods. I was then provided with a special programme which involved changing my diet completely. I felt so awful the first week, which they said I would, I actually wondered if it was worth continuing. One morning at the end of the first week, I woke up feeling terrible, I made breakfast and crawled back in to bed. I stayed there all day, and when I woke up the next morning I felt fantastic. I hadn't felt that good for ages. I couldn't believe it. It was as if a dark cloud had been lifted from me.

The longer I was on the programme the better I felt. It has been five years now, and I feel wonderful. I'm lively, energetic and those horrendous and unpredictable mood swings have gone completely.'

PHOBIAS

The difference between phobic disorders and general anxiety is that the symptoms are intermittent and relate to specific situations. Phobias like agoraphobia (fear of open spaces), and claustrophobia (fear of closed spaces), can limit the ability of the sufferer to work or socialise easily. Possible phobias are many and varied. Some people are afraid of heights or needles, others are too nervous to socialise or attend a social gathering, and others are afraid to leave home or get into an elevator.

The most common phobias we see at the WNAS are agoraphobia and to a lesser degree claustrophobia. Sufferers feel terrified and threatened at the prospect of going out of the house, in the case of the agoraphobic, or being in a confined space, in the case of the claustrophobic. The fear is usually characterised by a panic attack with palpitations, dry mouth, muscle tremors, and in severe cases, fear of a heart attack.

Interestingly, almost 90 per cent of agoraphobic sufferers are women. We had contact some years ago with a marvellous woman who ran a national group for agoraphobic sufferers. From her research data we discovered that 91 per cent of her sample of 94 also suffered premenstrual syndrome.

Susan's story

Susan was a 20-year-old single woman who was suffering from claustrophobia. She worked at the House of Commons as a chef and found it particularly difficult to carry out many of the functions of her job because of her symptoms.

'My health had deteriorated over a period of years. My most frightening symptom was claustrophobia – I was particularly afraid of tube trains, lifts and the walk-in fridges at work which I needed to use on a regular basis as a chef. I also suffered with craving for sweet food, especially before my period, chocolate-related migraine headaches which meant I felt awful after bingeing, and I experienced panic attacks and depression.

My doctor had prescribed anti-depressants over a period of years, the last one I was given was Prozac. He also referred me to a psychiatrist for phobia therapy. I came across the book No More PMS! *and was encouraged to read that other women experience phobias, especially in the two weeks before their periods. The book suggested the WNAS could help women with symptoms similar to mine, so I contacted them for help.*

After completing a long questionnaire and diet diary I was asked what seemed like hundreds of questions at my first consultation. I was told to eat little and often and to cut out all junk food, including chocolate, cakes, biscuits, sweet foods and cola-based drinks. Additionally I cut out caffeine and wheat. I took supplements of Optivite and Normoglycaemia and started to exercise.

Within three months I was off the anti-depressants, my phobias had completely gone and so too had the migraines and the premenstrual cravings for food. Lifts were no longer a problem and I had no trouble going in and out of the fridges at work. I felt so well, better than I ever hoped. I also lost just over 6 kilos in weight without dieting. I started my treatment four years ago. I must admit I have had a few lapses along the way, particularly when I'm on holiday, but at least I know how to get myself back in to tip-top shape again afterwards.'

What your doctor can do

He can refer you for some behaviour therapy. This is the usual treatment, and there are a variety to chose from, including desensitisation and cognitive manipulation. Essentially there are different methods of getting the sufferer to confront their phobia, either by talking to themselves, or by facing the phobia head on in the company of a therapist, or others who have no such phobia.

In addition he may offer you some of the options listed for general anxiety (see page 67).

Harriet's story

Harriet was a 41-year-old mother of three who had been taking anti-depressants for 24 years to ease her agoraphobia and panic attacks.

'I first had my first panic attack when I was 16 following a dental abscess. Looking back, that was the start of my agoraphobia, although I didn't realise it at the time. First of all my doctor put me on iron pills – but when my test came back in the normal range, I was then given tablets for my nerves. I can't remember the name of the first two, but they seemed to make my panic attacks worse. Within a short time I was prescribed Valium, at first 15 mg per day, increasing to 30 mg per day, which I stayed on for 24 years. The Valium knocked me out, I was like a zombie. They seemed to ease the panic attacks initially, but gradually I needed more and more pills to keep the symptoms at bay.

For the rest of my teenage years my social life was affected as I was unable to go out unaccompanied. I had a boyfriend for a while, but the symptoms of agoraphobia made me afraid to go out and he got fed up waiting around for me. I met my husband at a dance when I was 19. He didn't mind staying in, and we eventually got married when I was 21.

I had our first child when I was 23, and the pregnancy was followed by postnatal depression. I had such severe panic attacks after the birth every time I went into town, my horizons got smaller and smaller until eventually I was housebound and frightened to go through the front door. I couldn't even go out to do the food shopping. When our son was five he developed cancer in his leg, which I obviously found very stressful. He did survive thank goodness, but the stress of it left me with obsessional neurosis, on the top of my agoraphobia. It was a turning point for me. I just sat in a chair all day, didn't bother to cook or clean the house.

I eventually had two more children – but I was so afraid during my pregnancies as I felt the Valium might harm the unborn children. I managed to cut down to 20 mg of Valium per day during my pregnancy, but I was too scared to cut down any more as I didn't know how to do without them. I was prescribed a hormone, Duphaston after the third child, but it did not make any difference.

My husband resorted to working long hours as he couldn't cope with me. Fortunately the children's school was over the road from our house – I could just about manage to get to the pavement, but I couldn't cross the road as I felt so dizzy. The Valium prescriptions

*just kept coming, I'd be given 100 pills at a time without ever being
seen by the doctor.*

*After 24 years, in desperation, as my symptoms had become
worse before my period was due, I sent my husband out to find a
book on premenstrual syndrome, and he came back with* No More
PMS! *My doctor then offered me beta blockers and said they
weren't habit forming, but I didn't want to take any more drugs.
I decided to follow the recommendations in the book and to
come off the valium. I contacted the WNAS and had a telephone
consultation.*

*Coming off Valium was hell. The withdrawal symptoms were like
nothing I had ever experienced before. Within six weeks of following the WNAS programme I was feeling human again, and much
more like my old self. I even made an appointment to get my hair
done. I felt on top of the world. Then I woke up one day feeling
really angry and resentful, as I realised I had lost 24 years of my life.
I can't even remember the children growing up and I feel so sad
about that. My doctor was clearly ignorant, which upsets me
greatly, as I can never replace those years.*

*I have been better for three years now. I am still having some
counselling to deal with all the traumas in my life, but the end is in
sight. I now cope well with my family and my home, and am getting
involved with a local medical charity. Today I am catering a party
for 100 guests to celebrate my father's 90th birthday tomorrow – I
couldn't even have dreamt about doing that four years ago! I am so
grateful to the WNAS and am trying to persuade them to open a
centre in Glasgow as, in my experience, most women don't know
that there is help available.'*

PANIC ATTACKS

These can be very frightening episodes, which come on suddenly, apparently unprovoked, unlike phobias. The symptoms can be similar to the
general anxiety symptoms, but in addition are usually accompanied by
palpitations, which often cause additional anxiety about the possibility of
heart disease. In the past this disorder was referred to by heart specialists
as a heart condition know as 'effort syndrome'.

Prior to the panic attack the brain sends a message to the adrenal
glands which causes an adrenaline surge, sometimes known as the 'flight
and fight' mechanism. The anxiety that a medical emergency is impending is so severe that it sets up a vicious circle, leading to physical symptoms, which then justify the fear of physical problems, which then lead to
more anxiety, which causes the panic attack.

Once again panic attacks are suffered by many women in their premenstrual phase. In a survey the WNAS conducted on 1,000 patients it emerged that 91 per cent had previously suffered with anxiety before their periods, and in severe cases, sufferers often had panic attacks leading up to their periods.

Adrienne's story

Adrienne was a 22-year-old student nurse who was very frightened by the onset of severe anxiety and panic attacks. Her mother brought her to the clinic after seeing a television programme that featured the work of WNAS.

'My symptoms came on suddenly when I was 21. We had moved to Sussex and so I was feeling a bit isolated from my friends, plus I had begun a nursing course during that year which necessitated living away from home. My Grandad died that year, too, which I found upsetting as we are a close family.

At times my symptoms were uncontrollable. I became very depressed, withdrawn and anxious. I just felt like hiding in my room. I was verbally aggressive towards my family and refused to eat when I was depressed. My head used to pound so much it felt like it was going to explode. I was very afraid, and dreaded my symptoms which were considerably worse for two weeks before each period.

At first my doctor suggested vitamin B6, which didn't help. Then I was put on the Pill, which made me feel bloated and weird in the head. I was also given Duphaston and antidepressants, and eventually Estraderm patches which made my symptoms worse, and I now discover are for menopausal symptoms.

I had to give up nursing as I couldn't concentrate or absorb anything. I returned to my family home where I either sat on the sofa all day, on a good day, or hid away in my room. My family were clearly distraught by the situation, but at a loss to know what to do for me. One day whilst sitting on the sofa I happened to see a WNAS patient on a TV chat show. When she described her former symptoms it sounded just like she was describing me!

My mum went straight out and got me the book they mentioned, which I read from cover to cover without stopping. I got started on a self-help programme immediately and made an appointment to attend the WNAS clinic. I stopped all the hormones and antidepressants and was given a diet, exercise and supplement programme to follow, which was very different from my previous way of eating. My mum helped with the shopping and the cooking which made it a lot easier for me.

Within a month my depression and anxiety had vanished which was such a surprise. Unfortunately, as I thought I was better I didn't follow the programme strictly for the next month and ended up feeling almost as bad as ever. I realised I had to follow it to the letter and got my act together again. Within two months all the symptoms had disappeared again. I decided not to return to nursing for the time being, but instead got a job with an Insurance company, working with lots of other young people in the area.

That was a year ago, and I haven't had a bad day since. I keep to my diet, still take some supplements, regularly exercise, practice relaxation, and every fortnight I have some reflexology. Without my symptoms I felt more like socialising, so I have developed a circle of friends. I feel like a completely different person, with a future, and am so grateful I found the WNAS.'

What your doctor can do

- Offer the options discussed for general anxiety.
- Prescribe high doses of benzodiazepines, like Valium. Prolonged treatment is unwise though as it leads to dependency, as you will see from Harriet's experience.
- Give antidepressants such as one of the Tricyclic group or paroxxetine (seroxat) are used to control symptoms in the longer term, but it may be given in high doses with the risk of many side-effects. The problem with this treatment is the relapse rate has been found to be high when the medication ceases.
- Refer you to a psychologist or psychiatrist for some cognitive therapy, designed to change the fears and physical symptoms, which predispose the panic attack. This involves coming to terms with the irrational basis for your fears over several sessions.

What you can do

- Follow the instructions for The Simple Exclusion Diet on page 460. This will keep you busy for at least eight weeks.
- Take regular exercise, at least four good sessions per week to the point of breathlessness. If you can't manage to get out of the house use a skipping rope and an exercise video to build up your stamina.
- Try to practice relaxation each day, deep breathing, meditation, yoga, or anything you find therapeutic (see page 29).
- Take a generous dose of multi-vitamins and minerals daily, plus extra B vitamins, and vitamin C.
- Get some help to sort out the stress in your life, either from a friend or a therapist.

- If you suffer with premenstrual syndrome, follow the instructions on page 394, plus refer to the book *No More PMS*.
- Take a herbal 'tranquilliser' like Valerina Day which is an age-old herb used for the symptomatic relief of tension and irritability and helps cope with the stress and strain of modern living.
- Kava kava is a herb historically used for inducing a calming and relaxing effect. As noted above, kava has been found mostly to help reduce tension and improve mood in people who complain of stress, anxiety or certain phobias. The herb appears to relieve mild anxiety in less than one hour, but studies have found that it typically takes a week to exert a meaningful effect. In Germany, Kava remains one of the most popular doctor recommended remedies for anxiety.

Complementary therapies

There is a good chance that you will find additional help from many of the complementary therapies, and again it is a matter of choice. There are numerous homeopathic remedies to try, depending on which type of anxiety you suffer from. A medical herbalist will mix a prescription to suit your symptoms if you feel you need more than the herbs mentioned in the self-help section.

Acupuncture is particularly good at slowing down the energy flows in your body, and is undoubtedly worth a try (provided you don't have a phobia relating to needles). Other therapies well worth a try would be cranial osteopathy, to ease the tension within your body, and any sort of gentle massage, preferably with relaxing aromatherapy oils. Yoga, meditation and any of the techniques mentioned in the information on stress (see page 25).

See also: References.

Arthritis and Musculo-skeletal Problems

There are many different types of arthritis and conditions affecting muscles, ligaments and bones. We do not intend to cover them all but will deal with the common ones and those where nutritional factors seem to play an important part. From the early part of the 20th century, many arthritic conditions have been treated by dietary change by both conventional medical practitioners and naturopaths. The last 50 years have seen the development of many drugs – anti-inflammatory agents, steroids, immune-altering drugs and others. These are effective but often only partially so, and frequently cause side-effects. Non-toxic effective treatments such as dietary change and nutritional supplements are not only popular but can be highly effective. The last ten years have seen the publication of many studies re-investigating the worth of the older dietary and nutritional treatments which have proven to be effective (surprising to the conventional doctors only).

There are also many rare types of arthritis that are associated with a variety of other illnesses, including psoriasis, colitis and Crohn's disease, some types of gastroenteritis and other infections. Treatment both medical and nutritional is very much as for rheumatoid arthritis. Exclusion diets are an unknown quantity in such patients.

RHEUMATOID ARTHRITIS

This is a common type of chronic arthritis where there is much swelling and pain in both small and large joints. The hands, especially the large knuckle joints, are most commonly affected and this usually involves both sides in a symmetrical pattern. Stiffness of these or other joints, which is worse in the morning, is a typical feature. In other patients one or more of the larger joints are involved, such as an elbow, wrist, knee or ankle joint and this pattern of arthritis may be less aggressive than that in the hands.

The joint swelling, which is often warm to the touch, is due to considerable inflammation of the synovium. This is a thin layer of tissue that surrounds many joints and is responsible for the production of the lubricating synovial fluid. Thus in rheumatoid arthritis much of the swelling is due to an increase in this fluid. Sometimes other parts of the body such as the lungs, eyes and skin are involved in this. The inflammatory process involves a mixture of white cells and proteins called immunoglobulins. These are antibodies which, instead of being directed at infecting organisms, are actually directed at each other. A sort of immune mutiny. The 'fight' as it were, takes place mainly in the joints and involves many other inflammatory chemicals: the equivalent of the body's police. The real question is what triggers this fracas in the first place, and why it becomes so chronic. Tests for rheumatoid arthritis check for the presence of these 'self-directed' immune proteins.

Possible triggers are infections, food allergies and genetic factors.

Who gets it?

About 1 per cent of the population world-wide suffer from this form of arthritis, with women being three times more likely than men to suffer. The commonest age of onset is in the forties, and it is more likely to start in the winter months. The onset is often gradual, with stiffness present for several months before the arthritis is obvious. Sometimes there is a sudden and severe onset.

There can be a strong family element especially for the more aggressive forms of this arthritis. Some groups are especially vulnerable e.g. some American Indians probably because of genetic factors. As a rule the cause remains an enigma. Though a recent study suggested that consumers of cooked vegetables and olive oil were less likely to suffer.

What your doctor can do

Investigations to determine the type of arthritis, the presence of any associated anaemia or other problems are all important and are easily assessed by the use of blood tests and X-rays. Treatment is usually considered on a step-wise basis, with simple treatments being used first and the more powerful drugs being reserved for aggressive disease. Often the side-effects of these drugs limit their long-term use.

- Painkillers such as paracetamol and codeine are used for mild disease.
- Anti-inflammatory drugs called NSAIDs (non-steroidal anti-inflammatory drugs). There are many types, including simple aspirin, all of which are of similar efficacy. Delayed release preparations and suppositories are useful. The most serious side-effect is bleeding from the stomach which is much more likely in older patients. This type of medication does not stop the progress of the disease, however, and it is worth noticing that aspirin may increase the need for vitamin C.
- Gold, D-penicillamine, hydroxychloroquine and sulphasalazine are all termed second-line drugs, used when NSAIDs are not effective enough and if many joints are involved. D-penicillamine may cause deficiencies of zinc and vitamin B6.
- Steroids are very effective but high doses produce many unwanted effects especially osteoporosis or bone thinning and depression. Low doses, 10 mg or less per day of prednisolone, are effective and much less risky. Eating The Very Nutritious Diet (see page 437) that is low in salt and high in calcium, possibly with supplements may reduce the side-effects of long-term steroid use.
- Other drugs include immune altering and anti-cancer drugs. These were considered to be heavyweights and have the ability to alter the progress of the disease, but if used in small doses and carefully monitored, have the potential to produce considerable benefit.
- Surgery is sometimes needed to repair or replace damaged joints and tendons.
- Antibiotics are perhaps worth a final note as recent scientific research has lent support to the old idea that tetracycline antibiotics are some-

times helpful in this condition. The original theory put forward over 30 years ago was that the arthritis was due to an infection. Further research will hopefully tell us more.

What you can do

A lot, so don't give up. Rheumatoid arthritis is often a long-term condition and usually a conventional or complementary treatment will work. The real difficulty is knowing which is right for a particular individual. There is much merit in combining approaches, especially use of a NSAID with either low-dose steroid or a second-line drug and dietary manipulation and use of nutritional supplements especially fish oils.

In approximate order of importance consider the following:

- Lose weight if you are obese. Very few dietary treatments will work if you are significantly overweight and nothing will help your knees and hips as much.
- Consider an exclusion diet. Allergy to some foods is now widely accepted as occurring in rheumatoid arthritis. Reactions to milk, cheese, wheat, other grains and artificial colourings are all documented. You could follow The Simple Exclusion Diet yourself for three weeks or go through The Strict Exclusion Diet with supervision (see pages 460 and 466). If there is a good response, then the careful re-introduction of foods at possibly weekly intervals is needed to determine which, if any, contribute to the disease process.
- Supplements of fish oils have been shown to be effective in several trials. Large doses need to be taken for three or four months. They should provide 1.3 g of DHA (Docosahexaenoic acid) and 1.3 g of EPA (Eicosapentaenoic acid) per day. This approach is best combined with either The Very Nutritious Diet (see page 437) or The High Essential Fatty Acid Diet (see page 446).
- Supplements of zinc (30 mg per day) or selenium (100-200 mcg per day) have shown some benefit in some but not all studies. Again they are most likely to help if you are deficient in these nutrients and are best combined with a multi-vitamin supplement and a good diet.
- A vegan diet can be helpful, possibly because it reduces the intake of saturated fats. One of the reported successful vegan diets also excludes wheat which may explain some of its benefit.
- Other supplements might benefit. They include calcium pantothenate 2.0 g daily, New Zealand green lipped mussel extract, and possibly some plant extracts with anti-inflammatory effects such as pine bark extract, pycnogenol.

Most of these treatments will take several weeks if not two or three months to be effective.

Juliet's story

Juliet was a 35-year-old professional woman whose psoriasis had begun several years earlier. The arthritis had only begun in the last year, but she remembers that her joints had often been stiff as a child. Now she had painful swelling of the small joints in her hands and pain in her feet that limited her social activities, but had not stopped her from working. She had to take an anti-arthritis drug every night to help to get a good night's sleep and to minimise the degree of stiffness in the morning. The psoriasis was relatively mild, and she only used occasional ointments to control it.

She had observed that a number of foods appeared to aggravate the arthritis including red wine and cheese. She was advised to begin an exclusion diet taking care that she had a good overall nutrient intake as her weight was low at under 50 kilos. These measures led to further improvement in her joint pains, and the careful re-introduction of foods identified several that caused her symptoms to worsen, including beef and dairy products.

She had to avoid these long-term and therefore took a calcium supplement, which was vital in view of her low body weight and her intention to become pregnant.

She was further helped by taking regular supplements of high strength fish oils. Tests had shown that her blood levels of these anti-inflammatory agents were low. She took them in conjunction with supplements of multi-vitamins and selenium. These needed to be modified later on when she became pregnant. She also took a supplement of folic acid before conceiving.

Her arthritis was very well controlled by changes in her diet together with nutritional supplements. Eventually she had a very successful pregnancy. She continued to take supplements of vitamin B, fish oil and calcium during pregnancy and when breast-feeding to ensure a good balance of these nutrients.

OSTEOARTHRITIS

This is a common type of arthritis where there is loss of the protective surface of cartilage over the ends of bones, with subsequent changes to the underlying bone. This usually involves an increase in the amount of bone, leading to swelling and distortion of the joint, most easily seen in the joints at the ends of the fingers and in the knees. As well as these joints, the hips, base of the thumbs and the spine are commonly affected.

Pain and swelling are the most noticeable complaints and stiffness in the hands is usually less of a problem than with rheumatoid arthritis. The arthritis is often mild and limited to the fingers where despite a degree of deformity there may be little disability. When a hip or knee are affected the loss of mobility may be considerable, especially if the sufferer is over-weight.

Who gets it?

Age is the main risk factor with some 10 per cent of the over-60s being affected. Osteoarthritis of the fingers is more common in women than men, and is particularly likely to run in families. Damage to a joint at any time in the past, excessive sporting activity or repetitive occupational use can all increase the risk of this type of arthritis, though this only applies to a minority of cases. Obesity is strongly linked to osteoarthritis of the knee and to a lesser extent of the hip. This type of arthritis is thus often considered as a degenerative disease which slowly evolves over many years rather than one where there is a clear-cut trigger to the inflamma-tory process.

What your doctor can do

There is no cure for osteoarthritis. There are, however, many ways to control or lessen the pain and reduce the degree of disability.

- Assessing the disease and disability normally involves a few simple blood tests to exclude other types of arthritis and X-rays to assess the damage to the most problematic joints.
- Pain control using NSAIDs (non-steroidal anti-inflammatory drugs) can be highly effective. Their use is often limited by the gastro-intestinal irritation and internal bleeding that they may cause. Paracetamol is a less effective alternative.
- Physiotherapy, use of a walking stick, adapting shoes, and a splint to support a joint such as the knee are all useful measures.
- Surgery is needed for those with advanced disease of the knees and hips where joint replacement can be highly successful. It should be remem-bered that the success rate is not 100 per cent. Other surgical measures are useful for deformed joints.
- Other measures to control pain are important especially when there is widespread joint involvement. Sometimes the pain comes from the muscles around the joints, especially in the spine and lower limbs. In spinal arthritis, use of a Trans-Dermal Electrical Nerve Stimulator (TENS) machine may help reduce the pain, in much the same way that acupuncture does.

What you can do

- Lose weight if you are overweight and especially if the knees or hips are involved. The improvement from this can literally be (un)staggering.
- Exclusion diets are not as a rule helpful in the way they are with rheumatoid arthritis. Occasionally they are worth considering in younger people with recent onset of their disease, and where there is a lot of swelling around the joint. This picture would suggest a high degree of inflammation rather than degeneration. The authors have seen both sensitivity to wheat and dairy products in such patients.
- Improve muscle strength and reduce muscle pain. This is an under-emphasised aspect of care and applies especially to those patients where the hip and spine are affected. The pain of the arthritis leads to inactivity, which results in more muscle weakness leading to increased disability and pain. The solution involves increasing physical activity (despite the pain) and improved nutritional state to help muscle function and strength. The most important nutrients in regard to the latter are magnesium and potassium, lack of which leads to muscle weakness and spasms, and vitamin D, a deficiency of which is most likely in those aged over 75 years and the housebound. To improve the balance of these nutrients try eating The Very Nutritious Diet (see page 437), and take supplements of a multi-vitamin and 250 mg of magnesium per day.
- One study suggested that supplements of ginger may be mildly effective. Other supplements could be beneficial for some but there are few studies. As in rheumatoid arthritis, correcting a deficiency of zinc or selenium, and providing a supply of fish oils and antioxidants such as vitamin E and beta-carotene could have anti-inflammatory effects.

Latest research looks at the benefits of glucosamine, a substance that occurs naturally in the cartilage. As we age we lose some of the glucosamine and other substances which results in joint aches and pains, and in more severe cases, arthritis. Part of the function of glucosamine is to enhance the synovial fluid, which lubricates the joints, and it is also responsible for joint repair. It therefore has an essential role in the structure and function of the 'glue' which holds cartilage tissue together, and its deficiency can lead to cartilage degeneration.

Several clinical studies have shown that glucosamine sulphate, which is the most effective form of glucosamine, taken at a dose of 500mg three times a day, produces significant improvements in the symptoms of pain, joint tenderness and swelling.

The evidence for the use of glucosamine in the treatment of arthritis is now so strong that the World Health Organisation has accepted glucosamine as a superior long-term strategy and officially classified it as a slow acting drug in the treatment of osteoarthritis.

Glucosamine needs to be taken daily in conjunction with another substance known as chondroitin, which attracts nutrient-rich, shock-absorbing fluid and stimulates the production of cartilage and collagen. Chondroitin works by protecting the cartilage from breakdown by certain enzymes, which cut off the transport of nutrients necessary for healthy joints.

Other supplements to reduce the inflammation and swelling are favoured and include boswellia, bromelain (an enzyme naturally occurring in pineapple), curcumin (the active ingredient in turmeric) and ginger. Boswellia has a particularly beneficial anti-inflammatory action similar to conventional non-steroidal anti-inflammatory drugs, without the side-effects. Curcumin is a potent anti-oxidant that reduces inflammation by lowering histamine levels.

Noreen's story

Noreen had to give up her work as a cleaning lady at the tender age of 64 because of increasingly severe pain and swelling in the small joints of her hands. This had begun over the previous year and investigations by her own doctor had not shown any gout or rheumatoid arthritis. The picture of change was typical for osteo-arthritis for which she had been prescribed a NSAID drug. This had helped but had not controlled her pain and discomfort.

She ate an excellent diet, was a non-smoker and a non-drinker and the only abnormality was that she was a little overweight at 76 kilos. She was asked to begin a weight-reducing diet and take some cod liver oil supplements whilst WNAS awaited the results of some nutritional investigations. These showed a surprisingly low level of zinc, 7.6 mmols per litre (11.5–20). Supplements of zinc and multi-vitamins were added to her diet and within three months her zinc level had returned to normal. There was a surprising degree of improvement in her pain eventually getting to a point where she was able to stop her anti-arthritis drugs completely. She continued on a small dose of zinc, multi-vitamins and fish oils as well as keeping her weight below 76 kilos.

See also: References.

GOUT

Though less common than rheumatoid arthritis and osteoarthritis, gout is still an important cause of joint pain and swelling. It effects both men and usually only relatively older women. It is highly responsive to treatment. Gout is due to an accumulation of crystals of sodium urate for uric acid, which is derived from the breakdown of certain foods and chemicals in the body called purines. The level of uric acid rises in the blood and then precipitates out around various joints, often as a result of relatively minor trauma, and set up an inflammatory reaction. Typically it is the big toe joint that is first affected and the ankle, wrist, elbow, knee and hands are often involved later on.

Who gets it?

It is more common in men who may be affected at a relatively young age. Obesity and alcohol consumption play a large part in its development. In older people, deteriorating kidney function and use of diuretics (water tablets) increase the risk. Accumulation of the toxic mineral lead and certain chronic blood and other diseases are also known predisposing factors.

What your doctor can do

Firstly treat the acute attack, which can be severe.

- Drugs such as NSAIDs (non-steroidal anti-inflammatory drugs) in large amounts or colchicine, a drug derived from the crocus, are very effective.
- Aspirin, except in high doses, can actually make matters worse.
- In the long term, after the acute attack is over, use of the drug allopurinol, which prevents the build up of uric acid, is needed especially when the attacks are recurrent and there is an inadequate response to self-help measures. Occasionally damage to the kidney also occurs and more specialised treatment is needed.

What you can do

- Drink plenty of liquid, preferably water, during an acute attack.
- Lose weight if you need to. Take care, as crash or starvation diets can raise the level of uric acid.
- Cut down on alcohol especially beer, as this is rich in the purines that are converted into uric acid.
- Avoid purine-rich foods: liver, kidneys, sweetbreads, fish roe (including caviar).
- Supplements of vitamin C, at a dose of 4 g per day, help lower blood levels of uric acid and increases its loss in the urine.
- Eicosapentaenoic acid (EPA) derived from the Omega-3 series of essential fatty acids limit the production of pro-inflammatory mediators otherwise known as 'leukotrienes' which are responsible for the inflammation associated with this condition.

- Supplements of zinc and magnesium should help in theory, but their effect is probably not great.
- For some, further dietary advice and restriction of fructose, fruit sugar, might be needed.

ANKYLOSING SPONDYLITIS

This is a type of chronic arthritis that affects mainly the spine and lower back area. The sacro-iliac joints where the spinal column joins the pelvis are frequently affected. The illness may be accompanied by inflammation in other parts of the body notably, the eyes and the bowel.

Who gets it?

Mainly men, but a few women do too. It usually first affects patients between the ages of 20 and 40. Symptoms of low back pain and increasing stiffness may be present for several years before a diagnosis is made.

What causes it?

The cause is unknown except that there is a strong association between this type of arthritis and several genetically determined markers that are present on white cells. The chemical nature of these particular markers called HLA-B27 (Human Lymphocyte Antigen -B27) is similar to chemicals produced by a certain bacteria called *Klebsiella* which can be present in the normal human gut.

What your doctor can do

There is no cure. Usually treatment centres upon anti-inflammatory drugs, and physiotherapy and exercises to maintain mobility of the spine.

What you can do

This is at present uncertain. There has been a suggestion that dietary changes that would discourage the growth of the *Klebsiella* organism in the gut could be helpful. Such a diet was low in certain carbohydrate-rich foods, but more work is needed before we know if it is effective.

Anti-inflammatory supplements and a diet rich in EFAs would seem to be a reasonable and not too arduous an approach. Try multi-vitamins with zinc and selenium. Supplements of fish oils might help as they do for rheumatoid arthritis.

FIBROMYALGIA

Fibromyalgia is a relatively new term which replaces the old term fibrositis. It is a common condition characterised by tender painful muscles, most usually those around the shoulders and neck. Tender nodules or lumps can sometimes be felt in the affected muscles. Examination of these nodules reveals muscles whose regular anatomy is distorted with a mild degree of inflammation. Part of the problem appears to be a failure of the muscles to relax properly. This results in increased tension and pain in the muscles. Some research suggests that a relative lack of growth hormone factors from the pituitary gland may be to blame.

Who gets it?

It most commonly affects young to middle-aged women. It does not follow trauma, nor is it related to excessive use or arthritis.

What your doctor can do

- Prescribe simple painkillers but these are not very effective.
- Prescribe a small dose of an antidepressant called amitryptilline. This has pain-killing properties and is reasonably effective. Worth considering if sleep is disturbed by pain as it can help sleep if taken in the evening.
- Test to exclude other types of muscle inflammation or arthritis.

What you can do

- A massage often helps; try using some relaxing aromatherapy oils as well (see page 31).
- Heat is also helpful, such as a hot water bottle, a hot towel or a hot pad which can be easily applied to the painful area, or sunbathing.
- Supplements of magnesium can be very useful. We think of muscles as being able to do work by contracting. Every time a muscle contracts it then needs to relax before it can contract again. Muscles are not like pieces of elastic, as the process of relaxation is an active one needing energy and the mineral magnesium. Low levels of this mineral are known to occur in those with fibromyalgia. So you can try supplements of magnesium, about 300 mg per day, in combination with The Very Nutritious Diet, which is low in salt and reduced in calories if you need to lose weight (see page 437).

- Exercise helps. It may not feel like it initially, but provided your symptoms are not too severe, gentle exercise, especially swimming, can be very helpful. In the long term, those who do exercise regularly suffer less from this painful condition.
- Osteopathic or chiropractic treatment can be helpful to correct any displacement in the spine that may be triggering the problem.

These treatments often take several months to work. You can combine the self-help measures with painkillers if necessary.

Jacqueline's story

Within the two years before her 40th birthday Jacqueline was diagnosed as having an early menopause needing HRT, had a low bone density and a tendency to develop osteoporosis. She had experienced excessive weight gain with fluid retention, but all this was not bothering her as much as her feeling of fatigue and muscular aches and pains. Eventually an under-active thyroid was diagnosed and treated, but the level of fatigue and muscle pain continued unchanged. Her HRT was well managed, her osteoporosis treated and though on paper she should be doing well, still her symptoms of fatigue and muscle pains continued.

Her weight blossomed to 79 kilos from previously having been below 70 kilos.

Some nutritional tests showed that she had a very low red cell magnesium value of 1.82 mmols per litre (2.08–3.00). Her levels for a number of other minerals including zinc and potassium were borderline. It appeared she was not just having difficulty hanging onto calcium which is important for her bones, but the low magnesium almost certainly would be affecting her muscle function and fatigue.

A weight-reducing, low salt, high calcium, high magnesium nutritious diet was followed together with substantial supplements of calcium, magnesium and multi-vitamins. There was no quick improvement. However, over four months there was a gradual improvement in her energy level and the muscle aches and pains diminished significantly. She was still predisposed towards getting fluid retention too easily, developing fluid retention if she consumed any salt in her diet.

Her need for thyroid hormone and HRT continued and probably will for many years, but now she experiences the full benefit from them, perhaps because some of these nutrients interact with the action of these hormones. She will need calcium, magnesium and vitamin supplements long-term in order to maintain her health.

MUSCLE CRAMPS

These are simply episodes where a muscle, most often in the leg or hand, contracts and fails to relax. The sustained contraction causes a build-up of lactic acid which results in pain. Unlike fibromyalgia there is no change in the structure of the muscle or associated inflammation.

What causes them?

A lack of sodium, potassium or magnesium can lead to muscle cramps. Those who work in very hot environments and sweat a lot, the elderly, those on diuretics (water tablets) and women during pregnancy may suffer in particular. Those who do not have good amounts of potassium and magnesium in the diet from fresh fruit and vegetables are at risk, too.

What your doctor can do

- Check the blood levels of sodium, potassium and magnesium (a red cell level of the latter is perhaps the most useful).
- Occasionally disturbances in calcium level, too low or high, can be a cause.
- Prescribe quinine sulphate which is an old-fashioned but effective remedy.

What you can do

- Eat A Very Nutritious Diet (see page 437).
- Drink plenty and ensure a good intake of sodium salt if you are in a very hot climate.
- Try supplements of magnesium 300–400 mg per day, and a multi-vitamin supplement. Magnesium is a very safe supplement to try and has been used successfully to reduce muscle cramps in pregnancy.
- Avoid excess consumption of carbonated beverages especially cola and lemonade which are high in phosphoric acid even if they are the lower-calorie varieties. The high intake of phosphate lowers calcium and probably magnesium levels. A maximum intake of one litre per week is recommended.
- Gentle massage for painful muscle groups.

Complementary therapies

Acupuncture is worth considering. Homeopathy too has some remedies, and a popular one is Cuprum Met., a homeopathic preparation of the mineral copper.

Asthma

Asthma is a common condition characterised by shortness of breath and wheezing due to narrowing of the airways in the lung. This narrowing is to a large degree reversible, particularly in the early stages of the condition, and can be triggered by a variety of factors including allergies and irritants. Many of these are identical to those factors that cause or trigger rhinitis (see Hayfever and Allergic Rhinitis, page 226).

The airways are narrowed because of swelling of the tissues that line them, because of an increase in the production of mucus which may be hard to clear and because the ring of muscle around the medium-sized airway contracts, reducing the internal size of the airway. All this means that it is harder for air to pass in and out of the lung. A key feature is an increased lung sensitivity to many non-specific irritants which in normal individuals do not cause breathing difficulties: cold air, dusts, exercise and even laughter can all trigger wheezing in the asthmatic. There is almost always a noticeable reduction in the ease of breathing in the early morning or during the night in the untreated asthmatic. On top of these, there are three major triggers which often lie behind the more serious episodes: they include infection, allergy and pollution.

What are the symptoms?

Wheezing and a feeling of shortness of breath are the main but not the only symptoms of asthma. These are almost always improved by the use of drugs that open up the airways (called bronchodilators). A cough may be the sole complaint in children or mildly affected adults, and is often the reason for a sufferer seeking advice. White sticky phlegm may be produced too, and this may be discoloured if there is infection. Characteristically these symptoms vary. They are almost always worse in the morning and at times during the day when the individual may have been exposed to a triggering factor. The easiest way to observe this is by asking the person to record their 'peak flow measurement' several times each day. This is done using a simple light-weight peak flow meter, and recording three or four measures per day for a week or longer.

Who gets it?

More and more people, over the course of the last 20 years with the latest figures showing a doubling of asthma prevalence, especially in younger sufferers. Now about 5–6 per cent of children in the UK have asthma, with probably the same number again being undiagnosed sufferers. Many of these may only have a night-time cough as a symptom. This increase in prevalence has occurred in Europe, North America and Australasia. Fortunately the death rate which had risen throughout this century, has reached a plateau in the last 20 years, with 2,000 deaths being attributed to this condition per year in the UK. Asthma and bronchial hyper-responsiveness seem to be more likely in:

- urban dwellers
- middle-class families
- some polluted environments
- non breast-fed infants
- the children of smoking parents
- those who consume a lot of salt and salty food

Genetic factors are also relevant for both allergic and non-allergic asthma. In childhood-onset asthma there is often an allergic component, with an association with eczema, and often sensitivity to grass pollen, housedust and cats. If one parent is atopic (has allergic tendencies), the risk of a child developing inhalant allergies nearly doubles, compared with children of non-atopic parents, and nearly quadruple if both parents are atopic. The risk of developing these allergies is also greater for boys and if the child was born underweight.

What causes it?

In addition to the factors that contribute to bronchial hyperresponsiveness, the three main categories to consider are those already mentioned: allergies, infection and pollution. Recent research suggests that there are interactions between those whereby pollutants and viruses increase the magnitude of the allergic response.

Allergic causes

These are very similar to those that cause rhinitis (see page 226). They can cause both an immediate reaction with a peak effect at 5–15 minutes, and a delayed reaction peaking at 4–6 hours, and which can last for 24 hours. Thus daily exposure to an allergen may mean that there are nearly continuous symptoms with no discernible aggravations that would allow you to easily connect a possible allergen with the asthma. Possible allergens include:

- *Housedust mite* For control of the housedust mite, see Hay Fever (page 229).
- *Animals* Cats, and to a lesser extent dogs, birds (and feather-filled furnishings) and laboratory animals.
- *Grass pollen* An allergy can cause asthma as well as hayfever. Sensitivity to tree and weed pollen and, rarely, flower pollen may be minor triggers.

- *Mould sensitivity Aspergillus fumigatus* is a common garden and household mould which releases its spores in autumn and winter, and can produce chronic asthma in which the fungus actually infects the lung. Other mould spores are present in the atmosphere in the late summer and early autumn. They are more likely to be present in rural areas and some are released after rainstorms. Allergy to fungi that commonly cause skin infections such as athlete's foot or nail infections is another, albeit rare, cause of asthma.
- *Foods* Some of these may be obvious because they produce reactions within a few minutes or an hour or two of consumption. This probably applies to less than 10 per cent of asthmatics, and common culprit foods are nuts, eggs, milk, wheat, soya, fish and shellfish. Very delayed reactions to foods are notoriously hard to assess. Cows' milk products and wheat are possibilities. A reason that the role of these or other foods is unclear is that sensitivity to them may result only in an increase in catarrh, or produce biochemical changes in the lung that then require the presence of other more potent trigger factors before there is a discernible effect.
- *Health-food supplements* These are a rare possible cause, with asthmatic reactions and even death following consumption of royal jelly.
- *Artificial colourings* Notably Tartrazine E 102 and Sunset Yellow E110 in approximately 4 per cent of asthmatics.
- *Preservatives in food* Sulphites (E 220–E 227) in approximately 5–10 per cent of asthmatics. Sulphites are also found in many wines, and this beverage may occasionally trigger attacks.
- *Dust* From woods, wheat, other grains, tea, coffee, soya beans, and other foods.
- *Fumes* From soldering of metal and the soldering flux rosin.
- *Dust or fumes* From chemicals, medicines and enzymes in occupational exposure.
- *Chemicals* Those used in paint sprays.

Infective causes

These are an important possibility, and although antibiotics are often given during an acute episode, it is more often to cover the possibility than the actuality of infection.

- Viral infections seem especially common in children.
- Bacterial infections should be suspected if yellow or green phlegm is present. This is very relevant to older patients with a history of long-standing lung problems.
- Parasitic infection, not in the lung, but elsewhere may sometimes be a trigger due to the development of an allergy to the parasite's proteins which then cause a reaction in the lung. Only suspect if there are other symptoms of parasite infection or a history of foreign travel.

As a rule infections may be more likely if the diet is inadequate and there are deficiencies of certain key nutrients. Vitamins A, B complex and zinc may be especially relevant but there are no studies of their levels in asthmatic patients.

Pollution as a cause

- Smoking is the most obvious trigger factor, and this is nowadays very often another's smoke from passive exposure.
- Outdoor air pollutants include sulphur dioxide, nitrogen dioxide, chlorine and ozone. These chemicals are either released from industrial processes, are present in car exhaust fumes, are formed naturally by the action of lightning, or form in the photochemical smog that sits like a blanket over many large cities. A combination of bright sunlight and the right atmospheric conditions combine to create a chemical soup containing these potent lung irritants. Ozone seems often to be the most important, and levels of this chemical typically peak around midday. Weather forecasts now include warnings about poor air quality.
- Very fine smoke particles from fires of coal or wood, diesel engines and some industrial sources were once thought to be relatively harmless, but they do seem to cause problems. They may combine with allergens such as pollen and enhance their triggering effects.
- Indoor pollutants (is nowhere safe?) include paint strippers, oven cleaners, spray polishes and others. Sunlight may contribute to an indoor photochemical smog effect.

Other possible causes

- The most serious are a group of drugs called beta-blockers used in the treatment of high blood pressure and angina, and in the form of eye drops in the treatment of glaucoma. No one with asthma or a history of asthma should use these drugs.
- Aspirin and occasionally other analgesics may trigger an attack. There may be some association with nasal polyps or a family history of aspirin sensitivity. This may affect 2 per cent of asthmatics.
- Rarely, asthma is much worse premenstrually. The exact cause for this is not clear. It may respond to either the use of steroids or hormonal treatment. Treatment of associated premenstrual symptoms might be beneficial (*see* Premenstrual syndrome, page 394).
- A certain amount of asthma at night and in the early morning is due to the near silent regurgitation of acid secretions from the stomach and their passage in small amounts into the lung. This happens most easily at night when the person is lying down and the reflux of acid from the stomach into the oesophagus or gullet goes unnoticed. Coughing episodes at night with a burning sensation in the central chest would

suggest this possible situation. Treatment involves a dietary measure to help reduce acid reflux (see page 247) and use of drugs to suppress excessive acid production. They can be highly effective.

What your doctor can do

The management of asthma has undergone a substantial review in the UK, Australasia and elsewhere in the last decade. This came about because of a continuing high mortality rate which is now beginning to fall, and the realisation that a high percentage of these deaths was preventable. Management depended upon:

- Adequate treatment of acute attacks.
- Detection of precipitating cause(s). In some instances this may mean either skin or blood tests for possible allergies.
- Assessment of the degree of lung impairment. Most often regular use of a simple 'peak flow meter' will give good information about the severity of the asthma and its variation at different times. More detailed lung function tests are used by chest disease specialists.
- Drawing up a treatment action plan based upon the above information, the patient's needs and following recognised guidelines.

Most treatment centres upon the use of drugs most commonly given by inhalers. The main types are:

- Bronchodilators such as salbutamol (Ventolin); these produce a very quick response but need to be given several times per day. Mild asthmatics may not need any other therapy. Excessive use of these inhalers has in the past resulted in an increased risk of death. It is important that the recommended intake and prescribed pattern of use are followed.
- Steroid inhalers which come in a variety of strengths. They are useful when the asthma is not controlled by simple bronchodilators. They reduce the swelling and inflammation that narrows the airways, and are most usefully combined with a bronchodilator. Very potent inhaled steroid preparations are now available, and are used for more severe cases. Side-effects such as oral thrush may develop, and continued use may reduce growth rates in children.
- Sodium cromoglycate is a drug again given by inhaler, that has a unique action, blocking the allergic reactions that take place in the lung. It is most successful in young children and often should be tried before long-term steroid inhalers are used. The inhalers are less effective in adults, but are worth considering when allergy plays a major role.
- Oral steroids are used initially as a short high-dose course for severe attacks in either children or adults. Courses lasting seven days or so are

relatively free of side-effects, are life-saving, and frequently reduce the time spent in hospital. For those with severe asthma that requires maximal doses of inhaled steroids or repeated short courses of high-dose steroids, then long-term use of daily doses of steroids are worth considering. These are not without side-effects, most usually if the dose of prednisolone exceeds 10 mg daily. Weight gain, high blood pressure, muscle loss, osteoporosis and development of diabetes may all occur, but are perhaps less likely if the patient is encouraged to eat very healthily and has no associated nutritional deficiencies.

• Other drugs are sometimes used by specialists, and include long-acting bronchodilators (Salmeterol and Oxitropium) given by inhaler, preparations of Aminophylline, antihistamines and immune-altering drugs. All of these except the last catergory are usually tried before long-term steroid tablets are used.

When any of these treatments are first started it is a good policy for the patient's response to be carefully monitored. Recording the peak flow readings in the morning and at a further time later in the day, as well as the level of symptoms, can help decide on the best type of treatment and its dosage. This is important, as potentially many treatments will continue for years.

The drugs for inhalation can be given by a number of devices including metered dose inhalers which use chlorofluorocarbon propellant, dry powder devices and nebulisers for the severe attack. Large spacer devices attached to the inhaler may improve performance and reduce side-effects in the mouth.

• Desensitising was once a popular treatment, though it is now rarely used because of occasional deaths. Patients who were strongly reacting to housedust mite or pollen could be made less sensitive after being given a series of injections. Each injection contained a very small but increasing dose of the allergen which, instead of causing an allergic reation, stimulated the body to produce other antibodies that blocked the action of those antibodies involved in the asthmatic reaction. Thus the allergy was side-tracked. Such treatments may return in the future and be used at specialised centres.

What you can do

The importance of involving the sufferer in the care of their asthma is becoming increasingly recognised. The variable nature of this condition means that the asthmatic needs to know which changes can be made to their treatment and be familiar with what the possible triggering factors are for any acute episode. Avoidance of these triggers is important, especially if escalating doses of drugs are to be avoided.

- *Take your medication regularly* It sounds simple and it is. Regular use of the agreed medication should mean better lung function, fewer severe attacks and less disability. Better medical treatment plans may well be behind the recently reported falls in deaths from asthma in the UK.
- *Avoidance of known inhalant allergens* This applies particularly to those who need to use steroids in any form. The need for avoidance of housedust and other inhalant allergens will depend on documentation of the allergy, usually by use of skin prick tests, and recognition that the asthma is to a substantial degree influenced by them. The measures detailed under Hayfever and Allergic Rhinitis (see page 226) for the avoidance of the appropriate allergen should be followed. Prolonged avoidance of the allergen can, after a number of months, lead to a reduction in the individual's degree of sensitivity.
- *Avoid pollutants* Firstly do not smoke. Try not to use wood and coal fires in the home unless they are very well enclosed. You may need to avoid going outside during the time of the day when air quality is at its worst.
- *Reduce the chances of chest infection* Damp in the home is still a major risk factor for chest infections, and this is in turn related to social class. Treating damp areas and providing adequate heat and ventilation are important. These measures will help limit housedust mites and some moulds.
- *Improve your nutritional state* Mild nutritional deficiencies and a poor diet certainly influence resistance to infection and the rate of chest infections and possibly the development and severity of asthma. Eat The Very Nutritious Diet (see page 437). Certain nutrients may be especially important, and they include vitamins A and B complex and zinc.
- *Eat certain protective foods* A high intake of fresh fruit and vegetables may be desirable. They are rich in magnesium and potassium, and low in sodium. Onions have been shown to have anti-asthmatic properties. Certain chemicals called thiosulphates and cepaenes, which are formed when the onion is crushed or chopped, seem to inhibit the production of pro-inflammatory chemicals involved in asthma. Apparently you'll need to eat one medium-sized onion per day. Perhaps a bowl of steaming hot onion soup for the acute attack?
- *Avoid common food additives* These include artificial colourings and sulphites. Watch out for the latter in squashes and wines which do not list them on the label within the European Community. Australians are better informed, as these additives are detailed on the label.
- *Cut down on salt in the diet* High normal intakes might enhance the bronchial hyper-responsiveness that develops.
- *Take regular exercise* Provided that necessary care is taken, the asthma is stable, and medication is taken regularly, this can improve

the situation over time. Many sports people with asthma take a squirt of their bronchodilator just before exercise.
- *Protect yourself from cold air* This commonly triggers wheezing. Do so by wearing a scarf and even placing this over your mouth. Alternatively you can wear a face mask, especially if you are cycling in a city and are exposed to traffic fumes.

Nutritional supplements
- Vitamin C, 1g twice daily, has an antihistamine effect. Try it for six to eight weeks.
- Magnesium is a mineral that has mild anti-allergy and bronchodilating effects. It is not as strong as the equivalent drugs. Two recent pieces of research have revealed that the white cells of asthmatics are low in this mineral, and that a poor dietary intake in adults is associated with an increased chance of wheezing. The effects of supplements are awaited, but are unlikely to be very strong. A supplement of 300–400 mg per day for at least four months, together with a high-protein low-salt diet, is suggested.
- Vitamin B6, pyridoxine, was shown in one small trial to help reduce the asthmatics' dependency upon steroids. This supplement has been shown to enhance magnesium balance in women with premenstrual syndrome.
- Multi-vitamins and antioxidants such as beta-carotene, vitamin E, selenium and zinc might protect the lung from chemical assault. Lowered blood levels of this latter mineral have been linked with asthma and sensitivity to aspirin and salicylates. Vitamin A is important for the health of the mucous membranes lining the respiratory tract.
- Fish oil supplements have been tried in asthma with the expectation that their anti-inflammatory effects would reduce the degree of wheezing. In fact some of those who took part experienced a deterioration, and this type of supplement, including cod liver oil, should not be taken by the severe asthmatic without medical supervision.
- The bioflavonoid quercetin has been used successfully to reduce inflammation of the lungs and respiratory tract.
- Bromelain, an enzyme derived from pineapple, also possesses powerful anti-inflammatory properties.

As before with drug medication, evaluation of benefit is important. Monitoring the response to self-help measures, dietary treatment and use of supplements is best achieved by recording peak flow daily. Other measures of improvement include general well-being, need for medication, dosage of steroids or bronchodilators, and use of antibiotics. For many of these non-drug measures, improvement is likely to take three to six months, so be patient.

Complementary therapies

- Acupuncture can help with feelings of shortness of breath, and thus might be of benefit to some sufferers.
- Relaxation therapies such as massage and aromatherapy could help, especially where stressful incidents are a frequent asthma trigger.
- Herbal medicine is worth consideration, as there appear to be a number of plant extracts with the power to alter lung chemistry. Sanitised extracts of these may appear or pharmacological equivalents may be developed in the near future.

See also: Allergy, PMS, Indigestion, High blood pressure, What's wrong with present-day diet and lifestyle?, Nutrition is the key to health, The simple exclusion diet, References and Recommended reading.

Back Pain

Back pain is a common complaint with a variety of causes. The pain may vary from intermittent discomfort to severe pain that requires complete bed rest. At one end of the spectrum continuous pain may be caused by a disease in the back itself or as referred pain from some other part of the body that is diseased or infected, and at the other extreme the pain may be related only to pulled muscles or ligaments, and may only be a short-term problem. The sensations can vary from a dull aching feeling to sharp, shooting sensations.

What causes it?

There is an almost endless list of causes for common back and neck problems, and they include:

- muscular strain from moving awkwardly or lifting heavy items
- tearing of a ligament or tendon, or inflammation of the synovial fluid which surrounds the joints
- long-standing displacement or curvature of the spine
- arthritis of the spine
- prolapsed (slipped) disc
- vertebral collapse from osteoporosis
- infections such as viral infections
- kidney stones
- pressure on the nerves as in sciatica
- bad posture when sitting or standing
- a gynaecological disorder, like fibroids or cysts

- period pains
- ill-fitting or high-heeled shoes
- obesity or pregnancy placing strain on the spine
- injuries or accident
- bowel or intestinal problems
- depression and fatigue
- occasionally disease of the internal abdominal organs

What your doctor can do

Severe back pain lasting for more than a few days will require assessment by a doctor. All the patients with weight loss or severe persistent pain should be looked at particularly carefully, and this may well involve blood tests and X-rays. When underlying medical conditions have been eliminated, your doctor may refer you to an osteopath or a physiotherapist for a course of treatment. Osteopaths are particularly adept at treating pain of musculo-skeletal origin (derived from muscles, tendons, ligaments or bones). They are also trained to detect more common serious disorders that may present with back pain and often they, in turn, can refer you to your GP. Cranial osteopathy is a particularly effective and gentle form of treatment that is well worth investigating if you suffer with back problems, (see page 38).

What you can do

The simplest and most important message for those with back pain is that much of the pain is actually due to muscle spasm. Sometimes this is the only problem or it is secondary to painful skeletal conditions such as vertebral collapse or displacement. Muscle spasm can be relieved by a number of self-help measures, including:

- rest
- local heat or cold application
- gentle massage when the acute episode is over
- ordinary pain killers
- small amounts of alcohol
- supplements of magnesium, a simple cheap and at times surprisingly effective treatment (but which is unlikely to be effective for the control of severe back pain associated with arthritis). Supplements of between 200–400 mg of magnesium taken with multi-vitamins will help raise magnesium levels, in blood and muscle over a two-week to two-month period.
- The amino acid DL-Phenylalanine (DLPA) is used for pain relief. DLPA works by inhibiting the enzyme which normally inactivates the

pain relieving endorphins produced by the brain. *Do not* take if pregnant or breast-feeding, or suffering from panic attacks, diabetes or high blood pressure.

- Vitamin C and the mineral zinc work by enhancing protein synthesis and collagen formation.
- If the back pain is arthritic, introduce glucosamine sulphate to enhance cartilage formation and refer to the chapter on arthritis for more information.
- The Very Nutritious Diet (see page 437), low in salt and sugar, as this helps magnesium retention.
- The Alexander Technique is particularly good at re-training us to hold our bodies in an optimum way, thus preventing future back or neck problems.

Many back problems could be prevented by improving posture and by taking adequate exercise. The following points are worth implementing for long-term back health:

- Make sure you have a comfortable mattress to sleep on which is turned regularly. So many back problems occur gradually as an ageing mattress fails to support your back in the optimum way.
- Ensure that you have a comfortable working chair that supports your back fully and that your desk or table is the appropriate height.
- When you walk be aware of your posture, keeping your shoulders down and your head high. Imagine you have a piece of string coming out the top of your head which is being gently pulled from above.
- When bending, bend from the knees, rather than stooping over.
- Take regular exercise, but be careful not to cause any further back problems. The YMCA back-care video, *The Back and Beyond*, provides a useful healthy back maintenance programme for sufferers. It is worth a try in the comfort of your own home.

Complementary therapies

Osteopathy and chiropractic are now established to be of value. It is helpful to have a local therapist with whom you have good rapport, especially if you have repeated need of their services. Vigorous manipulative techniques are inappropriate for many older patients, and you may need to enquire of the therapist what type of approaches they use before seeking their advice. Cranial osteopathy is our preference because it is effective and non-invasive.

Homeopathic remedies for pain relief are a useful tool, and magnesium phosphoricum is particularly helpful.

See also: Recommended reading, References.

Breast Problems

Up to 60 per cent of working women have experienced breast pain at some time which is, surprisingly, a good sign, as pain is not usually associated with anything sinister. Breast cancer is a great concern to us all, though, especially as it is on the increase. Despite the fact that breast examinations and special X-rays, mammography, are now available to detect early breast cancer, there are still some 20,000 new cases diagnosed each year in the UK. England and Wales come top of the league for breast cancer, followed by Denmark and Scotland. New Zealand comes in eighth, the USA in eleventh place and Australia in fourteenth. Having begun in such an alarmist fashion, it should be said that for every patient with breast cancer, ten others will have a non-sinister breast lump or breast tenderness.

What are the symptoms?

There are various conditions that cause breast tenderness, pain (otherwise known as mastalgia) and lumps, and they are generally covered by the term 'benign breast disease'. This may sound unduly frightening, but non-cancerous lumps, bumps and cysts are quite normal and should not be regarded as disease. The word 'benign' means non-cancerous, and indicates that lumps will not spread and grow to invade other tissue, or affect other parts of the body. Even so, they can be very uncomfortable and a continuing source of worry.

Breast pain can be divided broadly into two categories. In approximately one-third of cases, breast tenderness and discomfort occur throughout the month, whilst in the remaining two-thirds, breast tenderness and pain tend to worsen before the onset of a period. The premenstrual pattern of breast tenderness that occurs for up to two weeks before the period, tends to occur in younger patients in their twenties to forties, and can usually be alleviated by natural means.

All women with breast tenderness or a breast lump should have a physical examination to determine the nature of the problem. Mild breast tenderness that occurs premenstrually, and clears completely without the presence of any breast lump, is rarely indicative of anything sinister. Persistent pain, alteration in the shape of the breast, or a discharge from the nipple, are all symptoms that should make you seek an early appointment with your doctor.

What causes it?

- In recent years, there has been some evidence to link breast disease with the type of diets we eat. Breast cancer, for example, is more common in countries with a high animal fat intake. Countries such as Japan, where fat intake is extremely low and the diet is composed mainly of vegetables, fish and rice, there is a low incidence of breast cancer and benign breast problems.

- Other scientists in the field have suggested that cigarette smoking and caffeine intakes from tea and coffee, chocolate and cola, may be linked with breast discomfort. This is not absolutely proven, but it may be helpful to reduce your consumption of these if breast tenderness is a problem.
- Hormonal factors are also important. The oral contraceptive pill, with its content of progesterone, may help to reduce some types of benign breast disease. Giving birth to a first child prior to the age of thirty is associated with a slight reduction in breast cancer risk.

What your doctor can do

- Examine your breasts and take a history of the problem. If you feel it is a recurring cyclic problem, in that it occurs monthly before your period is due, you should make this known.
- If your doctor is not unduly concerned, the next step is to prescribe evening primrose oil, Efamast, at a dose of 3,000–4,000g for at least four months. This has been shown to help with benign breast problems.
- Your doctor should tell you to eat a low-fat diet, see page 102, but may be unaware of the research published in this area.
- If your symptoms are not sinister or cyclic, then your doctor may prescribe either painkillers or an anti-inflammatory preparation.
- Should the pain or tenderness persist, your doctor may then prescribe powerful hormones, like Danazol, which will stop you ovulating or, as a last resort, Bromocriptine, another powerful drug, which blocks the hormone, prolactin, from the pituitary gland. Both of these drugs have a long list of side-effects which may be unacceptable and should be carefully considered.

What you can do

A carefully conducted study published in the leading medical journal, *The Lancet*, in 1988, showed that women with premenstrual breast tenderness, could benefit from a low-fat, high-fibre, high-protein diet. The diet requires a substantial reduction in overall fat intake to a level that would mean most of us reducing our fat intake by nearly 50 per cent. To achieve this, the following changes would need to be made:

- Eat leaner cuts of meat and trim all visible fat from meat.
- Don't eat meat products, such as pies, sausages, and pâté, which are high in fat.
- Don't eat the skin from fish, chicken or other poultry.
- All meat and fish should be grilled, steamed or baked, and not fried, or prepared with rich creamy sauces.
- Dairy intake should be limited, replacing full cream milk with skimmed or semi-skimmed milk. Cheese can be replaced by those with a low-fat content, such as Edam, and using low fat polyunsaturated spreads, instead of ordinary margarines or butter. Cream is to be avoided too; and low fat yoghurts or fromage frais, are good alternatives.
- Where possible eat organic food, especially dairy products and meat which can contain hormones, antibiotics and other synthetic chemicals.

Other dietary guidelines that are also of benefit in helping to reduce premenstrual breast tenderness include the following:

- Eat plenty of vegetables and fruit, which are low in fat.
- Aim to consume one portion of green vegetables, a portion of root vegetables and some salad every day.
- All green leafy vegetables, potatoes and other root vegetables should be consumed without butter or margarine.
- Eat at least two to three portions of fruit daily.
- Eat at least three servings of oily fish each week, including mackerel, pilchards sardines and salmon. These contain EFAs which have powerful anti-inflammatory properties, especially important for reducing breast tenderness.
- Have a daily serving of unsalted nuts and seeds, including pecans, almonds, walnuts and Brazil nuts and sunflower and pumpkin seeds. These are also rich in EFAs and form part of a very nutritious diet. Eat them sprinkled over your cereal or yogurt or eat them as a snack.
- Avoid wheat and bran which can encourage water retention. When the body sees a food as 'toxic', such as wheat the cells fill with fluid in an attempt to dilute the toxins, manifesting as fluid retention causing breast swelling and tenderness.
- Severely reduce or avoid salt and salty foods. Salt drags fluid into the cells and exacerbates breast tenderness. Use herbs and spices to enhance the flavour of food rather than disguising it with salt.
- Alcohol, sugar, confectionery and other foods rich in sugar and honey, should be severely limited, as they provide empty calories.

All these measures are particularly important if you are overweight. It has been shown that such diets may help bring down excessive levels of the hormone oestrogen, which may stimulate breast tissue. A high-fibre diet may help combat a tendency to constipation, which itself has been associated with hormonal abnormalities and even some breast conditions. Overall, the effects of this diet in the study group were very gratifying, but the benefits took some six months to become fully apparent. There was a substantial reduction in both premenstrual breast swelling, tenderness and discomfort, and it may be that these beneficial changes could eventually lead to a reduction in breast cancer risk.

Other potentially beneficial measures include:

- Reducing consumption of cigarettes and alcohol, as well as caffeine from tea, coffee, chocolate and cola-based drinks.
- Taking the supplement evening primrose oil, Efamol. This is widely available in chemists and health-food shops. The full dosage is six to eight 500 iu capsules taken daily through the menstrual cycle. It is best combined with the above dietary measures.
- Taking natural vitamin E, 400 iu per day, has also been shown to help with breast tenderness in one trial.
- Wearing a firm, supportive bra. Some women find a sports bra particularly comforting and helpful during the night.

Self-examination

It is important to have regular breast examinations, especially if you are prone to tender, lumpy breasts. Make sure you examine your breasts yourself on a regular basis to check for any lumps or changes in shape. Many women will notice that their breasts become lumpy and tender in the two weeks before their period, and that this disappears when the period has begun. These symptoms are not a cause for alarm, but should be treated, see page 101.

When to examine

Some doctors recommend examining your own breasts thoroughly at a regular time each month, after your period has finished. However, if you happen to be one of the 10 per cent of women who do self-examine, you will know that your breasts may sometimes alter in density and texture at different times of your cycle. It is important to get to know your breasts, and get in tune with your cycle, especially if you are of child-bearing age. It is probably a good idea to examine your breasts on a fortnightly basis – preferably at a regular time. If there is a set time, perhaps at the weekend, when you have a leisurely soak in the bath, maybe that would be the best opportunity, and one that you would not forget.

How to self-examine

- First have a good look at yourself undressed in the mirror. Check to make sure there are no changes in shape or colour.
- Next take each segment of your breast, like the segments of an orange,

and with one hand supporting the breast, probe and massage the section to check for lumps and bumps.

- Finally lie down, with one arm above your head, and check the circumference of the breast, including the section that merges with your underarm. Sometimes glands under the arm may be tender and swollen, indicating that there is some extra activity occurring in the area for some reason.
- If you have any concerns or confusion, it is best to get your doctor to examine the breast for you.

Most women who self-examine never find a lump, and the vast majority of lumps that *are* found are normal and harmless. Cysts, solid lumps, and discharge from the nipple are all things that occur from time to time, and which are usually hormonally related and with no sinister underlying cause. Be positive about examining your breasts on a regular basis. A lump detected early, which did turn out to be cancerous, would not be life-threatening if treated quickly. The medical profession are extremely efficient when it comes to breast cancer.

Never forget, if you have a pain or lump in your breast, you should be examined by your doctor. If neither the doctor nor the specialist can find nothing wrong, then taking care with your diet and using Efamol or Efamast, helps many women with benign breast disease. You would also be advised to follow the suggested menu on page 471.

Complementary therapies

Homeopathy, herbal medicine and massage would be the preferred choices of complementary therapies for breast problems, once it had been established that there was no underlying sinister cause. There are a number of homeopathic remedies worth trying, such as Natrum mur, Nux, Kali carb or Silica. Herbal medicine may also be worth a try.

Geraldine's story

Geraldine was a 42-year-old mother of two grown children who worked as a secretary. She suffered from painful breasts to the point where even walking hurt.

'My problem began when I was 33 and would occur every three months. Within three years the frequency and the pain had increased so that for three weeks out of four I was in agony. My doctor suggested vitamin B6 which helped for the first few months, but the symptoms returned. I was instructed to increase the dose, and ended up taking seven pills per day, which I thought may be dangerous. He then suggested I try some evening primrose oil which helped ease the pain a bit, but not completely.

That year my husband was killed in a road accident. My children were fourteen and ten at the time and life was extremely stressful. My breast pain grew worse until, by 1984, I was in pain for the majority of the time. My breast regularly swelled from 34B to 36B, and the skin was tight and shiny. I even wore a maternity bra in bed because I felt so heavy and uncomfortable. I went to see several doctors, one of whom suggested that perhaps I had strained my muscles driving a car!

Eventually I was treated with several powerful hormonal drugs. The medical theory was that the shock and stress of my bereavement had brought on an early menopause. I didn't believe this because I knew my symptoms had been just as severe, although less frequent, before I was widowed. When the drugs lost their effect I was prescribed new ones. I gradually put on 4.5 kilos and developed severe back pain. When the doctor eventually told me that my back pain was a side-effect of the drugs I went home and threw them all down the toilet. Within a week my back was as right as rain.

It was at this point I saw a magazine article about a woman with symptoms similar to mine who had been cured by changes to her diet. I really didn't have much faith in this, but I was so desperate I was ready to try anything. I phoned the WNAS and made an appointment. My first consultation was long and probing. I was given a strict diet to follow with no dairy produce, tea or coffee or added salt, no more than two slices of bread per day, and lots of fruit and vegetables. I was also given supplements of Optivite, vitamin C and Efamol, and told to follow an exercise programme.

Within a week I was a different woman. I felt so much better I could hardly believe it. It took just four months for the breast pain to completely disappear. I've been pain free for six years now. I still follow my programme and feel completely in control. Being free of breast pain has changed my life. I've been able to take swimming lessons and judo classes which would have been out of the question before. I feel like socialising and am thrilled about finding an answer to the problem that made my life a total misery for so many years.'

See also: Mastitis, Cancer, PMS, Recommended reading, and References.

Cancer

Cancer is one of the most common diseases of our time, and probably the most feared illness. Rightly so, for according to a World Health Organisation study on populations of some 50 countries, the incidence of cancer is much higher in industrialised Western societies when compared to the Asian populations. For example, depending on which western country you reside in, your chances of dying from breast or prostate cancer are between ten to 20 times greater than those consuming a typically Asian diet, whilst living in countries like Japan, China or Thailand. At present at least 20 per cent of the UK population will die of cancer, and it is thought that one in three will be affected by cancer in the UK, at some stage in their lives. More than one in four people will have cancer during their lifetime and, after heart disease, cancer is the most common cause of death in western countries. Statistics are on the increase because of the ever-expanding population. The peak incidence of adult cancer is after the age of 45. Sadly, we have reached the point where most of us have either a family member or friend who has become a cancer victim.

However, research is now showing that cancer is not inevitable, and it seems to be related more to diet and environmental factors than genetic disposition. To support this theory, let's look at what happens to the incidence of breast cancer when women move from Asia to the west and adopt the local diet. Ten times more women currently die of breast cancer in England and Wales than in Korea, and Japan loses one quarter of women to breast cancer compared to the USA. Research shows us that when Asian women migrate and adopt western eating habits, their statistics for cancer mimic those of the western world in a relatively short period of time. In fact, the rate at which the statistics change is directly related to the speed and extent to which the dietary changes are made.

How does cancer develop?

The cells in our body are constantly dividing and reproducing. The approximately 100 trillion cells in the average body are likely to reproduce 10,000 billion times in a lifetime, which means that in every minute of every day about 10 million of your cells divide. Healthy cells are incredibly intelligent. They know precisely when it is time to grow or divide, and when to stop, and this wisdom is known as 'the cell cycle'. These microscopic cells are also exceptionally astute as they are able to differentiate. They know how a kidney cell should act for example compared to a brain or a breast cell.

Not all cells have the potential to become cancerous, only those known as stem cells are candidates, and although stem cells usually divide correctly, sometimes things go wrong. Unlike normal cells, cancer cells lose their ability to differentiate; they return anonymous looking cells that instead of performing the particular function of the parent cell simply grow and disrupt the activity of healthy cells around them. The rapidly developing mass is known as a tumour which may either be benign (non-cancerous) or malignant (cancerous). When tumours or masses become sufficiently large, the adjacent organs fail to function properly, and if untreated, eventually death results.

The genetic material at the centre or nucleus of the cell determines our characteristics and is known as deoxyribonucleic acid (DNA). Its job is to give cells instructions about the production of proteins, including enzymes, without which we could not survive. When a cell divides it usually makes an exact copy of the DNA to pass on to the daughter cell. Usually this process progresses without problems, but in somewhere between one in a million and one in 100 million events a mistake occurs and the result can be a cancer cell. A damaged cell may lay dormant for many years or months before it is triggered to multiply. There is now strong scientific evidence to suppose that oestrogen encourages these 'damaged' cell's to start dividing. Many studies have shown that when oestrogen attaches itself to the receptor site within a cell, it can stimulate the cell to divide and grow abnormally. It speeds up the cell cycle and interferes with the cell's normal growth mechanism. This theory is not new, however, as in the 1880s doctors observed that women with breast cancer, who had their ovaries removed, subsequently had shrinking tumours.

Whilst it is thought that in some cases cancer may have a genetic element, for example, breast cancer is more likely to affect daughters of victims, and colon cancer can pass through families, the majority of us are not genetically fated to become cancer victims. Instead, the diet, lifestyle and environment will determine how our cells reproduce and whether or not they become cancerous.

What are the symptoms?

- *A lump* This may be the initial growth itself or a secondary deposit. New lumps or bumps anywhere should be taken seriously by your doctor. They do not have to be painful to be cancerous.
- *Pain* This is not usually an early symptom. Cancer in the bones or where the lump presses on a nerve in a confined space may lead to pain.
- *Weight loss* This is often the feature of an advanced cancer, but may also occur in the early stages of cancers affecting the stomach or other digestive organs.

- *Fatigue* This has many causes, but in patients with cancer this can be due to the associated anaemia or other affects on general metabolism.
- *Fever* Although usually caused by an infection, even in patients with cancer, this may sometimes be a feature of certain blood and glandular growths.

Risk factors for cancer

What causes it?

- Surprisingly, increased age is about the greatest risk for cancer. Of course some cancers occur in childhood, especially leukaemia and those related to certain rare genetic disorders. The majority of common cancers however occur over the age of 40. The good news is that in some very old populations the risk seems to fall, but from middle age onwards the risk is rising. This is perhaps because it takes time for some of the other causative factors to have an influence upon cells in a way that will make them change into cancerous ones. A few cancers do occur at a younger age and these include carcinoma of the cervix, some types of breast cancer and cancer of the lymph glands, Hodgkin's disease.
- Cigarette smoking is probably the next most easily identifiable factor in cancer. Its association with lung cancer is well known. What is not widely appreciated is that it is also associated with an increased risk of many other cancers, including the mouth, throat, oesophagus, the pancreas, the bladder and others. It is estimated that approximately one-third of all cancers are linked to smoking. Smoking switches off the 'guardian angel' P53 gene which checks our DNA to ensure that it has not been damaged. Smoking also increases free oxidising radicals (FORs), responsible for damaging our DNA.
- Fluid intake is a risk factor too. Smokers who drink a lot of fluid – not alcohol – halve their risk of bladder cancer, probably because the levels of cancer-causing chemicals in the urine are diluted.
- Increased risk of breast cancer is sited in women who have never had a pregnancy, have given birth late or have not breast-fed. Nuns, in fact, have one of the highest rates of breast cancer.
- Certain viral infections are associated with change in cells that may lead to cancer. This is true in a variety of conditions, including cancer of the cervix, in some blood cancers and in patients with the HIV virus. Stomach cancer is associated with chronic infection by the bacteria *Helicobacter pylori* (see page 371). These forms of cancer are potentially avoidable or preventable. Reducing the number of sexual partners a woman has, if her partner is circumcised or perhaps uses a condom, may all be associated with a lower risk of cervical cancer. Eradication of the Helicobacter germ associated with peptic ulcers may lead to a lower risk of stomach cancer.

- Environmental pollution probably plays a relatively small part, except in certain situations where there may be high exposure to a variety of industrial chemicals in either air or water.
- Radiation is a factor. In certain parts of the world, and even in certain parts of the UK, there are significant levels of natural radiation. This powerful invisible force can disrupt the structure of cells, precipitating cancerous change. Radioactive gas, radon, is found in trace amounts throughout the UK, but at high levels, in Devon and Cornwall particularly. There is a small contribution from the radiation involved in medical procedures. Local areas of pollution from nuclear reactors and more widespread radiation exposure following the Chernobyl disaster will continue to be the subject of medical research, though of only small relevance to the majority of us.
- A variety of chemicals used in industry are connected with increased cancer risks, and these include rubber, industrial dyes, asbestos, glues and varnishes, cadmium, nickel, and some rare metals.
- Scientists now believe that repeated exposure to xenoestrogens is related to the increased risk of breast tumours in women, and this is borne out by many studies including an Israeli study. In Israel breast cancer fell sharply between 1976 and 1986. The dramatic fall in death from breast cancer was due to a ban in 1978 on the use of three organochlorine pesticides. The chemical structure of environmental oestrogens is strikingly different from both oestrogen found in the body and oestrogen found in plants. Xenoestrogens interact with the receptor sites within a cell, but they block normal hormone activity.
- Exposure to sunlight or ultra-violet light in white, especially fair-skinned, individuals is associated with an increased risk of melanoma and other skin cancers. Melanoma has become one of the commonest causes of cancerous death in young people in Australia and South Africa as well as in the UK. The recent increase in line with the desire for increased sun exposure has prompted campaigns such as 'Slip Slop Slap' (*Slip* on a T-shirt, *Slop* on high factor sun cream, *Slap* on a hat). Heavy sun exposure before puberty in children with red hair, seems to be a particularly unwise combination. In older people, other types of less malignant skin cancer, especially rodent ulcers, also develop. These are influenced by sunlight exposure, especially on the face and hands.
- Finally, and importantly, poor diet is a major causative factor. High intakes of fat, especially saturated fats, are associated with increased risks of breast cancer, as well as cancer of the colon, endometrium (lining of the womb), pancreas and prostate. Lack of fibre may also increase risk of colon cancer. Research conducted in many countries around the world, including Australia, Europe and the USA, shows quite clearly that a diet rich in fruit, vegetables, fibre, combined with

phytoestrogens, and low in saturated animal fats, offers us a great deal of protection against most forms of cancer. The amount we eat, and not being overweight may be important factors, especially with regard to breast cancer in women and testicular cancer in men. A healthy diet is certainly necessary for normal immune function. Several studies have shown that vegetarians have higher levels of immune system cells, which are capable of killing both tumour cells and viruses.

The role of diet

It has long been established that those consuming a diet rich in animal fats and low in fibre are more likely to develop cancer than those consuming a wholesome diet, rich in antioxidants. However, until relatively recently the medical profession has had their attention focused firmly on drugs to kill off cancer cells and possibly to boost the immune system. Whilst we have come to accept that we treat cancer, if and when we unfortunately become victims, some very exciting research has been taking place. Surprisingly, significant research looking at the role of phytoestrogens in the prevention of cancer has been conducted by highly respected scientists, in reputable research units, around the world. In fact, there is a vast amount of research material available, much of which until now has not been translated from 'medicaleze' into ordinary language for the public.

Research has confirmed that the plant lignan and the isoflavanoids are converted by bacteria in our intestines to hormone-like compounds, with weak oestrogenic and antioxidative activity. They have been shown to influence many key functions within the body including:

- sex hormone metabolism
- biological activity
- enzyme function
- production of protein
- growth factor action
- malignant cell proliferation
- cell differentiation
- and angiogenesis – the development of new blood vessels.

Very recent research is suggesting that the dramatic reduction in cancer, which has been observed following the regular consumption of phyto-estrogens, may not be directly attributable to the foods themselves, but possibly to the chemical reactions that they bring about within the body.

There are literally hundreds of studies using phytoestrogtens on animals, aimed at reducing the incidence of cancer; two-thirds of which show a dramatic reduction in both the occurrences of cancer, and also the tumour size in those who had established cancer. Over two hundred of these studies have looked at genistein, the soya isoflavone, as it seems to be able to influence many of the fundamental aspects of the cancer process. For example, one of the common enzymes produced by the genes that cause cancer, the oncogenes, is known as protein tyrosine kinase. In 1987, it was discovered that the isoflavone, genistein, in the form of soy, was actually a naturally occurring tyrosine kinase inhibitor, which means that it is able to prevent the activation of the specific genes that cause cancer. This it seems is just one of the counter-productive enzymes involved in the cancer process that genistein is able to constrain. It is interesting to note that Oriental populations, that have low rates of breast and prostate cancer, consume between 20–80 mg of genistein per day, almost entirely derived from soya products. Conversely, daily intakes of soya products in western countries like Australia, the UK and the USA are almost negligible, between 1–3mg per day.

Another attribute of genistein, is that it seems to be able to inhibit the growth of blood vessels on which tumours depend for their supply of nutrients and oxygen. So as well as being a useful tool in the prevention of cancer, genistein may also have a part to play in treatment. In fact it has been suggested that genistein may become one of the first of a new class of anti-cancer drugs. We don't have to wait for this particular new science to evolve since we can get our daily genistein fix in the form of foods containing soya products.

In addition to the animal studies there have been over 30 population studies conducted around the world looking at a wide variety of cancers and the response to many types of soya foods. The overall consensus is that those consuming soya products on a regular basis, probably daily, are likely at least to halve their chances of getting cancer, compared to those who only eat soya products once or twice per week. The studies show that the soya foods used were able to inhibit the growth of many types of cancer, including breast, prostate, colon, rectum, skin, lung, stomach as well as leukaemia. The vast majority of the studies identified the protective effects of soya products and golden linseeds (flaxseed) in particular, and it is reassuring to note that there was no evidence reported in any study to suppose that these phytoestrogens could increase the incidence of cancer of any type. One Japanese study showed that a whole range of soya products, including soya milk, soya protein, miso and tofu, were also able to block the formation of nitrites, the chemical compounds that are carcinogenic.

Golden linseeds, or flaxseeds as they are sometimes known, are the richest source of lignans, and a regular intake has also been associated with low levels of cancer of the breast, the ovaries, uterus, prostate and the colon. Following consumption, they are readily excreted in the urine, which indicates that they are metabolised by the body. Researchers have shown that much higher levels of lignans are excreted by vegetarians than meat eaters, and in fact one study found that very low levels of lignans were excreted by older women with breast cancer. Animal studies, in primates show that those that excrete high levels of lignans rarely experience breast cancer. As well as containing anti-cancer properties, lignans have been found to contain antifungal, antibacterial and antiviral properties.

So it seems that research of recent years on phytoestrogens has provided us with the key to lower our risk of cancer, therefore making the cure a less urgent issue for many of us. However, as well as consuming a daily serving of soya and regular amounts of other foods that contain phyto-estrogen, which are outlined in Part Three – Eating for Health, it is impor-tant to ensure that other aspects of your diet and lifestyle are in order.

BREAST CANCER

Breast cancer has historically been the most common fatal cancer affect-ing women between the ages of 40–55, and in recent years it has almost reached epidemic proportions in western countries. In the USA for exam-ple, whereas in 1950 there was a one in 20 chance of women becoming breast cancer victims during their lifetime, today it has become a one in eight chance. This increase, makes it now the leading cause of death in women between the ages of 40–55 years of age, and approximately one quarter of the women diagnosed with breast cancer each year will die. In Australia in 1990, breast cancer was the most commonly diagnosed cancer apart from skin cancer. The highest breast cancer rates in the world are in North America, Northern Europe, Australia and New Zealand.

There are a number of contributory factors that have been shown been found to be associated with breast cancer:

- A high consumption of animal fat and low fibre diets, as found in many western countries. Although the additional animal fat in our diet increases our intake of oestrogen, it is unlikely that this factor alone could account for such a consistent increase in breast cancer statistics.
- The absence of pregnancy or pregnancies after the age of 35. The risk is reportedly less likely with increasing numbers of pregnancies and episodes of breast-feeding.
- Obesity, particularly in women after the menopause, as oestrogen is stored in the fat cells. Obesity is also reaching epidemic proportions. In the UK it is estimated that one in four people are overweight, one-third of the white adult population in the USA and Canada are obese, and according to a 1993 report, the direct cost of obesity in Australia in 1989–1990 was $672 million. Even more frightening, is that children of obese parents are 70 per cent likely to be obese themselves.
- Early onset of menstruation, which in theory means more hormonal cycles, which mean more oestrogen production, increases the chances of cancer.

- A family history of cancer, especially in a close relative like a mother or sister. Many researchers have been concentrating their efforts on a search for a 'breast cancer gene', but this is not likely to apply to more than 5 per cent of victims.
- Fibrocystic disease of the breast.
- Constipation, which may affect hormone metabolism and our excretion of oestrogen.
- The oral contraceptive pill and injectable contraceptives carry a small increase in risk after prolonged use.
- Hormone Replacement Therapy (HRT) appears to increase the chances of suffering breast cancer by approximately 35 per cent following long-term usage, over five or ten years.
- Lastly, and probably most importantly, exposure to xenoestrogens – the environmental oestrogens, see page 109.

It is thought that early life exposure to phytoestrogens may be critical for breast cancer prevention. Specifically, it is thought that genistein exposure prior to puberty may decrease risk of tumours in later life. There has been concern that soy isoflavones cannot yet be clearly stated as protective for breast cancer. This is mainly the result of laboratory work on rats using high levels of concentrated soya protein.

Recent research presented by Cline et al (3rd International Symposium on the Role of Soy in Preventing and Treating Chronic Disease in Washington DC, 1999) looking at the effects of dietary soy on the uterus and breast of female Macaque monkeys, concluded that soy phytoestrogens do not stimulate the breast or uterine tissue. These monkeys are an accepted model for human female reproductive studies. These postmenopausal monkeys were fed either 148 mg of soy phytoestrogens per day for three years, or given oestrogen (1.25mg per day). Cell proliferation was induced in monkeys given oestrogen but not soy phytoestrogens.

Phytoestrogens – some better news

Phytoestrogens are able to compete successfully for the oestrogen receptor sites within the body, over and above both normal oestrogen and xenoestrogen. It seems that they raise levels of sex hormone binding globulin, and are thereby able to block out the excess levels of oestrogen which are thought to precipitate breast cancer. Many published studies show encouraging results. One study in Singapore compared 200 women who suffered breast cancer with 420 who did not. It emerged that those with the lowest risk of breast cancer consumed about 55 grams of foods containing soya per day, and concluded that those with the highest soya consumption had less than half the risk of breast cancer of those who rarely consumed soya products. In another study, 142,857 Japanese women were studied for 17 years, and it emerged that those regularly consuming soybean paste soup had a much lower risk of experiencing breast cancer. Linseeds (flaxseed) have also been shown to reduce the inci-dence of breast cancer.

Current research shows that phytoestrogens are unlikely to be suffi-cient to inhibit the growth of mature, established breast cancer cells, but it seems they will regulate the proliferation of the cancer cells, thereby having a chemopreventive effect. Research is in its early stages, and much still remains to be learned about the influence of specific dietary constituents and cancer risk, but it is clear that our diet does have a signif-icant impact in cancer prevention and control.

Carla's story

Carla was a 32-year-old mother of three from Bradford, who had a history of breast cancer. She approached the WNAS for help, as she was not a candidate for HRT.

'I lost both my mother and my grandmother at the age of 56 from breast cancer. My own breast cancer was diagnosed at the beginning of 1994 for which I underwent a mastectomy. Following my chemotherapy I was put on a drug called Tamoxifen designed to prevent new cancerous cells, but unfortunately one of the side effects I experienced were hot flushes. In June 1995 I was advised to have a radical hysterectomy, which involved removing my ovaries, to lower my chances of contracting other female cancers.

I was relieved to have lowered my risk of cancer, but after the operation felt very tired, with little vitality, and noticed that my hot flushes had become severe and debilitating. I knew that I was not able to take HRT because of the cancer, and therefore set about find-ing an alternative. I found the first edition of Cruising Through the Menopause *in my local bookshop, and decided to contact the Advisory Service for some personalised help.*

I had my first telephone consultation at the beginning of April 1996, and within six weeks of following the recommendations my flushes had greatly reduced and I was feeling more energetic. Unfortunately, in June of 1996 I discovered another lump in my remaining breast and, after careful thought, decided to have a second mastectomy.

I got through the operation with lots of family support and by August I was feeling brilliant. I was pleased to report to the WNAS that I had no remaining symptoms, and that I felt I was in control of my health. My husband is amazed and has even said I'm like a new woman. I am so pleased to be able to assume the role of a caring mum to three small children. I feel 100 per cent well – it's brilliant.'

Phytoestrogens and other hormonally-related cancer

The womb

The endometrium, which is the lining of the womb, is particularly sensitive to oestrogens, and some of the risk factors for the development of cancer in this area are similar to those for breast cancer.

The cervix

Cancer of the neck of the womb is closely connected with sexual activity, and is more likely to occur in women who had many sexual partners at a young age. There is now clear evidence that cervical cancer is associated with certain viruses that cause change in the cells covering the neck of the womb. The more prosperous individuals within a community, who probably have a better nutrient intake, seem to be less at risk of developing this type of cancer. Disturbed levels of nutrients have been detected in women with cervical cancer, but it not clear whether supplements of these would have any genuine protective effect at this stage. Irregular vaginal bleeding or bleeding after intercourse are two of the warning signs.

The ovary

Ovarian cancer is one of the most difficult cancers to detect and treat, which explains why it claims more lives than many of the other types of cancer. Again, some of the risk factors are similar to those of breast cancer, including the family history factor. Women with a family history of ovarian cancer should be screened regularly. Early detection, using ultrasound and blood tests, and subsequent removal of the ovaries would prove to be lifesaving measures.

The general consensus from the wealth of studies that have been published on hormonally related cancer, indicate that in order to drastically reduce our chances of cancer we should be eating one serving of soya based food per day, regular amounts of organic linseed, and as many other fruits, nuts, seeds, beans and berries as we can manage. Refer to the Sample phytoestrogen-rich menu on page 480.

Colon and rectum

Cancer of the large bowel may also run in families, especially if the cancer develops at a young age, usually under the age of 45, and can also be associated with cancer of the womb, ovary or bladder. Whilst colon cancer is more common in women, cancer of the rectum claims more male victims. Those consuming a diet rich in meat and animal fat, and low in fibre and starch are more at risk. Low intakes of the mineral calcium are also thought to be associated with a higher risk of this type of cancer, or at least more rapid growth. Early detection by colonoscopy examination, X-rays and testing the stool for the presence of minute quantities of blood are all important, and blood tests for detecting early tumours are currently being developed.

Once again, the research using phytoestrogens to prevent bowel cancer are showing very positive results. A Japanese study showed that eating soybeans or tofu cut the risk of rectal cancer by more than 80 per cent. Those who ate soya products had one-seventh of the risk compared to those who did not. Soya products also lowered colon cancer risk by about 40 per cent. In this particular study just one or two servings of soya per week gave considerable protection. Researchers in the USA have found that those who eat tofu regularly cut their risk of colon cancer by half. The Chinese confirmed these findings as they discovered that those who did not consume soya products on a regular basis were three times more likely to develop rectal cancer than the soya consumers.

Several studies have found that a high level of urinary lignan excretion, found in those eating a phytoestrogen rich diet, correlates with lower levels of colon cancer.

Recent research presented in 1999 at the Third International Symposium on the Role of Soy in Preventing and Treating Chronic Disease, in Washington DC, concluded that subjects at risk of colon cancer who ate 39 gms of soy protein per day for one year had less cell proliferation in their colon and therefore a reduced colon cancer risk compared with those who consumed 39 gms per day of casein (cow's milk protein). It concluded that eating soy may delay the onset of colon cancer and lead to more cancer free years. Even if tumours develop while eating soy there are likely to be fewer tumours and they will grow more slowly.

STOMACH CANCER

One-third of Japanese Hawaiians consuming tofu were able to reduce their risk of contracting stomach cancer compared to non-consumers. In China, it was found that those who regularly consume soymilk had less than half the risk of developing cancer when compared to non-soymilk drinkers. In another Chinese study there was a 40 per cent reduction in stomach cancer statistics in those consuming soya products on a regular basis. However, it should be pointed out that negative results have been produced when using miso. The probable reason for this is that miso, unlike many other soya products, is fermented and is by nature rich in sodium (salt). As sodium is thought to be risk factor for stomach cancer and possibly for other cancers as well, this may well explain the increased risks with miso. On the positive side, it is thought that miso may protect

us from radiation damage. Studies have shown that medical profess-
ionals tending atomic bomb victims did not develop tumours themselves
because they regularly drank miso soup. Animal studies show that miso
increases the radioactive discharge from the body.

PROSTATE CANCER

Until recently, prostate problems, particularly prostate cancer were, like
bowel problems, not a subject on the social agenda. It took the deaths of
some men prominent in the public eye, like Frank Zappa, Telly Savalas
and Francois Mitterand, to increase public awareness about this
potentially fatal condition. Nearly half of all men over the age of 50
develop an enlarged prostate, known as benign prostate hypertrophy,
and prostate cancer kills four times as many men as cervical cancer kills
women. The prostrate gland is a reproductive gland that is wrapped
around the urethra between the bladder and the penis. It is about the size
and shape of a walnut, and is responsible for secreting the fluid that
combines with sperm to form semen. Prostate symptoms include the
frequent need to urinate, especially at night, an inability to empty the
bladder fully, sometimes leading to infection, and pain with an erection
or orgasm. Denis Norden, the TV presenter is reported to have said
following his prostate operation, 'when I was 20 my heart ruled my
head. When I was 40 my head ruled my heart. But when I was 60 my
bladder ruled both!'

Apart from skin cancer, cancer of the prostate is the most common
form of cancer in men over the age of 55. If caught in time it is treatable,
and as some of the tumours are slow growing, the medical profession
often carefully watch the progression rather than offering radical treatment. Screening tests are available in the form of a physical examination
via the rectum, which can detect whether the prostate is enlarged, infected
or indeed whether there are any signs of a tumour. There are also
prostate-specialist antigen blood tests available, and ultrasound is often
used before a diagnosis can be made.

Whilst Japanese men have the same prostate cancer rate as men in the
west, they have the lowest death rate in the world from this particular
cancer. As with other cancers, the growth of prostate cancer may be
stimulated by hormones such as oestrogen and testosterone. Although
oestrogen works in different ways in men, it can be equally destructive.
Oestrogen, being a precursor to androgens, the male hormones, can
trigger the production of testosterone, and studies have shown than men
with prostate cancer seem to have higher levels of testosterone than their
cancer-free counterparts. Once again phytoestrogens, particularly soya-
based foods, seem to help moderate hormone levels, thus slowing down

the growth at which the tumour grows. Test-tube studies on genistein have managed to show growth of prostate tumour cells being inhibited.

Professor Hermann Adlercreutz reported recently that in laboratory studies genistein and lignans, the fibre layers of grain, berries, seeds (linseeds), some vegetables and fruits, all inhibit prostate cancer cells to varying degrees. Studies on mice implanted with human prostate cancer cells who were fed rye bran, heated rye bran, as well as soy, had slower onset of palpable prostate cancer tumours. Furthermore, the tumour volume was smaller. Rye bran also caused increased cancer cell death. He concluded that isoflavone and lignan containing foods may be protective with regard to prostate cancer.

Since prostate disease is considered to be sex hormone dependent, an Australian study at Deakin University looked at the male sex hormone responses in men after eating either a tofu, lean meat or fatty meat meal. They found that sex hormone binding globulin (SHBG) significantly increased testosterone levels after both the tofu and lean meat meal, but not in the fatty meal. An increase in SHBG is considered positive as this helps 'mop up' excess testosterone which at higher levels is a risk factor for prostate cancer. Lower levels of sex hormone concentrations like testosterone may provide long term benefits in reducing the risk of a disease like prostate cancer that appears to be sex hormone dependent.

See also: Prostate cancer, page 406.

LUNG CANCER

Lung cancer is often precipitated by cigarette smoke, active or passive, and to reduce your chances of becoming a victim it is advisable to live and work in a smoke-free environment. However, there is evidence to support the fact that once again certain phytoestrogens may help to protect us. A study of over 200 Chinese women in Hong Kong, found that by consuming soya products, including tofu, on a daily basis they were able to cut the risk of lung cancer by half, compared to women consuming soya products less than three times per month. Another Chinese study, this time on almost 1,500 men, found that the risk of lung cancer was reduced by 50 per cent with frequent tofu consumption.

SKIN CANCER

Although research in this important area is young, animal studies have been done to show that soybeans were able to delay the onset of skin tumours by 100 days and topically applied genistein reduced the number of skin cancers in mice.

What your doctor can do

- Take your symptoms seriously. Because of the many different types of cancer, and the different ways in which it may present, early diagnosis is not always easy. This must however still remain an important goal as only early diagnosis will lead to a better outcome.
- Investigate for cancer, which includes:
  - a thorough physical examination
  - blood tests
  - x-rays or an ultrasound examination of the pelvis, liver or abdomen
  - specialist investigations, especially CT (Computerised Tomography) and MRI (Magnetic Resonance Imaging) scans. These are specialised X-rays which allow visualisation of internal abdominal organs and the nervous system. Specialist blood tests are also being evolved to allow the early detection of what are termed 'tumour markers'. This will tell us there is a cancer somewhere but won't tell us where it is.
  - Finally, a biopsy or a small sample of the suspected cancerous tissue is taken and usually allows identification of the cancer type by examination under the microscope. This then leads to decisions about treatment.
- Treat the cancer. This essentially involves the use of chemotherapy, radiotherapy and surgery. These treatments require special medical skill and indeed many types of cancer are now referred to specialist centres. Further treatment for the control of individual symptoms such as pain with painkillers, removing fluid that may have built up in the abdomen, and nutritional support as well as psychological support should all be part of standard cancer care. Greater awareness is now mindful of the broader needs of the cancer patient and this may involve a number of self-help approaches.

What you can do

Gone are the days when the patient was just simply a passive recipient of therapy. There is much that you can do.

- Learn about your type of cancer and how it affects your body. This you can do either via your own specialist or by contacting one of a number of support organisations, especially BACUP (see Useful addresses, page 512).
- Make adjustments to your diet. This will depend upon the type of cancer, the type of treatment you are receiving, and whether you are likely to have developed nutritional deficiencies. You may well need further advice and support from your doctor or the dietician attached to the hospital that is treating you. Some of the likely dietary changes that may be worthwhile are as follows:

- ○ Consume a diet rich in phytoestrogens, with a daily serving of soya based food and as many other foods from the Phytoestrogen-rich menu on page 480 that you can happily fit into your diet.
- ○ Eat organically grown food when possible.
- ○ Limit your intake of fat, especially that of saturated animal fat, and use foods containing Omega-3 and Omega-6 EFAs, see page 489 for the listings.
- ○ Do not smoke, minimise your exposure to cigarette smoke, and ensure you have a high fluid water intake.
- ○ Minimise your consumption of pickled and smoked foods.
- ○ Eat plenty of foods containing antioxidants, like fruits, vegetables and salad, particularly yellow vegetables like carrots and peppers, and green leafy vegetables. Aim to have at least five servings of fruit, vegetables and salad daily.
- ○ A high-protein, high-calorie, easy-to-digest diet is suitable for those who have experienced significant weight loss and have difficulty maintaining calorie intake. Supplemental feeds, high in protein, based on milk or soya, may be required. For those with swallowing or digestive difficulties, especially in older patients, putting main meals through a liquidiser may be useful. Particularly good foods in this situation include all dairy products, eggs, meat, stewed fruit, home-made ice cream and nuts and seeds if these latter two can be digested.
- ○ Reduce or, even better, avoid salt in the form of table salt and heavily processed food. Salt actually blocks oxygen from entering the cells, which is perfect for cancerous cells because we know that they thrive in the absence of oxygen.
- • Vegetarian and vegan diet regimes are recommended by some complementary therapists, and in theory they could be effective. Recently there have been one or two reports of benefit after many years of unsubstantiated or poorly substantiated claims. At present however, they cannot be broadly recommended for the general patient with cancer. In theory a high fruit and vegetable diet with a limited amount of protein might retard the growth of some cancers. However, in a patient who is seriously ill and rapidly losing weight, this could be a disastrous choice. The skill required to match these sorts of diets to a patient's individual needs will be as great as that required to determine effective chemotherapeutic regimes. This is a situation where expert medical and dietetic research needs to address some of the ideas of complementary therapists.
- • Take nutritional supplements. This is as contentious as recommending a diet for cancer. Those who have lost weight because of their cancer, who have digestive difficulties or have recently completed a course of radiotherapy or chemotherapy, are likely to have a number of nutritional deficiencies that need correcting with a better diet and nutritional supplements. Thus there is a dilemma.

○ Vitamin E and beta carotene capsules applied topically can alleviate mouth ulcers which are often caused by chemotherapy.
○ Vitamin E has been shown to reduce hair loss associated with chemotherapy.
○ Selenium reduces toxicity of chemotherapy drugs without reducing their anti-tumour ability.
○ A good intake of EFAs, particularly those from the Omega-3 series are necessary for strengthening cell membranes, therefore protecting them from free radical damage.
○ Avoid toiletries, particularly deodorants containing aluminium and parabens, synthetic chemicals which have been shown to bind with DNA and cause mutation.

Increased research is needed into the use of nutritional therapy as adjuncts to chemotherapy and radiotherapy, on the grounds that nutritional supplements can greatly reduce some of the worst side-effects of these treatments.

A reasonable mid-way course might be only to give nutritional supplements to those who have, or are likely to have, deficiencies, and not to give them to relatively well patients who are receiving anti-cancer treatments, especially if they are likely to have a high degree of success as in Hodgkin's disease, leukaemia and others. Often chemotherapy regimes are pulsed, that is, given every few days or at weekly or monthly intervals. If nutritional supplements need to be taken, then they could be stopped while the chemotherapy or radiotherapy is actually being given.

At the end of treatment there may be need for 'a nutritional rescue programme'. Equally some patients may be too unwell to tolerate the full course of radiotherapy or chemotherapy, and nutritional support before or during therapy may be necessary. Again this situation may require expert advice.

A further situation is in patients who have been 'cured' of a cancer. This now occurs with a variety of childhood cancers and happens more and more in the early treatment of adult cancers such as stomach, colon and breast. There is evidence that such patients, having survived one cancer, may be more at risk of a second type of cancer, either because of a cancer predisposition or because some of the anti-cancer drugs themselves may increase the risk of developing cancer in later life. For them eating The Very Nutritious Diet (see page 437) and perhaps taking supplements of strong multi-vitamins containing vitamins C, E, beta-carotene and selenium, would be advisable, but no firm recommendation can be made.

• Vitamin A as retinol and beta-carotene – the vegetable form of vitamin A – has been put forward as being cancer protective. Diets rich in beta-carotene derived from bread and red, green and yellow fruits and vegetables are associated with reducing the risk of cancer. The protective agent may not be just beta-carotene but may be other agents such as vitamin C, vitamin E and selenium. This group is known as the antioxidants because they may protect tissues from noxious chemicals which may 'oxidise' them, reducing damage and cancerous change. High dietary intakes of calcium may well be associated with a reduced risk of cancer of the large bowel.

- Maintain outside interests. There is increasing evidence that those who have a positive attitude, are socially active and continue a normal life, do better with their cancer. We have personally seen this with a number of patients. This does not just involve diet, supplements and exercise, but making the most of your time on a number of fronts. This may mean spending more time with your family, revitalising old interests and hobbies, beginning evening classes, or taking up outdoor activities such as walking or gardening. Just think back over the last years of your life and try and recall those things that you have enjoyed or have made you feel good. These are the sorts of things that you should concentrate on. Think also of the sorts of things that you really wanted to do but never did. Perhaps some of these are suitable for you to take up now. Pleasure obtained from personal achievement is good medicine.
  - Take regular exercise and make time for relaxation.
  - Keep the stress in your life to a minimum.
  - Drink filtered or bottled water rather than chlorinated water.
  - Do not use pesticides or herbicides.
  - Minimise your use of Hormone Replacement Therapy and the oral contraceptive pill.
  - Use alternatives to plastic containers for storing food, and steer away from plastic products where possible as they release chlorinated toxins into the environment.
  - Purchase non-bleached paper, including writing paper, toilet tissue, coffee filters etc to avoid unacceptable dioxin exposure.
  - Use tampons and towels made without chlorine. Organic sanitary towels, tampons and cotton wool are becoming increasing available in health-food stores and supermarkets.
  - Avoid aerosols and anti-perspirants – use natural underarm deodorants instead, including deodorant crystals and those without aluminium or synthetic chemicals such as parabens.
  - Use hydrogen peroxide as an alternative to chlorine bleach for household chores, for it breaks down to water and oxygen.

Complementary therapies

A number of these may appeal to you and are well worth considering.

Acupuncture may be helpful for pain relief and as a general tonic. Herbal medicine may help with a variety of persistent symptoms, massage and aromatherapy are a good way of relaxing, and homeopathy has a variety of specific anti-cancer remedies. These are prescribable and can be administered by qualified medical homeopaths. Again, there is some evidence that they may be helpful, but no large-scale recommendations can be made. You should consult a medically qualified homeopath specialising in cancer treatment.

The entire approach to cancer treatment should be person centred. Perhaps the most important factors in survival with cancer and a return to good health are the intangible factors residing with the individual – self-motivation, empowerment, and the decision to change oneself and take control. Disinterest and misery in following an unwanted dietary regime is not a desired goal, and without the enthusiastic co-operation of the person with cancer, there seems little justification in enforcing rules.

A word of warning on some complementary therapies

Beware of excessive or false claims. These are easily made, not necessarily with intent to deceive or defraud, but out of the therapist's desire to help. The fact that one or two patients have done well following a particular line does not mean that all will. In the end it is only good-quality research of the type performed by medical practitioners that will prove the case for or against a particular line of therapy. Fortunately, a number of conventional physicians are now looking seriously at the benefits of complementary medicine in cancer care.

Abigail's story

Abigail was a 41-year-old teacher who was experiencing menopausal symptoms following chemotherapy.

'I was diagnosed as having Hodgkinson's Lymphoma ten years ago and had both radio- and chemotherapy. I have been clear ever since but I really wanted to avoid Hormone Replacement Therapy because of my history. When my menopausal symptoms began I was aware I had to sort out an alternative. I was having 25 flushes a day at least and so I went off in search of a solution.

I managed to find the book Cruising Through the Menopause *at my local bookshop which I was delighted to discover outlined there was a scientifically based alternative. I made an appointment to visit the WNAS Clinic and was given a tailor-made programme to follow avoiding certain grains, alcohol, tea and coffee, and asked to concentrate on foods that contain naturally occurring oestrogens, oily fish and plenty of fresh fruit, salad and vegetables. Apart from my menopausal symptoms, I was very tired for much of the time and constipated. I had been living in the Middle East where my husband was working but felt that the hot flushes were so bad there that I came back to the UK. I followed the WNAS programme avidly and within just a few weeks the night sweats had stopped, the flushes were greatly reduced, and my constipation had gone completely. I found the exercise difficult initially as I felt so tired but persisted with my YMCA video and my Tai Chi which I feel helped enormously.*

I have been following the programme for three months now and all my symptoms have calmed down. I feel so much better and I am confident that I can manage quite happily without Hormone Replacement Therapy. I feel years younger than when I began the programme. I have been able to re-join my husband in the Middle East which was formerly too hot for me and I am really looking forward to the future.'

See also: Recommended reading, References.

Candida and Thrush

Candida is one of several types of yeast-like organisms that cause infections in humans. There are a number of different varieties of candida, the commonest being *candida albicans* which can cause infection in the vagina, mouth and skin. Infection with candida is commonly called 'thrush'. It is also the organism that plays a part in the development of nappy rash in infants. The organism grows best in warm, dark conditions and in the presence of sugar. Under these circumstances candida changes from small round dormant spores to a branching structure called a mycelium with the ability to invade and irritate tissues.

Candida is a very common organism that we have all had some contact with, and the majority of infections resolve themselves spontaneously. That said, some women experience repeated episodes of vaginal thrush, and there are usually a number of reasons for this (see opposite). In the last few years some doctors and complementary practitioners have put forward the idea that a number of health problems including chronic fatigue can be caused by infection with candida. The evidence for this is not strong.

What are the symptoms?

This depends on where the infection is. For women, vaginal thrush causes irritation and a thick, white, sticky discharge. This must be differentiated from the normal vaginal moisture that naturally increases at mid-cycle and is not associated with local irritation. Severe infections in women can cause swelling of the genital tissues and a rash can spread out into the groin.

In men, soreness or redness of the penis, sometimes with a sticky white discharge, may develop. However, many men and women may carry small amounts of candida in the vagina or on the penis without any ill effects.

Candida is often kept in check by the presence of healthy non-disease-causing bacteria in both the vagina and the bowel. Surveys reveal that about 20 per cent of the normal population carry candida in the digestive tract without it causing problems.

Thrush in the mouth, which mainly affects the ill, elderly or those using steroid inhalers for asthma, produces a very sore mouth and a white sticky deposit on the tongue and elsewhere. A slightly furred tongue without soreness is unlikely to be due to candida.

The skin can be infected, too, and this is usually in warm moist areas such as the groin, armpits or under the breasts. A red, sore rash with spreading little red spots or 'satellites' at the edge of the rash is the usual appearance.

Who gets it?

In short, we all do once or twice, but for those women who get repeated attacks of vaginal thrush there are often one or more predisposing factors. They include:

- *Being pregnant* Hormonal changes encourage thrush.
- *The combined oral contraceptive pill* Those with a high oestrogen content may increase the risk; this is rarely a problem with newer low-dose ones.
- *Steroid drugs* These, whether taken as tablets or as an inhaler, can encourage the growth of candida.
- *Antibiotics* By killing off the 'good' bacteria, antibiotics make it easier for candida to obtain a foothold.
- *Diabetes* The increased levels of sugar in diabetes make it easy for the thrush organism to grow.
- *Anaemia and lack of iron* These can reduce resistance to infection and lead to cracking at the corners of the mouth, making it easy for the infection to get started – one to think of in women with heavy periods.
- *Other nutritional deficiencies* Lack of zinc, vitamin B and even vitamin A have all been documented as reducing resistance to infection and leading to thrush.
- *A poor diet* A diet high in sugar and low in protein can probably make matters worse, though there is no direct proof of this.
- *Reduced resistance to infection* Anything that reduces your resistance to infection from stress, genetic and blood conditions to cancer, can be significant.
- *Hormonal disturbances* Thyroid, other hormone problems and low blood calcium can all (rarely) lead to episodes of thrush.

What causes it?

As you can imagine, anyone with one or more of the above predisposing factors is likely to experience thrush at some time. A common situation involves a sexually active woman, possibly on the pill, who may have a mild iron deficiency, and for whom treatment using over-the-counter creams has been only partially successful. Research suggests that, in recurrent cases, candida organisms on the skin or possibly from the bowel provide a source of re-infection. Sometimes this comes from the male partner, and intercourse or use of a tampon may be factors in causing a break in the delicate tissues lining the vagina and allowing infection to develop.

Wearing trousers, tights, and nylon underwear may all promote the conditions that encourage the growth of candida. Local irritation can be aggravated by use of some chemicals found in many toiletries, bath products, soaps and shampoos so it may be necessary to avoid these. Occasionally it appears that some sufferers are actually allergic to or react strongly against candida itself. In these cases, even a minor degree of infection can result in severe symptoms.

There is also evidence that reactions to foods or yeast in the diet may cause a vaginal discharge. This might cause symptoms similar to thrush without candida being present, or the reaction may encourage the growth of candida already present. So, for some, a change to a healthier diet that excludes some foods can help symptoms of thrush.

What your doctor can do

Your doctor can do one or more of the following:

- Examine you and take a swab from the vagina to assess the type of infection.
- Prescribe an antifungal treatment as a cream, pessary or tablet by mouth.
- Perform some tests to see why you have thrush. A urine test for diabetes and a blood test for anaemia and iron deficiency would be the most common and useful.

There is a wide choice of different preparations available that your doctor may prescribe. They can be creams, pessaries or tablets and they all have similar success rates. The main choices are:

- Nystatin as cream or pessaries. Once the most popular treatment, now largely replaced by other preparations. It is safe for use in pregnancy. Nystatin can also be given by mouth but as it is not absorbed this is only useful in clearing candida from the bowel. It is very useful for helping clear thrush in the mouth.

- Clotrimazole (Canesten) available as a cream or pessary and often this first-line treatment can be used as a one- or three-day treatment with similar high success rates of over 90 per cent.
- Miconazole (Daktarin) and Econazole (Ecostatin and Gyno-Pevaryl) also available as pessary and cream.
- Fluconazole (Diflucan) is a powerful anti-candida drug which is active by mouth and is highly effective after one single dose of 150mg. It is very effective against *Candida albicans* but not other types of candida.
- Itraconazole (Sporanox) is another anti-fungal agent which comes in tablet form. Two 100mg tablets twice a day for one day only will usually clear thrush and it has the advantage of being effective against different types of candida, not just albicans.

The key point to remember is that all these treatments have a small failure rate and that if one treatment is not successful then another probably will be.

What you can do

Many women do not go to their doctor but get treatment themselves from the chemist using a number of over-the-counter preparations. This is acceptable if you are reasonably certain that you do not have any other infection, and provided that your symptoms clear within three or four days. If not, see your doctor or attend a local STD (Sexually Transmitted Disease) clinic. Such clinics are particularly well equipped to identify the type of infection and the best form of treatment. You do not need to be referred by your doctor but can simply 'drop in'.

It is probably useful for you to know that some 50 per cent of women who think that they have thrush may have a different type of infection, and that the success rate for most standard anti-fungal treatments is 90 per cent. Consequently there will always be a significant number of women whose 'thrush' did not clear with the first treatment they try. In cases like these there is no substitute for an internal examination, a swab to identify the type of infection(s), and tests in the laboratory to find which anti-fungal agent is the most effective.

In addition to infection itself, the irritation may be due to some degree of allergy to candida itself, to local irritation from toiletries or occasionally to food allergy. There is no easy way for the sufferer to determine which of these might apply to them without expert assessment, so the advice given below is relevant for all eventualities.

- Avoid wearing restrictive clothing such as trousers, tights and synthetic underwear. Choose natural fabrics such as cotton or silk.
- Shower rather than bath, and do not use perfumed soaps and other toiletries that might come into contact with your tail end. If you do have a bath, do not wash your hair at the same time.

- Dry yourself thoroughly after a bath or swimming.
- Do wash and change your underwear every day.
- When washing your clothes and underwear it may be preferable to use a non-biological washing liquid just in case traces of soap remain and contribute to the irritation.
- Use sanitary pads rather than tampons.
- Always wipe yourself from the front to the back so as to reduce the chance of infection from the bowel. If you are very sensitive, white unbleached toilet tissue may be a good idea.
- Your diet should be low in sugar or sucrose, which means not adding sugar to tea and coffee, avoiding sweets, cakes, biscuits, chocolates and non-low-calorie soft drinks. For some a diet low in foods that are rich in yeast can help. Yeasty foods include alcoholic beverages (except gin and vodka), vinegar, pickled foods, yeast extract such as Marmite and many stock cubes, most packaged savoury foods including convenience meals and soups, and bread and buns and anything made from baker's or brewer's yeast. Occasionally it may be necessary for the diet to be even more restricted than this, but fruit restriction is rarely needed.
- Supplements may also be necessary. Consider a yeast-free multi-vitamin if you have recurrent thrush. A supplement of zinc, 20 mg per day can help, as can a supplement of iron such as ferrous sulphate, 200 mg once or twice a day, especially if heavy periods or anaemia are or have been problems.
- Capsules containing preparations of the healthy bacteria *Lactobacillus acidophillus* and related species are available and might help clear thrush from the gut (but not the vagina). Eating live yoghurt might also be helpful, and applying plain live yoghurt *to* the vagina is possibly beneficial but would be no substitute for anti-fungal medication.
- Caprylic acid is a naturally occurring fatty acid which has been reported to be an effective anti-fungal compound in the treatment of candida.
- Berberine containing plants, including goldenseal have shown natural antibiotic activity against bacteria, and fungi including candida.
- Grapefruit seed extract is another natural agent possessing antibiotic and anti-fungal properties.
- It is important to address digestive abnormalities when treating candida, and the first point of action is to improve digestive secretions. Hydrochloric acid (secreted by the parietal cells in the lining of the stomach), pancreatic enzymes (that ensure efficient digestion of proteins and carbohydrates) and bile (secreted by the gall bladder) all inhibit the overgrowth of candida and prevent its penetration into the lining of the small of intestine. Specific supplements of hydrochloric acid and digestive enzymes can be taken in conjunction with an anti-candida diet, but advice should be sought from a professional nutritionist.
- Garlic has demonstrated significant antifungal activity.
- Boosting the immune system by taking zinc, vitamin C and the herb echinacea can help with candida.

Sally's story

Sally was a 43-year-old headmistress who also had two young children of her own. She had been diagnosed as having thrush in her oesophagus, which was causing her great pain in the chest, particularly on waking.

'I had continued digestive problems which had become progressively worse. My doctor had sent me for investigations. I had an endoscopy, where a telescope is passed into the stomach, and a gall bladder scan, which were clear except for the thrush that was found in my gullet. My worst problem was the extreme pain I experienced on waking each day, and the indigestion. I also had an itchy bottom, so I presumed the thrush went right through my gut. Premenstrually I felt angry and clumsy and had experienced very sore breasts.

My job had become very stressful, I couldn't get on top of it somehow. To make matters worse I had developed panic attacks which I thought would subside during the school holidays, but they didn't. My libido had also disappeared and sexual intercourse had become painful as my muscles seemed so tight. A friend had recommended I consult a cranial osteopath for my back problem, and as luck would have it he referred me to the WNAS for help with my other problems.

I was quite sceptical about diet being the solution to what seemed to be extreme symptoms. I was so desperate that I was willing to try anything, so I went along for an initial consultation, which was very probing. I came away with a programme to start on which involved following an exclusion diet, particularly wheat, foods that contain yeast, caffeine and alcohol, plus I was asked to exercise and take some nutritional supplements.

At my second consultation, which was six weeks later, I was able to report that the pain on waking was only minor and had only occurred once in the last month. My itchy tail had cleared up, my period arrived unannounced with no symptoms or bloating and I felt that I was on the right track. I continued to make progress on all fronts, until Christmas. I was feeling so much better that I went for the dried fruit, chocolate, orange juice and wine. The symptoms flared up and it took a couple of weeks to calm down again, but it really brought home to me how sensitive my body was to these foods and drinks.

I have taken up jogging again, which I used to love, and I feel wonderful. All my gut symptoms have disappeared, I no longer feel like I have thrush, my PMS has gone and I am coping really well with situations at work and at home. We have been juggling with my diet for the last six months, and I have gradually been able to add things back without seeing a return of symptoms. I feel very *confident that I can manage my health myself now with my new knowledge, and be there for all those who depend upon me.'*

See also: The yeast-free diet, The very nutritious diet, References.

Carpal Tunnel Syndrome

This is a common condition where there is pressure on the nerves in the wrist, causing numbness and tingling in the hands, and typically affects the dominant hand. Symptoms are worse at night, or on waking in the morning, and the sufferer may have to get out of bed and shake their hands to achieve relief. The pain may also travel back up the arm.

What causes it?

The common causes include:

- fluid retention
- underactive thyroid
- in pregnancy, hormonal changes
- in obesity, additional strain on the joints
- arthritis of the wrist, particularly rheumatoid arthritis
- over-use during sports, such as tennis or squash.

The nerves that carry signals from the brain to the hand pass through a tunnel constructed by the carpals (wrist bones) on the way to the fingers. Sometimes when there is excess fluid in the area, or a change in the shape of the joints occurs, as seen in arthritis, then additional pressure may be placed on the nerves running through the tunnel, causing pins and needles, and numbness in the fingers and the arms. When the body is warm the blood vessels swell a little, which accounts for the fact that carpal tunnel syndrome is often worse during the night.

What your doctor can do

- Give injections of steroids at the wrist to reduce swelling.
- Prescribe splints to be worn at night – these can be surprisingly effective.
- Diuretics are sometimes recommended.
- If all else fails, recommend an operation to relieve the pressure on the nerves.

What you can do

- Lose weight if you need to.
- Follow a low-salt diet to reduce fluid retention (see page 449).

- Don't drink alcohol.
- Take supplements of vitamin B complex and B6. Several studies have shown that relatively high doses of vitamin B6 (100 mg daily) may help relieve symptoms. Not all studies have been positive. This is best taken as B complex (50–100mgs x 1 daily) for 3 months.
- Visit your osteopath for an assessment.
- As a temporary measure, raise your arms above your head at night, to allow the fluid to drain away from the carpal tunnel.
- Use ice packs on the wrists to reduce the heat, and subsequently the swelling.

The numbness and tingling very often disappear of their own accord after pregnancy, so it is unlikely that you will have to take any further action after the baby has been born.

Complementary therapies

Acupuncture is well worth a try, as are homeopathic remedies, but remember to follow the low-salt diet as well. Cranial osteopathy probably has more to offer than any other complementary therapy for this condition.

See also: Fluid retention, Obesity, Thyroid disease, plus References.

Cerebrovascular Disease

Cerebrovascular disease is a furring up and sometimes blockage of, or bleeding from, the major blood vessels that supply the brain. Commonly this causes what is termed a stroke or cerebrovascular accident where there is a sudden development of weakness, loss of sensation, loss of balance, vision or consciousness.

Who gets it?

The same people who are predisposed to ischaemic heart disease and peripheral vascular disease. The main risk factors seen in practice are:

- very high blood pressure 200/110 or higher
- excess alcohol consumption 28 units per week or greater
- obesity
- smoking.

If all four are present then it is simply a matter of time. Other important risk factors are.

- a family history of strokes.
- the presence of any heart abnormality that may lead to a blood clot forming in the heart chambers which can then break off and travel to the brain.
- a wide variety of blood-clotting problems and other rare conditions.
- Rarely, but worthy of mention – migraine headaches. Occasionally if these are very severe they may result in a small stroke with residual numbness or tingling in a limb as a consequence. The risk of this is increased for a woman if she is on the oral contraceptive pill and is a smoker. One suspected event like this means that oral contraceptives are to be avoided for ever more.
- Several recent studies have confirmed that elevated levels of the toxic amino acid homocysteine is a risk factor for stroke. *See* Ischaemic Heart Disease (page 277) for further information.

Prevention is the key, as damage to the nervous system from a stroke often leads to a degree of permanent disability. Large strokes and repeated small ones are frequently fatal. Warnings, however, do occur. Small strokes called transient ischaemic attacks (TIAs) commonly precede an impending major cerebrovasular accident. Warning symptoms include symptoms indicating a loss of neurological function which lasts for several minutes or hours and is followed by full or nearly full recovery. These warning episodes include loss of vision, loss of speech, weakness in a limb, loss of feeling in one side of the face, in a hand or a limb, transitory mental confusion or other unusual transitory feelings, or disturbed sensations. Combinations of these may occur often with a headache.

What your doctor can do

- Examine you and quickly assess the main risk factors. The blood pressure, the health of the heart, the presence of diabetes can all be checked quickly.
- Prescribe a daily dose of aspirin. This simple drug at a dose of up to 300 mg per day significantly reduces the risk of these warning episodes developing into a stroke.
- Treat any high blood pressure. This is probably the next priority.
- Assess the likelihood of a major narrowing of the carotid artery – the main artery in the neck. Listening with a stethoscope to the neck gives an idea of this possibility. Further specialist referral may lead to defurring of the artery by operation – worth it for severely narrowed arteries.
- Consider other treatments and assessments. Many of these, which are needed for young patients, those with a strong family history of strokes or high risk predisposing blood disorders, will mean specialist referral.
- For those who have had a stroke, hospital treatment is the rule for anyone other than the very elderly. Specialised x-rays help decide if the stroke is

due to a bleed, the formation of a clot or an embolism – a blood clot from a distant site, usually the heart – which has travelled to the brain.

What you can do

- See your doctor at the first sign of trouble.
- Do as he or she says and take any recommended medicines.
- Change your diet. Reducing weight, cholesterol and blood pressure by dietary change is very important.
- High intakes of fresh fruit has been known for years to be associated with a lower risk, and vegetables are protective too. Visit your greengrocer on the way home from the doctor and before you see your solicitor. Follow The Very Nutritious Diet on page 437 for a healthy dietary regime.
- Drink alcohol only very moderately.
- Do not smoke.
- Take some supplements. In theory there should be a substantial role for some supplements but large trials have yet to be performed. Poor dietary intakes of vitamin C, a low blood level of retinol (vitamin A) are risk factors for having a stroke or making a poor recovery from one. A reasonable suggestion might be a stronger multivitamin containing 200 milligrams of vitamin C and possibly vitamin E. Other supplements of fish oils, magnesium and vitamin B might also be worth considering on an individual basis.
- Take supplements of folic acid, B12 and B6 if the levels of the artery damaging amino acid homocysteine is elevated. Folic acid appears to be the most important vitamin to supplement with in order to normalise homocysteine levels.

Complementary therapies

One exciting development has occurred in the field of acupuncture. A London-based trial involving conventional doctors and traditional acupuncturists has apparently shown, at least initially, an improvement in the degree of recovery after a stroke in those patients who have received acupuncture. The full report will undoubtedly merit much study and attention. If this proves to be reliable then a long overdue role for the acupuncturist in the district hospital will come into being.

Coeliac Disease

Coeliac disease is a condition where there is marked sensitivity to a protein found in wheat and other grains. As a result there is damage to the lining of the small bowel, resulting in difficulty in absorbtion of a number of essential nutrients. There may also be a wide variety of other symptoms seemingly unrelated to the digestive system.

What are the symptoms?

Typical features of coeliac disease are weight loss, muscle wasting, diarrhoea, abdominal bloating, fatigue and anaemia. Other not infrequent problems include poor growth in children, delayed puberty, mouth ulcers, fatigue without other features, absent periods, infertility in the male or female and, rarely, heart or arthritic problems.

Under the microscope the lining of the small bowel is made up of tiny finger-like projections called villi. These become shrunken and finally disappear, with malabsorption resulting. The whole process takes many months, even years, and equally recovery on a specialised gluten-free diet can also take several months.

Who gets it?

- Coeliac disease is a disease of Caucasians. About one in 1,500 of the population in the UK are affected and many of these are undiagnosed.
- There is a strong genetic tendency, with a high risk, if you have an identical twin who is affected. Lesser degrees of sensitivity and change in the bowel may be present in many first-degree relatives of those who have this disease.
- A possible predisposing factor is the early introduction of wheat and other grains into the infant's diet. Since 1974 the recommendation has been that wheat should not be introduced before four months of age, rather than six weeks which was the norm previously. This may have resulted in a fall in the incidence of childhood coeliac disease.
- Infection with a virus may also be a trigger, perhaps only in predisposed individuals.
- Finally coeliac disease is also associated with diabetes, thyroid disease and some types of arthritis.

What your doctor can do

- Investigate suspected cases with:
  - Biopsy of the small bowel taken via a telescope. This usually gives a definite or near definite answer. Subsequent avoidance of gluten should result in marked improvement in the bowel appearance as seen on a second biopsy.
  - Perform blood tests to look for anaemia, nutritional deficiencies and patterns of antibodies that would support the diagnosis of coeliac disease.
  - Perform a barium meal x-ray of the small bowel, which doesn't confirm the diagnosis but may help exclude other conditions.
  - Sometimes challenge with a gluten preparation and repeating the bowel biopsy are necessary to confirm the diagnosis.

- Treat with a gluten-free diet (see page 442) which means not consuming wheat, oats, barley and rye, and any food made from them. The degree of sensitivity may be remarkable even with modified starch, communion wafers and some beers causing problems. The advice of an experienced dietician is invaluable, especially for those whose illness does not recover promptly.
- Correct nutritional deficiencies. Supplements of iron, folic acid and zinc may be needed. Those with severe malabsorption may also need calcium, vitamin D and multi-vitamins. Eventually long-term supplements should not be required. However there may be a slight relative lack of calcium, selenium and possibly other nutrients. Whether these are important is not certain.
- Very rarely patients do not improve with a gluten-free diet, and other treatments are needed. These include steroids and immune system altering drugs.
- In the long term other bowel problems may develop despite careful adherence to a gluten-free diet. Life-long follow-up is recommended and reinvestigation of those with a return of symptoms is needed.

What you can do

- Follow the gluten-free diet carefully. Keeping a diet diary for four weeks, which is then reviewed by the dietician, is a useful exercise. It allows assessment of nutrient intake, and may allow early identification of foods that may not be gluten-free.
- Other foods may sometimes need to be avoided. Sometimes milk products contribute to the diarrhoea, possibly because of their lactose (milk sugar) content. When recovery is complete, some of the eliminated foods may be able to be re-introduced into the diet. Sometimes other food sensitivities exist; soya is a particular possibility.
- If your bowel has recovered completely, there is recent evidence that some coeliacs are able to tolerate oats. This cereal is lower in gluten than the others. Discuss this possibility with your specialist or dietician.
- Take supplements of zinc if appetite is poor, there is poor resistance to infection or a poor response to a gluten-free diet.
- Supplements may have to be taken in a sublingual form because damage to the villi reduces absorption of nutrients in the small intestine.

Special note for mothers

It would seem prudent for all new mothers who are not coeliac not to introduce gluten-containing cereals, including oats, into their children's diet until at least after their first birthday, possibly even later. Refer to the Weaning Section in *Healthy Parents, Healthy Baby* (see Recommended reading page 490).

Constipation

Our bowels are not something we talk about in public, and yet a disturbance in bowel function, especially constipation, is a common affliction of those living in industrialised countries. A change in lifestyle and a relatively poor intake of fibre-rich foods are contributory factors. Constipation is the result of the bowel becoming sluggish and therefore not doing its job properly, due usually to a lazy bowel muscle which does not contract regularly and strongly, or bowel muscles that do contract, but in a poorly coordinated fashion.

There are two layers of muscle throughout the gut which extend from the throat. They are involved in swallowing, the passage of food through the gut, and the expulsion of waste from the the rectum and anus. They all work to propel food through the gut while it is being broken down, digested, and absorbed into the body, and while the waste residues are formed. The whole process normally takes between one to two days in most men and up to three days in women.

In order for food and digestive material to pass smoothly along the bowel, both muscle layers must work together in a carefully coordinated fashion. First, the ring muscles, which are found at the entrance or exit to the stomach, must relax. This relaxation is then followed by a wave of muscular contraction which pushes a ball of food along the gut and slowly down its length. Each muscle contraction is preceded by an area of muscle relaxation before it. The high pressure generated by the bowel contraction pushes the bowel contents forwards into the low-pressure area of the relaxed bowel. This is what would happen in a healthy gut.

What are the symptoms?

Apart from resulting in much attention being placed on the bowel, constipation can result in a most uncomfortable feeling in the lower abdomen, sometimes accompanied by wind and pain. Straining on the toilet can result in haemorrhoids.

When the bowels are working normally they are usually emptied daily, with perhaps one or two motions. Those who are constipated cannot seem to empty their bowels more than once or twice each week, and may take even longer in severe cases, usually with the use of laxatives.

What is not widely appreciated is that other disturbing health problems are also associated with severe constipation in young women. These include:

- hormonal abnormalities such as a low oestrogen level
- more painful and irregular periods
- breast lumps and pre-cancerous changes in breast tissue

- a greater chance of hysterectomy or operation for a cyst on the ovary
- pain on intercourse and difficulty achieving orgasm
- infertility
- hesitancy in starting to pass water
- cold hands and a tendency to faint.

Who gets it?

Women are more prone to constipation than men. Firstly the gut transit time is faster in men than women (the time it takes for food to be processed from one end of the gut to the other). Secondly, the bowel seems to be slowed by the presence of oestrogen, the female sex hormone.

In some women with constipation the muscles of the pelvic floor are tense and not able to relax properly. These muscles support our urethra allowing water to pass from the bladder to the outside world, and the walls of the vagina as well as the bowel. You can feel these muscles by pulling in your tummy and drawing your buttocks together, as if you were trying to stop the flow of urine in mid-stream. If these muscles are tense and do not relax then the motions cannot easily pass through.

Approximately 50 per cent of the women we see in our clinics each year suffer with constipation to some degree, and in many cases have done so for years.

What causes it?

Lack of fibre

A number of experts have recommended that the UK population as a whole should increase its fibre intake by about 40 per cent. This means that everyone, in theory, should eat on average 40 per cent more fruit, vegetables and cereals (bread and other foods containing wheat, oats, barley, rye and sweetcorn maize). The theory is the increased amount of fibre (and, if you remember, fibre is the food that does not get digested), would increase the stool output and reduce the gut transit time. But it doesn't work like that for all of us, unfortunately. In fact it is now acknowledged that some cereals can actually *worsen* constipation.

Wheat and other grains

Although bran has been heralded as the best remedy for constipation, and is still recommended by many doctors today, more recent evidence suggests that it may serve to worsen symptoms in some people. Early studies in *The Lancet* medical journal showed the benefits of bran in some of a small sample. (Interestingly, these doctors used Allinson's bran. Dr Allinson, the nineteenth century doctor was struck off the medical register for advocating the then controversial health benefits of wholemeal as opposed to white bread.)

More recently *The Lancet* carried a report from a group of specialists at Addenbrookes's Hospital in Cambridge, led by Dr John Hunter, which told a rather different story. Their observation was that the avoidance of certain foods helped two-thirds of their patients who had erratic bowel habit including constipation. Wheat was reported as the most common aggravating food, and subsequent work has confirmed this initial observation. Wheat and its associated grains – oats, barley and rye – which all contain the protein gluten, can cause either constipation or diarrhoea.

Tea

It seems that tea slows down gut-transit time for 50 per cent of people, according to a Scandinavian study. It can then aggravate constipation, having the opposite effect to coffee.

Dehydration

Lack of fluid is sometimes a cause of constipation, particularly in hot climates. If you take fibre supplements you will need to drink an extra two glasses of fluid per day.

Periods

It is now widely known that many women become constipated in the week before their period is due. The normal rate at which food moves through the gut slows down, and may well contribute to the abdominal bloating that many women experience premenstrually.

Magnesium deficiency

Magnesium is needed for smooth muscle control. As the lining of the gut is made up of smooth muscle, when levels of magnesium are low, as seems to be the case in over 50 per cent of women with PMS, the muscle groups do not contract and relax in their usual sequence, and constipation results. Taking supplements of magnesium, to correct levels, seems also to ease constipation.

Stress

Following the emphasis that many people have placed on stress, it probably won't come as a surprise to find that it affects the movement of food through the gut. Studies have shown that any stress can inhibit the normal regular contractions that occur spontaneously as part of the digestive system, and might aggravate constipation.

Pain

Understandably, any painful pelvic condition, including ovarian cysts, endometriosis, period pains, or post childbirth, can easily inhibit the urge to go to the toilet. In addition to these sources of pain and discomfort, piles (a tear in the margin of the anus or an anal fissure) are almost always associated with a powerful spasm of the muscles in the anus also, making it very difficult for motions to pass through.

Drugs

A number of drugs can cause constipation as a side-effect, the most common of which include antidepressants and painkillers.

Antidepressants are frequently accompanied by constipation, a dry mouth and sometimes blurred vision, especially at the start of therapy or if high doses are used. This effect is most noticeable with older types of antidepressants such as Amitryptiline and Desimipramine.

Strong painkillers

Painkillers which are derived from morphine, such as codeine, will invariably cause constipation. This means that when taking any pain killer that contains codeine or dihydrocodeine you can expect to become constipated.

Lack of exercise

As we get lazier as a nation, the incidence of heart disease, stroke and obesity increases. There is nothing like a good workout to get the bowels moving, so if you have a sluggish bowel and you are not exercising, turn to page 32 and get started!

What your doctor can do

- Recommend a diet rich in fruit and vegetable fibre, rather than bran or wheat fibre.
- Offer laxatives or a fibre supplement.
- If the onset of constipation is sudden in an older patient, and accompanied by bleeding or pain, your doctor should test for an underlying reason, like colon cancer. This may mean performing tests for hidden traces of blood in the stools, x-rays or arranging a specialist examination.

What you can do

- *Eat plenty of fibre-rich foods* These include fruit, vegetables, nuts and seeds, some cereals like brown rice, sweetcorn (maize), buckwheat, sago and tapioca. Take care, as some of these foods might make other symptoms worse, especially if you have bloating and wind.
- *Take a fibre supplement* This can be from your doctor or from a health-food shop. Good supplements include those containing ispaghula (Fybogel), sterculia (Normacol), linseeds (Linusit Gold), psyllium husks and, when tolerated, coarse oats. These are all highly water retentive and can be very effective, especially when combined with other measures to stimulate movement through the gut.

- *Ensure a good intake of fluid* This is very important if you are elderly or when taking a fibre supplement.
- *Avoid wheat, oats, barley and rye* Avoid too all foods containing them. This is a major change to your diet, and you will need to refer to the suggested menus on page 442.
- *Cut down or stop your tea consumption* Limit yourself to two cups of weak tea per day, or drink a herbal alternative (see page 7).
- *Drink one or two cups of coffee instead of tea* This may act as a laxative for some. The stimulating effect appears to take about 60 minutes before it is noticeable.
- *Have a cigarette!* Yes, if you are already a smoker, you may be aware that a few puffs – especially first thing in the morning or after your main meal – can stimulate your bowels. This is no recommendation to start smoking and no excuse not to give up, but if you do smoke you can sometimes help your bowels along.
- *Take some magnesium* This is particularly effective if you don't suffer with intermittent diarrhoea as well, and have premenstrual problems or suffer fatigue. Some women find that it is better for them to take magnesium last thing at night, gradually increasing the dose to what is called 'gut tolerance level'. This means that you will reach a level when the magnesium causes diarrhoea, and you will then need to cut back. A safe starting dose is between 200 and 400 mg per day. We frequently have patients who take a combination of linseeds with their morning cereal and up to 800 mg magnesium at night in order to control their constipation. We use magnesium amino acid chelate because it is gentle on the gut, but magnesium oxide or gluconate will do. Magnesium hydroxide, in the form of a white liquid and sulphate or in the form of crystals are available from some chemists, and are much more dramatic in their effect.
- *Take regular exercise* Try exercising three or four times each week. Choose a form of exercise that you have enjoyed in the past so that you continue on a regular basis (see page 32).
- *Avoid stressful situations whenever possible* Stress can cause muscles to go into spasm. Yoga is an excellent way of helping your body to relax and improve tolerance of stress. Listening to music, going for a walk, eating a good meal or just enjoying the company of family and friends, are all useful and effective ways of reducing tension.
- *Set aside time for your bowels* Some of us need peace and quiet and plenty of time to relax our muscles so that the bowels work properly. If you prefer to be undisturbed, choose a time when you can be alone, take the phone off the hook if necessary, and make a hot drink. A morning exercise session may stimulate the bowels too. Try to open your bowels at a regular time each day, like after breakfast or after your main meal. Our bodies like habits.

- *Use a suppository* If the other methods have failed try using a glycerine suppository to stimulate a bowel movement. They can be bought over the counter in any pharmacy. However do not use them in place of the above recommendations as your bowels might become dependent on them.

Complementary therapies

There are numerous treatment approaches to try to help relieve the symptoms of constipation. Massage is a favourite one, as it encourages peristalsis, which is the coordinated wave-like muscle contractions that take place in the gut, and will also release tension in those muscles. You should ideally have a regular professional massage, and do some self-massage of the tummy and lower back in between.

Colonic irrigation is said to be effective at flushing out the toxins in the bowel and some people swear by it. Always remember though that colonic irrigation is aiming at symptom relief rather than addressing the root cause.

Both acupuncture and herbal medicine are likely to be useful tools, helping to get your whole body functioning optimally. A herbal practitioner can also prepare a special cream for you to insert into your back passage to sooth piles and help to heal cracks and tears.

Taking time to relax formerly each day, perhaps combining relaxation with some self-massage is one way that you can help to speed up the recovery process (see page 29).

Nicole's story

Nicole was a 37-year-old doctor and mother of two children who had been suffering with constipation for many years.

'I had constipation for absolutely years to a point where I thought it was normal for me. I remember a representative from a pharmaceutical company raving about a product for constipation called Regulan which I subsequently tried. It did make a bit of difference to start with but not a great deal. I remember being constipated during pregnancy. I also developed haemorrhoids after my first pregnancy which were made worse by the constipation.

The doctors were concerned after the birth of our first child as they thought I had a prolapsed uterus which the piles and constipation aggravated. I usually open my bowels every few days and my motions were very hard and pellety. Because of the prolapse, in order to pass a motion, I had to actually stick my fingers into my vagina as everything seemed to be pressing on my bowel. I always felt as if 'everything was falling out'. I thought I was going to need major surgery at some point. After my second baby, the consultant

I was under decided I had a weak pelvic floor rather than a prolapse and that I must avoid being constipated at all costs!

I heard an interview with the WNAS on the radio and decided to get some advice about my diet. Even though I'm medically qualified I had had so little education on the subject of nutrition as part of my training. The WNAS recommended taking supplements of magnesium and organic linseeds to help combat the constipation. In addition I eliminated certain foods such as wheat, rye and oats from my diet. I must say I have not been constipated since the week after I began the programme. I have to watch my diet and the occasions when I eat foods I should not be eating I can feel some of the symptoms starting up again, but this time I know how to put it right. I don't have that falling out feeling any more or any pressure in the pelvic floor area. My bowels have calmed down and I feel a great deal better for it. I also had severe premenstrual syndrome which I have managed to sort out on the same programme. I now feel comfortable physically and mentally. I feel that I have had my eyes opened.'

See also: Irritable bowel syndrome (IBS), The Women's Nutritional Advisory Service.

Crohn's Disease

Crohn's disease is named after an American physician who, over 60 years ago, described, with others, this chronic inflammatory disease of the bowel. Its cause remains as elusive now as it was then. This condition can affect any part of the bowel from the mouth to the anus. Young adults are most commonly affected, and it seems to affect equal numbers of men and women. Typical features are diarrhoea, abdominal pain and weight loss. The affected parts of the bowel become swollen and inflamed, with large numbers of white cells being present, though what stimulates this reaction is unclear. Most usually the small bowel, which is primarily involved in digestion and absorption, and the large bowel, are the main targets for this disease. At times the inflammatory process extends to other distant parts of the body, namely the eyes, joints and skin.

What causes it?

This is a much debated subject, with a mixture of genetic and environmental factors at work.

- *It tends to run in families* In identical twins, if one has the disease, there is nearly a 66 per cent chance that the other will develop it. However, it is rare for both husband and wife to suffer.

- *Dietary factors are a possibility* Recovery from Crohn's disease can be achieved by the exclusion from the diet of a variety of foods. Whether this is due to an actual allergy or the influence of some foods upon the type of bacteria present in the bowel is uncertain.
- *Infection with either the measles virus, or a bacteria* that is a distant relative of that which causes tuberculosis, are two possibilities.
- *Immune system overactivity* is a possible factor, causing the body to over-react to the presence of bacteria or even to attack the body's own tissues.
- *Smoking,* antibodies against baker's yeast, the swallowing of tooth-paste, and not being breast-fed as an infant, are all possible contributing factors.

What your doctor can do

- *Assess the extent of the disease* Barium x-rays, examination of the lower or upper bowel with a flexible telescope called an endoscope, and use of radioactive white cells are all used for this.
- *Perform blood tests* These will assess disease activity, anaemia and nutritional deficiencies, especially iron, vitamin B12 and zinc.
- *Give advice on diet* Any one of the following types of diet may be appropriate. This is best determined on the basis of specialist recommendation:
  ○ a high-calorie, high-protein diet for those with weight loss and nutritional deficiencies
  ○ a low-fibre diet for those in whom the bowel is very inflamed
  ○ a diet that avoids milk and milk sugar (lactose) for those who are sensitive to it/them
  ○ an exclusion diet if multiple food sensitivities are suspected
  ○ a diet using only specialised pre-digested foods – an elemental diet – used in a hospital setting.
- *Prescribe drug therapy* Steroids are the mainstay of treatment, and high doses are required if the illness is severe. Other anti-inflammatory and immune system altering drugs are used, especially if the patient needs repeatedly high doses of steroids. Antibiotics are used for infective complications and sometimes to help with the bowel disease.
- *Consider surgery* This would be to remove severely affected parts of the bowel or to tackle the inflammation if it has spread to neighbouring areas.

What you can do

- Take your medicine regularly.
- Staying in regular and good contact with your specialist is very important. Crohn's disease is never cured, and the quality of care will depend on a good two-way flow of information.

- Stop smoking if you are a smoker.
- Avoid foods that aggravate your symptoms. This will for the majority of patients require some expert advice along the lines given above. It seems that the commonest foods to aggravate Crohn's disease are the same that aggravate irritable bowel disease. These are:
  - wheat and other grains and all food such as bread, cakes and pasta
  - milk and cheese
  - coffee, and possibly tea
  - some fruits, especially raw, with orange and tomato the most likely
  - foods that contain baker's yeast, e.g. bread and some buns
  - other yeast rich foods, e.g. alcohol, vinegar, pickled foods and yeast extract
  - foods that are hard to digest, e.g. sweetcorn and beans.

Many of these can be easily avoided without recourse to expert advice. You will need to avoid the foods for three or four weeks to see if there is any improvement.

- Take supplements. Probably the simplest supplement to take for those who are not receiving specific advice on this from their doctor is a strong multi-vitamin multi-mineral preparation. This may need amending if the following situations are present:
  - severe diarrhoea – a soluble vitamin supplement may be better absorbed
  - blood loss or anaemia – iron supplements may be needed
  - poor wound healing or reduced resistance to infection – supplements of zinc
  - prolonged bleeding in those with severe disease or receiving antibiotics – supplements of vitamin K
  - long-standing disease with osteoporosis – calcium supplements
  - sulphsalazine therapy – folic acid supplements
  - severe or long-standing diarrhoea and muscle cramps – extra magnesium or potassium supplements
  - severe disease and a restricted diet or special feeding regime – supplements of the mineral selenium
  - damage to the terminal ileum or its surgical removal – vitamin B12 by injection
  - severe or long-standing disease and poor night vision – vitamin A.
- Take a probiotic supplement like Acidophillus to repopulate the colon with 'friendly' bacteria. Crohn's sufferers have up to six times more 'bad' bacteria, (bacteriodes) present in the colon.
- Limit foods which contain the additive carageenan found in jelly, drinks and other manufactured foods. This additive actually stimulates the growth of bacteriodes and thus has an adverse effect on the friendly bacteria (bifidobacteria).

- Do not give time-release supplements as they rely on adequate hydrochloric acid (HCL) to break them down over a long period of time.
- If supplements are hard to take, try crushing the tablet and mix it with jam or honey. Buy capsules which can be opened and sprinkled on food or in a drink. They might not taste too pleasant, but absorbancy will be more efficient.
- Take some aloe vera, which can reduce inflammation of the gut lining and has a healing effect on the gastrointestinal tract.
- Zinc loss through the bowel is quite great, so supplementing with this mineral is fundamental.
- The amino acid L-glutamine helps to help the gut lining and reduce the risk of it becoming 'leaky' and setting up further reactions.
- Take a supplement of evening primrose oil and marine fish oil to reduce the synthesis of the pro-inflammatory prostaglandins.

If any of these situations apply then you should discuss the need for such supplements with your specialist. All of these nutrients can be tested for, though some require the use of a specialised laboratory. Correcting any nutritional deficiency can only help, and it is possible that doing so may positively influence the degree of inflammation, the rate of wound healing, resistance to infection, appetite, general well-being and possibly the future risk of cancer.

Complementary therapies
None are likely to control the disease.

Cystitis

Cystitis is an inflammation of the bladder caused by a bacterial infection or a mechanical disturbance in the area. Vigorous sexual intercourse can be a trigger, which is why it became known as 'the honeymoon syndrome'. Consequently it should come as no surprise to discover that cystitis is nearly thirteen times more common in the general female population than in nuns. Studies estimate that one woman in five will have had a recent episode of cystitis. A physician-based study conducted in London demonstrated that 52 per cent of women get cystitis at some point in their lives, but some 6 per cent suffer repeated attacks.

What causes it?

- In approximately 50 per cent of cases it is caused by the organism *E. coli*, which sometimes travels from the anus area. The bacteria

penetrate the urethra, via the perineum, and work their way into the bladder. There is a clear association between diaphragm users and cystitis, again because of the *E.coli*.
- Vigorous sexual intercourse can bring on symptoms.
- Tight clothing, which can put unacceptable pressure on the urethra.
- Vaginal deodorants and disinfectants can also bring on symptoms.
- A prolapse may restrict the urinary flow and predispose an infection.
- Caffeine affects the muscles of the bladder and aggravates symptoms of urgency.

What your doctor can do

- Test your urine to determine which sort of bacteria are present and whether they are sensitive to any particular types of antibiotics.
- Prescribing antibiotics is the usual method of treatment. However, studies have shown that approximately two-thirds of female sufferers recover naturally without antibiotics, and even after treatment with antibiotics symptoms can return.

Penny's story

Penny was a 37-year-old researcher who had been suffering with bouts of recurrent cystitis, which were becoming almost constant at the time she approached the WNAS.

'I had my first episode of cystitis three years ago. It was painful and unpleasant, but it came and went and I didn't give it much thought. The following year I had three separate bouts which I found alarming. I consulted my doctor and researched self-help methods to overcome the symptoms, but nothing really seemed to help. This last year I reckon I had cystitis every month, at period time. I really lived in dread of the symptoms as the month progressed.

I approached the WNAS for advice after reading one of their books as I was suffering with diarrhoea, and horrendous period pains. I completed their questionnaire and diet diary, and then made an appointment for a telephone consultation. I was given a programme to follow which involved changing my diet, taking regular exercise and some nutritional supplements. I also started being meticulous about my hygiene, and began using baby wipes after going to the toilet.

To my absolute delight I haven't had any cystitis since I began the programme, the diarrhoea has cleared up and I have now had several pain-free periods. I am amazed and relieved as I am due to get married in a few months time and we are hoping to start a family straight away.'

What you can do

- Drink plenty of liquids, particularly water, throughout the day. Aim to have the equivalent of a glass of water every hour whilst the symptoms are acute to flush your system through.
- Drink a few glasses of cranberry juice. Cranberry juice contains a compound called hippuric acid which actually inhibits the bacteria responsible for cystitis from adhering to the lining of the bladder and urinary tract. However, the caution with drinking too much is that most commercial varieties contain a lot of sugar to disguise the bitter taste of the fruit. Since sugar has a detrimental effect on the immune system, it would be more beneficial to take a concentrated cranberry formula in tablet or powder form.
- Strengthen the immune system to help prevent recurrent bouts of cystitis by taking garlic capsules and 25mg of zinc daily. Garlic, as well as being an immune enhancer, is also a natural antibiotic. Antibiotics are normally the first line of treatment given by doctors to clear up cystitis, but more natural means are healthier and safer in the long term.
- After sex and after a bowel movement wash yourself carefully with warm, unperfumed soapy water, wiping yourself from front to back to wash the germs away. Sit so that your anus is at a lower point than your urethra, and let the water run down to wash away any faecal bacteria.
- Choose unperfumed bath products, as allergies can develop, and the urethra may become inflamed as a result. Do not use feminine fresh sprays as the chemicals can cause a reaction.
- Organic tampons and sanitary towels are becoming widely available in health food stores and even supermarkets.
- Add a small amount of bicarbonate of soda to the water you drink; this can help to ease the symptoms by making your urine more alkaline.
- Avoid drinking caffeine, and use alternative drinks, as coffee can make the bladder irritation worse.
- If you use a diaphragm, and your symptoms are recurrent, try switching to an alternative method of contraception for a while.
- If there is blood in the urine, consult a medical practitioner for further diagnosis.

Complementary therapies

Homeopathic remedies like Cantharis, Staphisagria or Apis may well bring relief. Herbal remedies may also be helpful as an adjunct to the conventional methods of overcoming symptoms of cystitis. Aromatherapy can be useful and juniper oil can be used as part of a lower abdominal massage.

See also: Recommended reading and References.

Dementia

Dementia is the subject of many jokes, has numerous terms to define it, and is something we often casually admit to suffering ourselves. But true dementia is really no joke. It is characterised by a loss of cognition, which means a loss of the ability to use one's mind in a variety of ways; this includes memory, use of language, visual awareness of space, perception, thinking, problem-solving and personality. Significant loss of two or more of these functions in someone would qualify for a diagnosis of dementia. Underlying psychiatric problems such as depression or a physical illness that reduces the level of consciousness (e.g. heart disease) must first be excluded. One in five elderly people aged 80 years or more will develop dementia. There are in fact many causes, a few are treatable and there may be some with a nutritional element. Alzheimer's disease accounts for approximately two-thirds of cases.

How to recognise early dementia

This information is presented as an aid to relatives and friends of those who might be developing a problem. The majority of such cases present slowly, almost insidiously, and it is not usually until there have been several events that real suspicion should arise. Then only assessment by an experienced doctor will lead to a proper diagnosis. There are a number of questions to be asked, such as, 'Is the problem really dementia, or is there some other illness?', 'What is the likely cause?' and 'Is it treatable?'.

The most useful information for the health professional comes from a close relative or similar witness. They should be asked to describe suspicious events where the person's mental functions may have failed them. Then the following checklist should be appraised:

- memory, both for recent events and for distant ones
- use of language, finding and using words correctly, understanding what is said or written, reading and writing ability
- numeracy, especially with money when shopping
- perception: of self as in appearance and dressing; of nearby objects; and of where they are, and ability to find their way around
- thinking, planning and problem-solving
- personality and conduct toward others
- features of depression
- delusions or hallucinations.

Many other details are important to assess the general level of health including:

- consumption of alcohol and tobacco
- use of drugs
- past health, especially heart disease, and if there is a history of a stroke
- a recent fall or injury
- the presence of a severe headache
- loss of control over the bowels or bladder
- recent weight loss or fever
- type of diet consumed
- the cause of death or state of health of all first degree relatives.

What your doctor can do

After assessing the problem the next step is to examine and then investigate the patient. This will mean a number of tests including those for:

- anaemia and infection
- kidney and liver function
- calcium, sodium and potassium
- vitamin B12, folic acid and possibly vitamin B1
- thyroid function
- chest x-ray
- x-ray of the brain – CT scan.

The purpose of these tests is to exclude causes of dementia other than Alzheimer's disease, and identify those that are treatable. Particular thoroughness should be shown if the patient is young, the deterioration is rapid, there is an unsteady gait, loss of control of eye movement, a loss of bowel or bladder control, a tremor, or features to suggest repeated small strokes, infection or a disturbance in metabolism.

Treatment may involve drugs, surgery and occasionally correction of nutritional deficiencies or treatment of an infection or a metabolic problem. Very often the diagnosis is one of Alzheimer's disease which can only be confirmed by the exclusion of other conditions, as there is no test for it. The theories behind the causation of Alzheimer's disease include: genetic predisposition, aluminium accumulation, and past head injury. The greatest risk factor is by far and away age. Treatment is very unsatisfactory. Only one drug has had any real success and that is Tacrine which is of very limited benefit. It helps maintain the level of chemicals involved in the transmission of signals from one nerve cell to another.

What you can do

The information here tells you how you may help someone with dementia.

- Don't give up hope. The rate of decline is very variable. Join an appropriate support group.
- Get the sufferer to eat as well as possible.
- Cut down on their alcohol if this is excessive (more than two units per day).
- Get their doctor to check their drugs if they are taking some and decide whether they are all really necessary.
- Maintain a daily routine. This helps them to remember what they need to do.
- Label things and rooms if they are forgetful.
- Help keep them physically active. A 30–40 minute walk per day is ideal.
- Help them keep mentally active. This may help them preserve their faculties. Reading, watching TV (and discussing it), keeping up hobbies and socialising are all important.
- Supplements of vitamins may be appropriate. Vitamins B and C if deficient can have a small influence on concentration. There is no harm in giving a modest supplement of these especially if the diet is less than perfect. Expect no miracles.
- Inform the driving licence authorities.
- Make arrangement for the management of the person's financial affairs.

Complementary therapies

Complementary therapy is unable to reverse the process of dementia.

See also: References.

Depression

We all experience mood changes from time to time, which is a perfectly natural phenomenon. Bad news, the loss of a dear one, prolonged dull weather, financial problems and lack of sleep are a few examples of changes that may depress our mood. The majority of us bounce back relatively quickly, but for approximately one in ten people symptoms of depression become chronic, even when the apparent stimulus is long gone.

Mood swings are a lower harmonic of depression, and affect us at different times in our lives. Women experience numerous hormonal events which can leave them feeling drained. Childbirth is a good example. Before a period or during the menopause are other key times when extra nutrient demands are placed upon them. When they are unable to meet the demand, symptoms of depression and mood swings can result. From a survey conducted at the WNAS on 1000 patients with premenstrual syndrome, we discovered that 96 per cent of them suffered with mood swings in their premenstrual phase, 62 per cent severely. Ninety-four per cent of the women also suffered from premenstrual depression, 83.8 per cent severe to moderate. This, we felt, was a frightening high number, and in view of the possible consequences of depression, not something that should be taken lightly. As premenstrual depression is such a common condition, we will deal with the cyclic aspects of depression, before going on to examine the more chronic symptoms.

What causes premenstrual moodswings and depression?

Theories about the cause of premenstrual mood swings are similar to those that cause premenstrual anxiety as mentioned in the chapter on PMS. When there is an inadequate supply of nutrients and a disturbance in brain chemistry, our mood becomes volatile.

Depression is a common premenstrual symptom, and usually presents with other symptoms such an anxiety and breast tenderness. In 1959 Dr Katharina Dalton published a study in *The British Medical Journal* which showed that the time of admission to hospital for female depressed patients coincided with the menstrual period, the premenstrual phase, and ovulation. Our own research has shown that those most likely to suffer from premenstrual depression are more often overweight and do less exercise than non-sufferers.

The balance of certain nutrients has an important influence on both hormone and brain chemistry. Magnesium, for example, influences how the ovaries respond in the normal menstrual cycles, and many other nutrients are also important in this respect. It is also known that in people with severe depression the chance of finding some degree of B vitamin deficiency is much higher than would be expected in the general population. These nutrients have been used successfully in treating both PMS and depression.

The balance of hormones – or whatever determines their balance – seems to be crucial in controlling mood, and as the years pass by it becomes even more apparent that our diet and lifestyle can influence our hormones and our moods.

What your doctor can do

The average woman who complains to her doctor about fluctuating moods and depression in her premenstrual phase, or at the time of the menopause, will probably not have any physical symptoms. As the majority of family doctors lack information about nutrient levels, they will have a limited number of options on offer.

- First you would be given a physical examination, with routine blood screening to eliminate the possibility of an underlying problem.
- If nothing tangible is found, your doctor is likely to offer either hormone treatment or tranquillisers.
- An enlightened doctor would ask you about your eating and exercise habits, and about your stress levels.
- You may be referred for some counselling.
- Alternatively, you may be simply told to pull yourself together.

What you can do

- Follow the recommendations in Premenstrual Syndrome (see page 394), and the dietary recommendations on page 474.
- Use the Supplement Chart on pages 18–21 to work out which supplements you should be taking, and ensure that you take them regularly, at least until your symptoms have abated. The most effective are likely to be high doses of vitamin B – about 100 mg of B1, B2, B3 and B6 and magnesium.
- The herb St John's Wort, which is otherwise known as hypericum perforatum, has been successfully used to treat depression for over 2,000 years. In Germany, St John's Wort is prescribed by at least half of the doctors dealing with depression, and a study in the UK in 1997 found St John's Wort at a dose of three 300 mg capsule per day to be as effective as many standard antidepressants. (NB: see note on page 162.)
- Get some help to sort out any stressful situations that face you, including your current commitments, if you find them overwhelming.
- Never underestimate the value of exercise – it has been scientifically proven to influence your mood and helps to lift depression. You need to exercise for at least four good sessions each week (see page 32).
- Make some time for yourself, no matter what your schedule, and don't be afraid to indulge yourself in the odd treat now and then, most of us more than deserve them!
- Spend time with friends who like to laugh, and watch some comedy films.
- Hum in the bath, and at other convenient times. Sound therapists have discovered that humming alters our breathing pattern and as a result increases our energy levels and raises our mood.

Complementary therapies

Our recommendations are pretty good at sorting out premenstrual mood swings and depression, but it may take a few cycles before you feel the benefit. In the meantime, it is worth trying some herbal preparations, or a homeopathic remedy or two.

CHRONIC DEPRESSION

Unlike premenstrual depression, this true depressive disorder persists, and the symptoms are not linked to the menstrual cycle. True depression can accompany a physical illness or can be an illness in its own right. So the first thing a doctor has to do is eliminate an underlying physical cause before assuming that you are suffering with pure depression. One to two men per thousand suffer with depressive disorders, three times as many women.

Seasonal Affective Disorder (SAD) is another form of major depression, where sufferers are profoundly affected by the lack of sunlight that occurs in autumn and winter. This triggers biochemical changes in the brain, directed by the brain chemicals melatonin and serotonin, and leads to depression.

Men are slightly less likely than women to experience depression but there are certain problems that are more likely to occur in the male which will contribute to this problem. Alcohol excess is perhaps the most relevant. Consumption of four units (1.5 pints of beer or half a bottle of wine) or more per day is likely to have an adverse effect on many nutrients that influence mood. The B vitamins are particularly vulnerable as are the minerals zinc and magnesium, all of which are involved in the production of mood-altering chemicals in the nervous system. If you drink heavily or regularly, take a supplement.

Additionally, lack of vitamin C, even if mild, can contribute to depression. Requirements are known to be increased in those with large muscle bulk, as well as in smokers. A supplement of 500mg-1000mg is recommended.

An underactive thyroid is less common in men, but other hormonal changes could present with depression. Increased levels of prolactin – from the pituitary gland – can cause a reduced sperm count, loss of libido and depression in the male.

Finally some men just don't feel right unless they exercise regularly. Regular exercise even once or twice a week aids mood, physical fitness and sleeping patterns, as well as protecting against cardiovascular disease.

What are the symptoms?

The main features of a depressive disorder are low mood, lack of enjoyment, loss of interest in usual pastimes, and becoming generally withdrawn. Often people suffering with depression also have disturbed sleep and wake early in the morning, lack energy and find that their appetites for both food and sex are reduced. They seem to see life through dark grey glasses, and are pessimistic, regard most endeavours as hopeless, and often display suicidal tendencies. Even their physical appearance may be affected with a downturned mouth, frown lines on their forehead and a stooped posture.

Key features of depression

- depressed mood, or mood swings
- lack of energy
- lethargy and despondency
- inability to experience enjoyment
- pessimistic attitude
- suicidal thoughts
- regretful and guilty recollections
- disturbed sleep with early morning waking
- insomnia or somnolence
- reduced appetite for food
- loss of libido
- constipation
- weight loss or weight gain
- amenorrhoea (absent periods) in women

What causes it?

There can be many underlying causes of depression:

- Marital problems, bereavement, redundancy, financial stress and so on. Very often symptoms of depression can arrive as the result of an accumulation of stresses and strains.
- An under-active thyroid gland can produce symptoms of depression, and so too can other serious illness, like cancer, kidney, liver or heart disease, anaemia and diabetes.
- Serious infections
- Alcoholism – prolonged consumption of excessive amounts of alcohol.
- Repeated lack of food
- Chronic pain
- A drug side-effect
- Deficiencies of B vitamins, calcium, magnesium, copper, iron potassium, folic acid or EFAs. Numerous studies have shown that patients with depression commonly have low levels of one or more of these nutrients.
- Excessive consumption of caffeine, as heavy caffeine users have a tendency to be more depressed and have a lower academic performance.
- Food sensitivities

What your doctor can do

- Determine whether you are suffering with pure depression and that there is no underlying physical cause for your change in mood. This would be done by physical examination and routine blood tests, to check for anaemia, infection, thyroid function, and kidney and liver disease. There would also be a urine test to check for diabetes.
- Decide whether you need help from a psychiatrist, or whether you should be treated in the surgery. As a rule of thumb, those who are suicidal, not eating or hallucinating should be given specialist help without delay.
- Advise counselling that would help you deal with immediate problems, and come to terms with past traumas.
- Encourage you to take each day as it comes, and to temporarily relinquish some of your responsibilities.
- Prescribe antidepressants. There is now a bewildering choice. Remember that there is a lot of individual variation in response and several may need to be tried before one is found to be effective. A psychiatrist may use stronger drugs like Lithium, a mood regulator, or ECT, electro-convulsive therapy, which is not common these days because it causes irreversible brain damage.

What you can do

- Eat wholesome food regularly, and in particular avoid sweets and chocolate as these can worsen symptoms, especially when they are eaten in the place of nutritious food.
- Follow the recommendations for The Very Nutritious Diet on page 437. Nutrition can be very important in depression. Many nutrient deficiencies can result in depression, but some are particularly important nutrients for healthy mental function including most of the B vitamins, vitamin C, zinc and magnesium. Good food providing adequate calories and protein nourishes both the body and the brain. The brain has first call on the available supply of many nutrients, therefore, the first effects of nutritional deficiencies are often mental symptoms.
- There are also plenty of foods that should be avoided, such as 'simple', highly refined sugar in foods and drinks, which can affect mental symptoms by causing blood sugar swings.
- Excessive alcohol consumption can cause depression, as it substantially decreases the ability of the body to extract nutrients from the food we eat. Limit yourself to a maximum of two units per day.
- Spend some time in a stress-free environment with a companion who is willing to listen to you.

- Get some help to sort out the immediate stress or trauma you are facing.
- Ensure you get plenty of fresh air and sunlight, when available, each day.
- Exercise six days per week to the point of breathlessness, as this will induce an endorphin release, which helps to lift you out of your depression.
- If possible, arrange to have your nutrient levels measured so that you can determine whether you have any deficiencies.
- Take supplements of strong multi-vitamins, B vitamins, magnesium and anything else that may be indicated following your tests.
- Amino acids are the building blocks of protein, and precursors, or raw materials for neurotransmitters. Neurotransmitters are chemical like substances which are necessary for conducting messages. There are 3 amino acids that are most directly related to mood and depression: phenylalanine, tyrosine and tryptophan. Tryptophan helps to raise levels of a naturally occurring chemical in the brain called serotonin, which has been found to be abnormally low in depressed people.
- Vitamin B3 is a co-factor in the conversion of tryptophan to serotonin so a good dietary intake with the addition of a supplement is necessary in the treatment of depression. Some foods like milk and turkey contain an abundant supply of tryptophan and can act as anti-depressants.
- The herb St John's Wort has been successfully used to treat depression for over 2,000 years (see page 152).
- Spend 15–20 minutes each day relaxing to soothing music, or a relaxation tape, or perhaps try some yoga or meditation. Follow the recommendations on the role of relaxation (see page 29).

Essentially, what you need is good food, nutritional supplements, plenty of exercise, good company, a break from your routine, and time to reflect and reorganise.

Complementary therapies

Seek advice from a qualified homeopath if necessary, who will choose a remedy to suit your individual set of symptoms. Aromatherapy massage might help to ease the blues also.

Justine's story

It was clear from the outset that Justine was an unusual patient. She was intelligent, significantly depressed, but with very clear insight. At the age of 36 she had had ample opportunity after 20 years of depression to gain some understanding of her problems. In particular she had observed that throughout her large family virtually all the female members were miserable. She had coped with her depression well, only rarely making use of anti-depressants. She had managed to develop a career in administration which she continued with full-time even though she had a young child.

The pattern of her depression made her feel that there was some chemical basis for it and she thought that at least in part, this might have a nutritional component. She was a non-smoker and non-drinker, and ate a reasonably good diet, although occasionally convenience meals had to be used because of her busy lifestyle. Indeed there is research to support her suspicions. Sometimes depression does run in families and subtle changes in brain chemistry are known to occur with certain patterns of depression. The accepted treatment however involves anti-depressants.

In Justine's case nutritional investigations revealed markedly abnormal results. The levels for vitamin B1 and vitamin B6 were extremely abnormal putting her easily into the worst one per cent of results for patients we see. There was a reduced level for magnesium and a borderline level for vitamin C. Low levels of these nutrients are associated with depression, fatigue and increased risk of suicide. The severity could not be explained by her diet and thus it is possible that there was some genetically determined metabolic factor contributing to these abnormalities. Without investigating other members of the family it would be impossible to be certain about this.

She began an improved diet, together with supplements of high strength vitamin D, multi-vitamins and magnesium. Her day-to-day depressive symptoms lessened and in the next month her pre-menstrual mood changes also diminished. Episodes of stress and argument with her husband also reduced. She chose not to take the anti-depressant which had been described by her psychiatrist.

She was careful to limit her alcohol intake to 14 units a week as levels greater than this may indeed increase a demand for vitamin B. She may well prove to be the sort of person who needs to take vitamin supplements long-term in order to maintain good physical and mental health.

POSTNATAL DEPRESSION

This brand of depression occurs after the birth of a baby, and can vary from the 'baby blues', which may arrive in the first seven to ten days after giving birth , to a full blown psychotic disorder, with total rejection of the baby. The baby blues is very common and, in a well-nourished mum, should pass almost as quickly as they arrived. Severe postnatal depression is far less common, and needs immediate attention.

The most common symptoms of the baby blues include depressed mood, crying, insomnia and irritability, and are experienced to some degree by between 66–85 per cent of women, depending on the criteria used to define it. It is thought to occur in women who have a history of premenstrual syndrome. Postnatal depression is less common, affecting some 10 per cent of women, and it has been noted that there is often a previous history of depression in this group of sufferers.

What are the symptoms?

- mood changes that vary from depression to elation
- lack of interest in the baby
- withdrawn and tearful
- irritability
- extreme fatigue
- insomnia
- anxiety
- thoughts of suicide
- thoughts of harming the baby

What causes it?

- It is thought that fluctuating levels of the hormones progesterone and oestrodial, shortly after the birth of a baby may be an underlying cause. However, there are differing opinions amongst the medical fraternity.
- Thyroid insufficiency occurs in approximately 5 per cent of women.
- Low levels of nutrients, particularly vitamin B, calcium, magnesium and EFAs, may be factors.
- A unsatisfactory relationship or lack of support from family members.
- Disrupted lifestyle or status as a result of the birth.
- A difficult labour that did not fulfil a woman's hopes.

What your doctor can do

- Check your thyroid function, including a check for thyroid antibodies.
- Check your iron levels, and in an ideal world your blood levels of calcium, B6 and magnesium, all of which have been shown to be low in some women in clinical studies.
- Arrange for some counselling to help you talk through your emotions.
- If the symptoms persist, prescribe antidepressants.
- In a minority of cases of extreme postnatal depression the help of a psychiatrist and hospital treatment will be necessary.

What you and your family can do

- *Communicate* You should never feel ashamed of feeling low after the birth of a baby. Your family and friends will want to support you, so you must let them know how you feel.
- *Offload any responsibilities you can* In those first few weeks after having a baby Mother Nature prefers you to be supported, in a calm environment, and to take time to get to know your baby, whilst getting your strength back. Not so many years ago, women were expected to 'lie-in' for four weeks after having a baby. Translated this meant that everyone else rallied round to do the household chores and the new mum was left to feed, sleep and get to explore her new relationship with the baby.
- *Eat well* If possible, get your partner, friend or relative to prepare wholesome meals for you. If you are breast-feeding you will have increased nutrient demands which you need to bear in mind. Follow the recommendations for The Very Nutritious Diet on page 437, and refer to the Nutritional Content of Food lists starting on page 483. The nutritional demands that are placed on you during pregnancy and breast-feeding are greater than at any other time in your life – so make sure the cook knows that!
- *Take supplements* Research shows that many nutrients, including EFAs can be in short supply after the birth. Take a good strong multi-vitamin and multi-mineral supplement, and evening primrose oil combined with marine fish oil.
- *Get out regularly* Walk out with the pram in the fresh air every day, even short distances will make a difference.
- *Have time for yourself* Get your partner, friend or mum to look after the baby for a few hours on a regular basis, so that you can have some time for yourself. You may choose to sleep initially, especially if you are having disturbed nights. Take advantage of the time, get your hair done, buy some new clothes, or meet up with a friend for a bit of reassurance.
- *Take regular exercise* Six weeks after the birth you should be able to do a gentle workout. Stretching exercises will help to restore your muscle tone, and will make you feel better about yourself. Gradually, over the months, ease into low-impact aerobics, as this will encourage the release of the brain chemicals, endorphins, which help to raise your mood.
- *Try to socialise* Make every effort to attend social gatherings in your area, particularly those run by The National Childbirth Trust. It will be good for you to meet other new mums, many of whom will be experiencing the same problems as you. You could support each other.

A healthy diet, vitamin and mineral supplements, plenty of rest, adequate sleep and a supportive and loving environment seem to be good treatment for postnatal depression. It is noteworthy that during pregnancy and whilst breast-feeding, the demands for calcium, magnesium and the B vitamins are very high and a loss of most of these can cause changes in mood. It often is that simple.

Complementary therapies

There is no harm in trying a herbal or homeopathic remedy alongside the recommendations made here. A session with the cranial osteopath after the birth will help to realign the body, and massage, especially with relaxing aromatherapy oils, would be soothing. But remember that correcting nutrient levels and environmental stresses and strains has to take first place.

Linda's story

Linda battled with post-natal depression for two years following a very traumatic delivery.

'I only had one child – I could never face having another one, as it was such an awful experience for me. My husband particularly wanted children and so I agreed to have a baby, more to fulfil his needs than mine. The pregnancy was relatively uneventful although I don't remember enjoying it much and must admit I tried to disguise my shape for several months. I did all the right things during pregnancy though such as giving up alcohol, eating well, exercising and resting but the effect Caroline's birth had on me was overwhelming.

I found delivering the baby hard work and just after she had been born the cord ruptured whilst I was attempting to deliver the afterbirth. I remember blood pumping out everywhere and being given an emergency general anaesthetic to enable the doctor to manually remove the placenta. My husband was literally left 'holding the baby' while all this was happening before his eyes. I was given four units of blood and prayed that it was not contaminated – something that troubled me for years and years afterwards. When I came round I remember seeing tubes everywhere and felt so utterly sorry for myself. I was not interested in the baby at all. When the nurse asked if I wanted to feed the baby I felt like telling her to get lost.

I was in hospital for ten days and home for a week before we moved house. The move had been planned before Caroline was born. Although I did want to settle in the new house, with hindsight, moving so quickly was probably a very bad idea. My husband, sensing I needed help, offered to take extra time off work but being very independent I assured him I could manage. Consequently I was left at home attempting to go through the motions of looking after Caroline in our new house but spent most of the day crying while she cried. I can remember rocking the pram so hard to try and quieten her down that she almost fell out. I was forever shouting and screaming at her and would leave her crying in her room until she literally cried herself to sleep.

I did not go to see my GP as I was ashamed of my feelings and felt that I should have been able to pull myself together. I know I wasn't in my right mind at the time. All I could feel was the baby encroaching on my space, preventing me from leading my life. I remember one night when my husband was away, she was screaming with earache and I could not get her to take any medicine or calm her down. In the end I closed the door to her room and went off and left her. I felt so bad about it afterwards that I started drinking alcohol. I had a friend who was keen on the bottle and we used to get together about lunchtime each day and get through a couple of bottles of wine, lots of gin and really anything we could lay our hands on. I suppose I was trying to numb my senses.

My husband has since told me that he was convinced he would come home from work one day and I would have gone, leaving Caroline behind. I was awful and felt ill. I had diarrhoea at least six or seven times a day which was totally out of control and my wrist bones became so painful that I couldn't even lift the baby out of the bath. My Health Visitor suggested I take evening primrose oil which did help a bit. I made an appointment to see a psychotherapist privately and had three sessions of talking my problems through. This seemed to help a bit. With hindsight I realised I did not really feel anything for Caroline until she was about two – as she started to become less dependent on me and more communicative.

I eventually settled in to a routine of having horrendous pre-menstrual syndrome and this is what eventually drew me to the WNAS. With my new knowledge from the WNAS and a lot of hindsight I realise that a combination of being unprepared to the baby, lack of sleep once she was born and inadequate levels of important nutrients affected my brain chemistry, and as a result, badly affected my sanity. I had no training to be a mother and, it seems, no instinct. I feel looking back I could have looked after my cat better than I looked after Caroline. I feel so guilty about the way I treated her.

Thankfully I have really sorted myself out completely now. I don't have any more PMS, I don't drink alcohol and I absolutely adore Caroline. The WNAS was my refuge – I honestly feel it saved my sanity and since going on my programme I have been able to find my emotions and develop a very wholesome relationship with my daughter. There is nothing I wouldn't do for her and I would certainly like to make up for my lack of mothering in the past.'

A note about St John's Wort

St John's Wort is a potent herb, and should be used correctly and cautiously. The herbal preparation should not be taken in conjunction with anti-depressants, HIV drugs, the oral contraceptive pill or anti-coagulant medication. Consult your medical doctor before taking St John's Wort.

Dermatitis (Allergic)

Dermatitis literally means irritation of the skin and the term is sometimes used to mean the same as eczema. However 'dermatitis' is now used to describe an irritating red, sometimes scaly, rash that has followed contact or exposure to a number of possible agents. Usually it is the area of skin that is most exposed to the irritant that develops the rash. Common irritants include: washing-up liquid, acids, alkalis, many cleaning agents and glassfibre as used in insulation.

Sometimes an allergy develops to something that is in contact with the skin. In this situation even very small amounts of the allergen may cause a rash in some, unlike common irritants. The culprit agent may have been used without difficulty for years as sensitivity may take a long time to develop. Common agents causing allergic dermatitis include:

- Cosmetics, perfumes, hair bleaches and dyes, chemicals used in 'perms', lanolin or wool fat.
- Metal, mainly nickel, found in cheaper jewellery, studs in jeans, wrist watch bands.
- Rubber found in many items, from rubber gloves, scuba diving suits and elastic bands to condoms.
- Foods, when handled – garlic and citrus fruit are particularly troublesome.
- Medicines, local anaesthetics, antibiotic creams and even steroid creams.
- Other compounds – wood, plants, rosin from pine trees which is found in paper and glossy magazines, plastics, dyes used in leather, pesticides and other garden chemicals.

What your doctor can do

- Skin patch testing will help to identify the cause of the dermatitis. This is particularly important when employment is affected.
- Avoidance is always important and can not only resolve the problem but may after several years lead to a clearing of the sensitivity.
- Steroid creams are useful for severe acute episodes.

What you can do

- Make sure that your skin is as healthy as possible, as a dry, cracked or broken skin makes it easier for contact allergies to develop.
- Use cotton-lined rubber gloves when doing the dishes, or when your hands are in water.
- Use hypoallergenic soaps and cosmetics and wash your clothes in non-biological washing powder or liquid.
- A healthy diet and supplements of multi-vitamins and zinc might be useful if the skin is particularly poor quality, and you do not eat as well as you might.
- Supplements of evening primrose oil are worth considering if your skin is very dry.

Complementary therapies

These may not be very successful as the cause really needs to be addressed, and this is usually physical. Herbal treatments may be worth considering.

Dermatitis (Seborrhoeic)

This is a red, greasy, scaly dermatitis which develops usually on the face, especially around the sides of the nose and the ears, on the front of the chest or at the back between the shoulder blades. Dandruff, eyebrow and even eyelid scaling can also develop. Mild forms of this are often referred to as 'combination skin', with some parts of the face being greasy and others dry and scaly. In some cases the rash is worsened, possibly caused by the presence of a superficial yeast infection with *Pityrosporum ovale*. Anti-fungal treatments can be very effective.

What your doctor can do

- Ointments based either on mild steroids or salicylic acid can be used on the face and trunk.
- An ointment of lithium and zinc (Efalith) can be quite effective.
- Scalp scaling can respond to tar-based shampoos, and antifungal shampoos (Nizoral).
- Anti-fungal creams are sometimes helpful.

What you can do

In certain deficiency states, very similar skin problems develop. This applies to deficiencies of vitamin B (especially pyridoxine, B6, riboflavin, B2, and biotin) as well as zinc. So try the following:

- Eat The Very Nutritious Diet (see page 437).
- Take a strong vitamin B supplement providing 50 mg of B6 and B2, a supplement of biotin, at least 300 mcg per day, and 30 mg of zinc.
- Sunbathe. This sometimes helps.
- Try using some plant oil extracts, some of which come as shampoos, as these may have anti-scaling and anti-fungal properties. Tea tree oil and juniper berry are two suggestions.
- Possibly try dietary exclusion. Probably only worth considering as a last resort or if there is an element of eczema present as well. True sensitivity to yeast does seem particularly likely if there is facial eczema.

Complementary therapies

Try homeopathy and herbalism. Some plants and plant oil preparations could have anti-fungal activity and be quite effective.

Raylene's story

Raylene looked every year of her 48. Her red puffy face was covered by a fine, dry, scaly rash. This was bad enough, but it was her severe scalp scaling that really troubled her. Scalp irritation had been unrelieved by many types of shampoo, nor even a steroid scalp application. The cause of the rash was unclear. It had possibly been triggered by a reaction to a hairdye applied six months earlier, but this did not explain why it was persisting so severely. She had been under considerable stress over the past year and as a consequence had been smoking 20–25 cigarettes daily, and drinking perhaps up to 20 units per week.

The failure of her scalp and skin conditions to respond to more standard treatment suggested that there may have been an untackled nutritional cause. Investigations revealed evidence of moderate deficiency of the vitamin biotin and there were reduced levels of some of the essential fatty acids derived from vegetable and fish oils.

She was asked to halve her cigarette and alcohol consumption, eat a healthier diet and to take supplements of high strength vitamin B with biotin, together with evening primrose oil and fish oil.

The response was gratifying. Over six weeks her scalp irritation diminished considerably, the rash on her face and scalp scaling improved markedly. Over the next three months the transformation was nearly complete.

On reflection it was felt that her increased alcohol intake had placed a great strain on vitamin B metabolism that had cost her her previously good complexion.

It is interesting that how in the development of a deficiency the body will probably, quite correctly 'sacrifice' the nutrient levels in the skin before other parts of the body are affected. This has good survival potential for vital organs such as the liver, kidneys and brain, but does mean we become less beautiful. At least this gives us some outward sign that all is not well internally.

Diabetes Mellitus

The term diabetes, used without qualification, is taken to mean diabetes mellitus. In this condition there is a chronic rise in the level of glucose in the blood which routinely spills out into the urine. This gives the condition its name: diabetes meaning 'a flowing through' and mellitus 'sweet'. Thus the urine is passed in excessive amounts because the high level of sugar in the urine pulls water along with it. Thus the typical presenting symptoms are:

- increased passage of urine
- increased thirst
- a craving for sweet foods
- fatigue due to the effects of this upon the body's metabolism.

Other features include changes in visual acuity, recurrent thrush, muscle cramps, tingling in the feet and hands and constipation.

Blood glucose levels are controlled by what we eat, a careful balance of two primary hormones, insulin and glucagon, and the function of the liver and muscles. In medicine there are in fact a wide variety of situations, many of which are rare, where blood glucose control is disturbed. Understandably this happens with liver and muscle disorders and a number of exotic hormonal conditions, as well as in some pregnancies.

The most important hormone in blood glucose control is insulin, which is produced by alpha cells in the pancreas, a gland situated in the abdomen. The role of insulin is to help glucose pass from the bloodstream into cells, especially the nervous system, muscles and the liver, and increases entry of glucose into insulin sensitive cells. Insulin also binds glucose with phosphorous turning it into glucose-6-phosphate – the form in which it is used in the cells and prevents it from leaving. Glucagon has an opposing effect, releasing glucose from the cells when blood sugar levels are low. To all these organs glucose is a source of energy, and uniquely for the nervous system it is the only source of energy that it can use. When glucose is not available it has to call on other sources of fuel, primarily fats and proteins. This can lead to complications in the long term, so it is important to control blood-sugar levels through life-long healthy eating.

Insulin does not affect insulin insensitive cells. Some tissues allow free access of glucose by diffusion, including the eyes, liver, kidney, brain and intestine wall. These tissues are liable to damage in poorly controlled diabetes. Glucose enters the cells and is converted into fructose, then to an insoluble sugar, sorbitol which cystallises, increasing the risk of cataracts.

Diabetes used to be simply divided into two main types – insulin dependent (IDDM) and non-insulin dependent (NIDDM). In the insulin-dependent variety there is a lack of the hormone which must then be given by injection. In the non-insulin dependent form there is plenty of insulin or related forms of the hormone, but the tissues of the body are relatively insensitive to it. This type does not need insulin but a diet and drugs that improve the body's response to insulin.

There is now a more complicated classification based upon not only the need for insulin but the probable cause(s) of that type of diabetes.

What causes it?

This is one of the great questions of twentieth-century medicine, and it is being answered in a curiously piecemeal way. The pieces of the jigsaw include:

- Genetic factors, which are particularly important for the insulin-dependent diabetic. It is predominantly a disease of Caucasians, but not exclusively from the northern parts of Europe. There are many environmental factors too: if members of a low-risk population, such as the Japanese, emigrate to a high-risk country like the USA, their risk pattern follows that of USA residents.
- Genetic factors also appear for the non-insulin dependent diabetic. This, usually the adult onset form of diabetes, seems to run in the female line of the family, may be linked with other conditions affecting muscles, and also with a tendency to high blood pressure and raised blood fats.
- Immune changes causing the body to produce antibodies that attack the insulin-producing alpha cells in the pancreas. This may be genetically determined and triggered by some viral infections.
- Food allergy! This is a possibility, as some researchers report that the antibodies involved in cow's milk allergy can also react against the insulin producing alpha cells in the pancreas. This seems particularly relevant to children. Cow's milk should be avoided until a baby is at least a year old.
- Being overweight is an extremely important risk factor especially for the elderly with NIDDM.
- Smoking in some studies slightly increases the risk of NIDDM.
- Being small at birth has also been shown to be a risk factor, perhaps reflecting a reduced ability to produce insulin in a form that is

functional. This risk does not appear until later life, and can become marked if the individual is obese, has high blood pressure and elevated blood fats.

- In association with various types of malnutrition in third world countries.
- In association with a number of other hormonal problems affecting the adrenal glands, the ovaries (see Polycystic Ovaries, page 368).
- Rare genetic disorders.
- Triggering incident including viral conditions like mumps.
- Following drug therapy especially thiazide diuretics if deficient in potassium.
- In pregnancy resulting in the birth of a large baby.
- Another theory as to the cause of NIDDM suggests that a high fat and sugar diet reduces the 'friendly' bifidobacteria, allowing E. coli, a harmful strain of bacteria to proliferate. E. coli produces an insulin-like substance, which it is suggested may block the insulin receptor cells, producing adult onset diabetes, in spite of normal insulin production.

This is a fantastically diverse list. In practice, for the majority of those with, or at risk of developing, diabetes, dietary factors are the most important area that we can do something about on an individual level.

In 1917, John Harvey Kellogg wrote about the role of the soybean in the control of diabetes. At about the same time two researchers with an interest in soybeans, published a paper in the *American Journal of Medical Science*, which outlined how diabetic patients who consumed soybeans regularly, passed less sugar in their urine; a marker for the control of diabetes. There has been more recent interest in the role of soy fibre and the control of diabetes, as this fibre, which helps to control cholesterol levels, also seems to be able to regulate glucose levels, and helps with insulin sensitivity. The high-fibre diet, consisting of oats, fruit, vegetables, and legumes including soya, appears to help the cells of the Type II diabetic to recognise insulin, and thus allow entry into the cell.

In 1987, a study published in the *American Journal of Clinical Nutrition*, compared using 10 grams of soy fibre at one meal, and then none at another sitting of the same meal. They discovered that when soy was included in the diet the blood glucose levels rose and fell at normal rates, compared to the non-soy sittings whose blood glucose rose to higher than normal levels, and stayed there for longer than usual periods. Another study used just 7 grams of soya and compared it to cellulose, the insoluble fibre found in wheat bran and vegetables. For the three hours following the meal, the soya consumers had notably lower levels of glucose in their bloodstream compared to those who had consumed cellulose.

Furthermore, it seems that not only does soy have benefits for blood sugar control and heart health, but kidney health as well. This is very important for people with diabetes, since nearly one-third of them develop renal disease.

Diabetic renal disease (nephropathy) is a major contributor to death in those with diabetes, mainly from end stage renal disease and cardiovascular disease. Nephropathy is damage to the tiny nephrons in the kidney, which act like tiny little filters. As a result of this damage, protein is filtered into the urine instead of being reabsorbed back into the bloodstream. This is a condition called microalbuminuria. The likelihood of nephropathy increases significantly after having diabetes for ten or more years. Early stages of nephropathy are an increase in protein leaking into the urine and an increased workload on the kidneys. Too much dietary protein can cause a faster decline in kidney function. However, it seems that not all proteins are created equal as recent research suggests that soy protein may be relatively protective for kidney health.

Research by the University of Kentucky presented at the 3rd International Symposium on the Role of Soy in Preventing and Treating Chronic Disease (1999) showed that changes in blood flow to the kidney following various protein meals was found to be greatest with beef, followed by poultry and fish. Soy protein does not significantly alter kidney function following a meal which is good news. Other work by Professor Anderson in a group of six patients with Type I diabetes, who have early signs of kidney damage, shows that soy may help conserve kidney health. Patients ate 55 gms of soy protein per day via a soy patty, soy beverage and soy pasta for eight weeks, then resumed their normal animal protein intake. After eating soy protein for eight weeks, these patients showed evidence of a decreased workload on their kidneys compared with that on their normal diet. Two patients who were previously losing protein in their urine also lowered the amount lost after the eight weeks of soy protein. Furthermore the average reduction in total cholesterol and LDL (bad cholesterol) cholesterol were 7 per cent and 13 per cent respectively. This is a highly positive outcome in reducing the risk of further health problems such as heart disease. This small study suggests that soy may be preventative for the early stages of diabetes, as well as the obvious heart health benefits.

Sally's story

Sally is a 24-year-old waitress who has been diabetic since puberty. She has also had a history of repeated viral infections, including meningitis and shingles, and there was a strong suspicion that a virus infection had triggered her diabetes. Once, before attending the clinic, she had another viral infection that was just a bout of flu, which left her feeling very tired indeed, so that she had to give up work. Her diabetic control had deteriorated and she had made several attempts to improve this by adjusting her dose of insulin.

Her fatigue every day was quite severe, with muscular aches and pains, and the diabetic specialist discovered that the sodium level in her blood was very low. Investigations also revealed low levels of many other nutrients, especially magnesium, zinc, and vitamin B.

She made some changes to her diet, took supplements of all of these nutrients, except for sodium, and also took a multi-vitamin preparation. Her energy level duly improved, as did her diabetic control. Low levels of magnesium are common in diabetes and may influence the balance of other minerals, especially sodium and potassium.

What your doctor can do

- *Make the diagnosis using blood and urine tests* Sometimes this is easy if there are large amounts of sugar in the urine or blood. The presence of ketones in the urine detected by a simple dip test means that insulin will need to be given.
- *Treat with insulin* This is necessary for the majority of young patients where the diabetes is due to a lack of insulin from the pancreas. There are a variety of different types of insulin and varying treatment regimes which may need to be adjusted to suit a person's lifestyle. Injections several times per day are usually required. Minute pumps that provide insulin on a continuous basis rather like the human pancreas are being developed.
- *Treat with drugs* There are two types of drug which are most suited to older patients where there is a supply of insulin but the tissues are relatively insensitive to it. One type, the sulphonylureas, act by increasing the amount of insulin released and is the main type used. The second, biguanides, are usually used in conjunction with the sulphonylureas and they act by altering the metabolism of glucose in the liver and other organs. Both are always used when diet alone has not worked.
- *Advice on diet* This has assumed increased importance over the years. It is clear that the control of blood glucose, the risk of serious and less serious complications, are to a large degree influenced by the diet. The standard recommendations are as follows:
  - Eat an appropriate amount of calories to achieve a reasonable weight. For most NIDDM patients this will mean losing weight. This may well be all that is required to normalise blood glucose levels.

- ○ Eat regularly. Consume three meals a day and where necessary snacks between meals. These are likely to be needed by children, those who are physically active, and pregnant women provided they are not overweight.
- Ensure a regular intake of phytoestrogens in your diet, in the form of soya products: milk, tofu and pulses, cereals and seeds.
- The diet should contain a large quantity of foods that are digested slowly and therefore cause only a small rise in blood sugar. This means excluding or severely limiting the consumption of sugar, cakes, biscuits, white, and to a lesser extent, wholemeal bread. Desirable foods are beans, peas, lentils, pasta, oats and oat products, whole-wheat cereals, sweetcorn and most fruits.
- High-fat foods are to be limited. Intake of saturated fats in particular should be curbed. This means consuming low-fat dairy products including low-fat cheeses, trimming all visible fat from meat before cooking (by grilling or baking), not eating the skin of poultry and fish and not eating fried foods.
- Suitable oils for cooking are those high in polyunsaturates, e.g. sunflower, safflower, corn and soya. Olive oil can be used in small amounts as can walnut oil. Butter should not normally be used and margarines high in polyunsaturates used in their place.
- High-cholesterol foods should also be limited, especially if the blood fats are high. Up to eight eggs per week can be consumed.
- Further dietary advice may well be needed for those with heart disease, kidney disease, in pregnancy or if the diabetes is particularly difficult to control.
- It is vital to monitor your progress. Regular attendance at a clinic based either at your general practitioner or at the local hospital will allow the early identification of problems and their treatment. These checks involve measurement of:
  - ○ weight
  - ○ blood pressure
  - ○ measurement of glycated haemoglobin which gives a good long-term measure of blood glucose control
  - ○ examination of the urine for sugar, protein and blood
  - ○ examination of the eyes for blood vessel changes
  - ○ examination of the heart, occasional checks on blood cholesterol and triglycerides
  - ○ examination of the feet to check circulation and nerve function.

These measures need to be looked at alongside your measures of progress in order to get the full picture.

- *Treat complications* as they occur, but hopefully at an early stage. Changes in the eyes, kidneys, nerves, blood vessels affecting circulation to the heart, feet and brain are all possible and may respond to treatment with drugs, surgery or better diabetic control.

- *Tackle special situations* such as infection, surgery, pregnancy and coma. These often require the services and expertise of several specialists in a hospital setting.

What you can do

- *Learn all about your diabetes* Join the British Diabetic Association. Be a professional patient.
- *Monitor your diabetes* This means regular, usually daily, tests of blood sugar for all those with IDDM, urine tests of sugar and sometimes protein. The intention is to keep the blood sugar level between 4 and 9 millimols/l, though this may vary from person to person. There should be no glucose in the urine if kidney function is normal.
- *Be strict with your diet* The high intake of beans may cause an increase in abdominal wind and bloating. Be patient, this should settle after two or three months. Ask your partner to be considerate too.
- *Control blood sugar levels* by eating low glycaemic index (GI) foods where sugar release is slower (see Glycaemic Index on page 172). Foods include wholegrains, pulses and fresh fruit and vegetables. Avoid high GI foods like white bread, rice, pasta and some fruits.
- A 2:1 balance of complex carbohydrates to protein may also facilitate a slower release of sugar and stimulate less insulin and more glucagon production.
- Small frequent meals maintain a lower, steady blood sugar level, decreasing the need for insulin.
- Essential fatty acids (EFAs) in the form of oily fish, and unsalted nuts and seeds increase cell membrane fluidity and sensitivity of the receptor sites, thus increasing the effectiveness of insulin. They may also reduce the risk of developing problems with the blood vessels and the back of the eyes. Fish oil might be beneficial too in reducing blood stickiness, but there could be a problem with this.
- Excess saturated fat from full fat dairy products and meat in the diet blocks EFA mechanisms and reduces the response of blood sugar levels to insulin.
- Excess sugar and saturated fat may lower bifidobacteria allowing E.coli to proliferate.
- Eating sufficient fibre in the form of fresh fruit and vegetables and wholegrains produces short chain fatty acids (SCFAs) which are necessary for healthy gut flora, raising bifidobacteria levels lowering E.coli.

Glycaemic Index Chart

Low		Intermediate		High	
Apple	38	Apricots	57	Bagel	74
Buckwheat	54	Wholemeal bread	69	Cornflakes	84
Butter beans	31	Couscous	65	Puffed wheat	80
Lentils	30	Sweetcorn	55	Corn chips	72
Orange	44	Pineapple	66	Potatoes	75
Pasta	55	Sweet potato	54	Watermelon	72
Pear	38	Raisins	64	Pumpernickel	80
Porridge	46	White bread	70	French bread	96
Rice bran	46	Oat bran	55	Rye bread	76
Skimmed milk	32	Digestive biscuit	59	White rice	87
Yogurt	33	Banana	55	Brown rice	76
Soya beans	14	Basmati rice	58	Parsnips	97

Research on the glycaemic index (what we call the GI factor) shows that different carbohydrates have different effects on blood sugar levels. There is a misconception that complex carbohydrates such as potatoes, wholemeal pasta and bread are broken down into sugar slowly, thus stabilising blood sugar. However, French bread has nearly the same effect on blood sugar levels as pure glucose!

Carbohydrate foods that break down quickly during digestion have the highest GI factor. Conversely, carbohydrates which break down slowly, releasing glucose gradually into the bloodstream have a low GI factor.

GI Scores

Low GI	less than 55
Intermediate GI	55 to 70
High GI	more than 70

Pure glucose produces the greatest rise in blood sugar levels. The GI is set at 100 and every other food is ranked on a scale from 0 to 100 according to its actual effect on blood sugar levels.

- *Exercise regularly* This helps keep weight down, reduces blood cholesterol, lowers blood pressure and may improve blood glucose control. The minimum is to walk for 30 minutes four times per week.
- *Don't smoke.*
- *Limit alcohol intake* This should be kept to an average of no more than two units per day, with up to four units on special occasions.
- *Be aware of hypoglycaemia* This is low blood sugar and could be dangerous! Symptoms include light-headedness, confusion, anxiety feelings, palpitations, hunger, shortness of breath and sweating.

Unfortunately some diabetics have little warning of these episodes and loss of consciousness develops quickly. This is very important if they are driving or in charge of machinery.

- *Take some nutritional supplements* This is a very difficult but potentially important area. There are many small reports that patients with diabetes especially if present for many years, if there is a poor response to insulin, in older diabetics or those with complications may lack a variety of essential nutrients. This lack may not be corrected by a standard diabetic diet.

Potentially important nutrients are:

- *Vitamin B1* Thiamine is needed to metabolise glucose. Those first beginning on oral medication, consumers of alcohol and the elderly are at risk. Fatigue, muscle pains in the legs and loss of feeling in the hands and feet are early symptoms.
- *Magnesium* Lack may develop with vitamin B1 deficiency, especially if the diet is poor. Lack of response to insulin and increased risk of damage to the blood vessels at the back of the eye can be features of a lack of this nutrient.
- *Chromium* This is a curious trace element worthy of a particular mention in diabetes. It is involved in influencing the tissues response to insulin which is clearly important in the elderly diabetic with NIDDM. So much so that marked chromium deficiency produces a state virtually indistinguishable from this type of diabetes and is also associated with an increased risk of cardiovascular disease. Potentially correcting a deficiency of this trace mineral could be beneficial to many diabetics. We will have to wait for more research to be performed to be certain about the role of chromium.
- *Glucose Tolerance Factor (GTF)* GTF contains chromium together with niacin, and amino-acids, and is believed to aid insulin entry to cells at the receptor sites. It is thought to be made by either liver or gut bacteria.
- *Zinc* This is easily lost in the urine in diabetics. Poor resistance to infection, poor wound healing and possibly reduced response to insulin may be features. Zinc is required for insulin production.
- *Vitamin B6* Pyridoxine has been used successfully to help control the diabetes that develops in pregnancy. Vitamin B6, in conjunction with zinc, is required for insulin production.
- *Vitamin B3* Niacin prolongs the life of the insulin producing alpha cells in the pancreas, and is a component of Glucose Tolerance Factor.
- *Antioxidants* These include vitamins E, C, A as beta-carotene and selenium, and they are all involved in minimising the damage to tissue that occurs as a part of ageing or with an altered metabolism. They may prove to be important in the progress of vascular disease, heart disease and cataract formation in the diabetic.

NB diabetics may not be very efficient at converting beta-carotene into vitamin A (retinol) in the body so a vitamin A supplement may be considered if needed.

Expert advice and individual assessment would seem the best way forward until there are large and long-term trials to assess the benefits of using these types of supplements. It should be remembered that they are no substitute for good dietary control and, where necessary, insulin and drug treatment.

> Do not take vitamin and mineral supplements, except perhaps for low-dose preparations, without the permission of your doctor. At times their use could alter insulin requirements and blood glucose control. Hypoglycaemia, a low blood glucose, could occur as a result.

Complementary therapies

There is no substitute for standard care. Some homeopathic remedies are reputed to affect blood glucose control but you need to see a medically qualified practitioner, especially if you are taking insulin. Acupuncture could be helpful when there are problems with the nerves, especially in the legs.

See also: References.

Diarrhoea

Symptoms of diarrhoea are frequent or loose stools. 'Frequent' means having more than three motions per day, and 'loose' means that the stools are not formed, and vary from a soft putty consistency to watery. Diarrhoea mainly occurs because food has moved too quickly through the gut, and there has not been time for the water in the bowel to be absorbed.

What are the symptoms?

Diarrhoea is usually associated with an urgency to go to the toilet, and is often proceeded by pain or waves of muscle contractions, often influenced by our diet or the environment. Most of us will have experienced pre-exam nerves, and had to rush off to the toilet. Some sufferers may not experience any pain before an episode, and in these cases there seems to be relatively little bowel muscle activity. The diarrhoea can therefore be due to over-sensitive bowel muscles or to the contents of the bowel irritating the bowel in some way. The gut transit time is increased in diarrhoea sufferers from the usual 48–72 hours to a mere 24 hours. Experiencing these symptoms every day may well leave the sufferer feeling washed out and nutritionally deficient.

Who gets it?

There is no age limit for diarrhoea. Young children sometimes have persistent symptoms which are often linked to food allergies. Adults may suffer similarly, or notice that symptoms of diarrhoea follow a bout of gastroenteritis or food poisoning. It is not as common as constipation, but still widely experienced by women, especially around the onset of a period, when there is a brief release of inflammatory chemicals as the uterus sheds its lining. Long-term symptoms should undoubtedly be investigated by your doctor, especially if self-help measures fail.

What causes it?

- *Food intolerance* This is often the underlying reason for diarrhoea, which can occur at any stage in life, particularly following stress or trauma, when the immune system is impaired.
- *Milk* Some people, especially children and infants, may react to the protein in milk and this can cause abdominal pain (colic in an infant) and sometimes diarrhoea. Drinking semi-skimmed or skimmed milk won't usually make a difference, as this only reduces the fat content, not the protein or milk sugar. Other signs of allergy that may be present are eczema, asthma or rhinitis.
- *Lactose* Milk sugar can sometimes cause problems. If there is an inability to digest lactose, then sugar passes into the small bowel and colon, where it acts as a potent laxative. The severely affected sufferer would be troubled with symptoms within an hour of consuming milk or soft cheese, although small amounts of hard cheese or milk itself may be tolerated. This type of food intolerance is quite common in those of Eastern European, Middle Eastern or Asian origin.

    People who are truly lactose intolerant may be able to tolerate lactose-free milk, which is available in some supermarkets; hard cheeses, as they contain relatively small amounts of lactose; and be helped by adding Lactaid (available from the chemists and health-food shops) to ordinary milk. A few drops of this preparation helps break down lactose into two component sugars, glucose and galactose, which are easily absorbed without causing diarrhoea.
- *Wheat and other grains* Sensitivity to wheat, oats, barley and rye has been recorded as a cause of diarrhoea, especially in women. It seems that very sensitive individuals do react to wheat which can cause some minor but definite damage to the lining of the gut resulting in

diarrhoea. This situation is similar to, but not so severe as, coeliac disease. This is by no means accepted as conventional medical wisdom, even though a group of ten such patients were described as long ago as 1980 by one leading group of gastroenterologists from Birmingham in the UK.

- *Eating a large meal* When the stomach becomes distended a reflex contraction of the muscles of the colon occurs which is known as the gastro-colic reflex. This explains why many people need to empty their bowels within an hour of having a large meal. It is not the meal we have just eaten coming through, but probably the meal of the day before moving on.

- *Fatty foods, too much and too little* When fat remains undigested in the small bowel it can be broken down into irritating acids by bacteria in the large bowel, which again can result in diarrhoea a few hours after eating a large or rich meal. This is most evident in those with digestive problems, and in the elderly, especially if there is weight loss.

   At the other end of the scale, fat in smaller quantities actually slows down the rate at which the stomach empties and food moves along the small bowel. As it takes time to digest fat from a meal, the gut may become sensitive to its presence. Certain foods containing oleic acid, such as olive oil, almonds, hazel nuts, Brazil nuts and avocado pears, are particular offenders. The low-fat theory may explain why toddlers and children who consume low-fat cow's milk products suffer with diarrhoea, and are more prone to acute gastroenteritis.

- *Coffee* This, unfortunately, is an excellent bowel stimulant. Both ordinary varieties and decaffeinated coffee can have the same effect on the gut. It stimulates a wave of contractions through the bowel, and whilst it is a useful tool for constipation sufferers, it should be avoided by those suffering with diarrhoea.

- *Hot drinks* These may also stimulate a wave of contractions through the bowel. If you enjoy hot drinks, leave them to cool a little first.

- *Artificial sweeteners* Sorbitol, an artificial sugar that cannot be digested, can cause diarrhoea. It is used in some 'sugarfree' chewing gums, sweets and mints. As it passes through the gut it attracts water in the same way that mineral laxatives do.

- *Spicy foods* These can have a laxative effect on some people as presumably they irritate the bowel. In others it seems that both red chilli pepper and cayenne pepper actually slow the rate at which food passes through the small bowel, allowing more time for digestion. This one is down to individual observations.

- *Smoking cigarettes* This can increase the contraction of the gut in sensitive individuals. For many a cup of coffee and a cigarette is their way of stimulating their gut into action, and thus is good for constipation.

- *Alcohol* Alcohol is only likely to cause diarrhoea in those who drink excessively, and if you fall into that category, you will have already discovered why you should be reducing your consumption from the advice on page 8.

What your doctor can do

If you have not already consulted your doctor about your diarrhoea, and it has persisted for some time, then you need to make an appointment, especially if you have lost weight, are aged over 50, or if the self-help tips that follow do not help.

- *Examination and investigations* These will look for a cause of the diarrhoea, and assess the likelihood of nutritional deficiencies. Blood tests for anaemia and measurement of vitamin B, iron and zinc are now widely available.
- *X-ray of the bowel* This is done using a barium meal or barium enema. Barium is a heavy mineral liquid which shows up as dense white on x-ray and allows a good impression of the bowel and its lining to be obtained.
- *Endoscopy of the bowel* This involves passing a sophisticated flexible telescope through the upper and lower gut in order to inspect the bowel lining for inflammation. Samples or biopsies from the gut lining can also be taken for further examination.
- *Arrange for a stool examination* This would show up parasite infections, blood in the stool or undigested fats. If the diarrhoea is due to poor digestion, and difficulty digesting fat, excesses of fat may be discovered in your stool, which if untreated might lead to nutritional deficiencies.
- *Prescribe a drug* Loperamide (Motilin) slows the passage of material along the gut, increases the amount of water absorbed by the gut and increases the tone of the anal muscles. Codeine phosphate is an old-fashioned drug derived from opium, which if taken in small doses, is relatively free from side-effects. Sodium cromoglycate (Nalcrom capsules) is an anti-allergy preparation used in spray form in the treatment of asthma. It can also be used in the form of capsules taken by mouth for those with true food allergies. One trial in Australia found that it also benefitted ten out of 20 patients with diarrhoea due to irritable bowel syndrome, in whom food allergy had not originally been suspected. This preparation is worth considering as it has very few side-effects, but it is expensive, although available on the NHS in the UK.
- *Prescribe a vitamin supplement* Certain nutritional deficiencies can occur in association with diarrhoea as the gut transit time is so fast the body does not have a chance to digest or absorb the nutrients. It may

be appropriate for your doctor to prescribe strong vitamin B complex or multi-vitamins, depending on the results of your investigations. Some standard UK NHS vitamin B and multi-vitamin preparations are not strong enough for the correction of severe nutritional deficiencies.

What you can do

- Consider avoiding wheat, oats, barley and rye.
- Consider avoiding milk, yoghurt, cream and cheese. Other foods containing these or lactose (milk sugar) should also be avoided.
- Eat moderate-sized meals and eat every two to three hours. This will prevent overburdening your digestive system.
- Eat slowly and chew your food well. This may give your stomach and digestive system a much better chance to digest food properly.
- Adjust your fat intake. It is a good idea for many to ensure that there is a moderate amount of fat in each main meal.
- Stop or reduce your intake of coffee. Both ordinary and decaffeinated can cause diarrhoea. Consider drinking ordinary tea instead, as this can slow the passage of food through the gut in about 50 per cent of people. Cut down on hot drinks generally if you think that they make symptoms worse.
- Avoid excessive use of the artificial sweetener Sorbitol. Watch out for 'sugarfree' chewing gum and mints that contain Sorbitol.
- Avoid spicy foods, if they upset you. In theory taking large amounts of chilli and other hot spices might slow the gut down and help prevent diarrhoea.
- Reduce or stop smoking. Try to pace yourself between cigarettes so that you gradually smoke fewer each day.
- Reduce or stop drinking alcohol. Try to cut down to no more than three drinks per week initially.
- Change drug therapy. If you suspect that a drug you are taking might be causing your diarrhoea, discuss this with your doctor or specialist. A change of drug therapy may be necessary.
- Take some strong yeast-free vitamin B complex. Those with a high alcohol intake or experience diarrhoea following antibiotic usage or following gastroenteritis are particularly likely to benefit. A dose providing 50–100 mg of most of the B vitamins, including vitamin B3 or nicotinamide, is recommended as a daily dose. This should not be taken without your doctor's approval if you are known to be anaemic, have recently lost weight or have had stomach or bowel surgery.
- Essential fatty acids (EFAs) can assist with healthy stool formation. Take a supplement containing evening primrose oil and marine fish oil for the best results.
- Take a probiotic supplement of acidophillus or lactobacillus bifidus to

repopulate the colon with 'friendly' bacteria which is often disturbed in cases of severe diarrhoea. Probiotic supplements are in fact routinely prescribed to travellers to exotic countries where they are susceptible to food poisoning, parasites and diarrhoea.

- Slippery elm bark as tea or in extract form is soothing to the digestive tract.
- Drink plenty of fluids, preferably water to replenish the body as long term diarrhoea is likely to result in dehydration and mineral loss, especially of the minerals sodium, potassium and magnesium.
- Avoid stress. Take steps to cope with stress, and avoid stressful situations if you can (see page 25).

If these tips are going to help you should notice some improvement within four weeks. If this is not the case, then you should check with your doctor.

Complementary therapies

Doctors have used hypnotherapy to assist with bowel problems with reasonably good results. It is worth having a session of hypnotherapy if you are a severe sufferer, or alternatively master the art of self-hypnosis to see whether this works for you. Acupuncture is very good at slowing down a rapid metabolism by addressing the root cause, and a herbal medicine practitioner will mix you a potion to try. Both of these avenues are well worth exploring.

See also: Irritable bowel syndrome, Coeliac disease, References, The simple exclusion diet or The strict exclusion diet.

Eating Disorders

A Gallup Poll published in January 1996 found that 28 per cent of men think they are 'a little bit overweight' and 6 per cent thought they were 'a lot overweight'. In total 34 per cent were dissatisfied with their weight, and that figure rises to 44 per cent for women.

Some 30 per cent of the Gallup sample were attempting to diet. More than half claimed to try a diet at least once a year; 41 per cent admitted the pounds piled on again pretty quickly. Some 79 per cent of the men said they went on a diet for health reasons; only 14 per cent admitted it was to improve their appearance. But, 61 per cent of women said they dieted to look better, with 37 per cent saying it was on health grounds.

The poll went on to confirm all our fears that it's the skinny bird that gets the worm. Most men prefer the slenderness of the supermodel to a plumper woman: 43 per cent of men prefer the thin silhouette and, more sadly, 48 per cent of women do, too. The poll also asked people to rate their own appearance, and 17 per cent rated themselves poorly, while only 9 per cent of the interviewees agreed with their rating – an example of poor self-image. Bearing in mind that women were far more critical of their own appearance, it's hardly surprising that large numbers of people suffer with eating disorders.

Women often downgrade themselves and think of themselves as far fatter than their friends. They see themselves out of focus, which perhaps accounts for why the anorexic can't perceive how painfully thin she actually is. The media and the fashion industry have been blamed for placing unrealistic goals upon people when it comes to weight and body shape. A Health Education Authority report in the UK in March 1996 highlighted fears about children as young as eleven, 50 per cent of the girls and one-third of the boys, having major anxieties about their weight and body image. Twice as many girls as boys wanted to lose weight and the researchers said the desire to be slim was influenced by images of the supermodels. Failure to live up to the image resulted in low self-confidence and self esteem.

The National Food Alliance, in February 1996, published a new report on slimming advertising which found 88 per cent of slimming aid and product adverts in women's magazines, slimming and teen magazines and papers breached advertising rules. Most omitted to state they could not aid slimming except as part of a calorie-controlled diet, and many made unsubstantiated 'miracle' claims, failing to state the time period over which weight could be lost. It is actually illegal to promote any slimming aids to the under-eighteens anyway, but this seems to be disregarded if the adverts in the teen magazines are anything to go by.

A report in *Labour Research* in March 1966 also commented that although the diet industry is aimed mainly at women, (50 per cent of whom are dieting at any given time and 90 per cent of whom will at some time in their lives), the board of directors of the companies are almost entirely men. They looked at twelve of the major companies in three main sectors of the industry – food and drink, magazines and slimming clubs. Of the 77 directors only four were women. At eight of the companies there were no women on the board at all. The meal-replacement market alone (products like Slimfast) was estimated to be worth £88 million in 1994. There are 5,000 Weightwatchers clubs in the UK with some 150,000 members – and Weightwatchers is run by Heinz, which also produces diet foods. There are some 1,000 Rosemary Conley Diet and Fitness Clubs and 560 *Slimming* Magazine Clubs. Yet there is plenty of new evidence to suggest that dieting makes you fat – the yo-yo syndrome.

According to the politician Tessa Jowell, the number of children being treated by the National Health Service for eating disorders is 5,000, with some as young as eight dieting because they think they are too fat.

Eating disorders can be broadly divided into two groups, anorexia nervosa and bulimia nervosa. Both are conditions found predominantly in women aged between ten and 40 years, and are seen particularly amongst those of middle-class origins. Both conditions can be regarded as diseases of 'society' as much as they are diseases of the individual.

ANOREXIA NERVOSA

Anorexia nervosa has three main features:

- Very low body weight, usually at least 15 per cent below the expected weight.
- Disordered attitude towards body weight. Despite their thinness, the individual considers they are overweight, or still needing to lose weight, in order to achieve a better shape. This disturbed thinking underpins the methods achieved to lose weight which may include fasting, exercise, self-induced vomiting and laxative abuse.
- Absence of periods in women who would normally be expected to menstruate, and who are not taking the oral contraceptive pill.

Other common co-existing features of anorexia include:

- depression
- mood swings
- obsessive behaviour
- thoughts of suicide
- limited outside interests
- being socially withdrawn
- disturbed relationships with parents
- as well as physical characteristics of malnutrition.

Physical features may include:

- muscle wasting
- abdominal bloating
- scalp hair loss
- a development of fine downy hair over the body – lanugo
- dry skin
- poor circulation in the hands and feet.

There are a number of secondary hormonal changes which are mild and reversible. These include changes in pituitary and thyroid hormone in particular. Mild anaemia, raised blood cholesterol and disturbances in the balance of certain minerals may also be present.

Laxative or diuretic use can lead to loss of potassium and magnesium in particular. Interestingly, delayed emptying of the stomach and delayed bowel transit times leading to constipation are present. These features may lead to the complaint of fullness after eating only small amounts of food. If untreated severe malnutrition may develop bringing irrevocable damage to organs, and in severe cases girls become so ill they die.

What your doctor can do

Usually people with anorexia nervosa do not present themselves for treatment. Invariably they are forced to do so by concerned parents or friends. All anorexics (and bulimics) require psychological treatment as well as nutritional support. The doctor must:

- Establish a rapport and relationship with the sufferer and family members and friends. This is a vital first step.
- Weigh the sufferer and test her blood for anaemia and mineral and vitamin deficiencies.
- Search for predisposing factors and explore the anorexic's perception of stress factors that may have contributed to depression and disordered eating habits. This may include being overweight in the past and needing to diet, relationships with boyfriend or partner, work or domestic stresses.
- Aim to educate about the dangers of low body weight. Explaining that nutritional deficiencies may influence mood and energy level, that hormonal disturbances may prejudice chances of fertility in the future and predispose to osteoporosis, may all be ways of promoting the patient's understanding and cooperation.
- Work to improve the anorexic's perception of her wellbeing and examine the stress factors that she perceives as playing a role in her condition.
- Consider in- or out-patient treatment, with the need for counselling and psychiatric support.
- Decide whether drug treatment is required. This is rarely the case. Anti-depressants are used, but should never be relied upon alone.
- Specialist feeding, feeding by tube or intravenous methods should only be required in the minority of cases who are severely malnourished.

What you can do

- Be prepared to discuss your feelings honestly with the doctor, psychotherapist and family members.
- Acknowledge that there is a physical and mental health problem.
- Attend your doctor or psychotherapist regularly. This may mean daily, or at least weekly, consultations.
- Make a list of those foods you like most and those you dislike. Discuss

this with your therapist who obviously will need to advise you which foods will be the most nutritious and appropriate for you to consume.

- Take some strong multi-vitamin and multi-mineral supplements initially. Other specialist supplements may be required when you get the results of your tests but consider the following:
  - Vitamin B1 – A severe deficiency of this causes a clinical picture indistinguishable from anorexia nervosa, with delayed gastric emptying, loss of appetite, weight loss, fatigue and depression. Supplements of 50 mg per day may be required.
  - Zinc – A deficiency is also reported in anorexia nervosa and correction might improve appetite.
  - Calcium – Supplements are probably prudent in all women with prolonged amenorrhoea. Five hundred to 1,000 mg per day may help minimise the future development of osteoporosis.
  - Even moderate dieting appears to lower brain tryptophan and serotonin levels which are important amino acids for stimulating positive mood and improving eating behaviour and feelings about eating. Supplements in the form of 5-HTP, the precursor of tryptophan can be introduced to influence normal brain function.
  - Anorexics can have essential fatty acid (EFA) deficiencies which explains the physical characteristics of dry skin, hair and hormone changes. EFAs are essential for normal hormone function and if they are severely deficient menstrual irregularities and in the extreme case, amenorrhoea can manifest.
  - Other deficiencies – Deficiency in the other B vitamins, in magnesium or the trace elements, chromium and selenium are all possible in malnourished individuals.
- Reduce your level of exercise if you have been over-exercising obsessively. Aim to restrict your exercise to three or four sessions per week.
- Recognise the support of close family members and friends and try not to be manipulative. Be honest and open with them or you will lose their friendship and support. Treat them as you would wish to be treated yourself.

Complementary therapies

Though none is of proven value, if you feel that one or more of these appeal to you or have been helpful in the past, then consider them now:

- Aromatherapy and massage may help relieve feelings of tension.
- Acupuncture might help balance the body's chemistry or nervous system.
- Some herbal preparations might act as a tonic.

In all these cases a good relationship with the complementary therapist is vital.

BULIMIA NERVOSA

Bulimia nervosa is now the most common eating disorder presented to psychiatrists and psychotherapists. It is not the opposite of anorexia nervosa, rather a variant of it. There seems to have been a genuine and substantial increase in its recognition over the last twenty years. There are three characteristic features:

- Binge episodes with the consumption of a large amount of food, most frequently refined carbohydrates, and usually accompanied by a sense of loss of control.
- Use of extreme behaviour to control body shape and weight, such as self-induced vomiting, often after a binge episode, and laxative or diuretic misuse.
- A disturbed attitude towards body shape and weight.

Again women predominate with bulimia nervosa. They tend to be slightly older than those with anorexia although there is considerable overlap. The prevalence may be as high as one or two per cent in both Britain and North America, with the majority never having sought medical attention.

The features that distinguish bulimia nervosa from anorexia are:

- The body weight is usually normal.
- Periods are not necessarily absent although they may be irregular.
- There are frequent bulimic 'bingeing' episodes. Considerable secrecy surrounds these episodes with parents or partners being often unaware of the problem.
- The binge episodes may lead to the consumption of massive amounts of carbohydrate, up to some 3,000 kc (approximately 2 days' energy intake).
- Occasionally alcohol bingeing or drug abuse are present.

Other features may include weakness and lethargy, erosions to the teeth because of the effect of vomited stomach acid, and signs of malnutrition, peripheral or facial swelling, enlargement of salivary gland or signs indicative of specific nutrient deficiencies.

Laboratory investigations may uncover low levels of potassium, especially in those who abuse laxatives or diuretics. Other possible nutrient deficiencies are magnesium, zinc and vitamin B. Prolonged repeated vomiting is a known and potent cause of vitamin B1 deficiency, as is a high intake of refined carbohydrates e.g. cakes, biscuits, chocolates, sweets.

What your doctor can do

As with anorexia, virtually all patients should be seen by a psychiatrist or psychotherapist specialising in this area. The doctor and specialist should:

- Establish a rapport with the bulimic and her family members.
- Examine for signs of nutritional deficiency.
- Assess the level of depression which, if severe, may require treatment with antidepressants or hospital admission.
- Perform tests to assess the level of electrolytes, especially potassium and vitamin B1.
- If there is prolonged vomiting, refer for psychological treatment which will usually involve several months of cognitive behavioural therapy. This is designed to encourage insight into the person's condition leading to changes in their behaviour.
- Explain techniques, such as keeping a daily diary of:
  - diet
  - behaviour and thoughts
  - setting of limits and goals on binge eating
  - advice and direction on healthy eating
  - the avoidance of stressful situations that lead to binge eating.
- Further exploration of the thoughts and attitudes that may underlie this disordered behaviour. Such an approach normally requires weekly consultations over several months and is tackled on a step-by-step basis.
- Anti-depressants can sometimes help but are less important than cognitive behaviour therapy.
- Set treatment programmes have a potentially excellent outcome in bulimia. Key elements include:
  - regular contact with the therapist
  - use of a written contract agreeing to maintain weight
  - agreeing to follow certain dietary goals about eating regularly
  - the amounts of certain foods eaten and recommendations on healthy eating
  - agreeing to maintain a regular food intake despite bingeing and vomit episodes.

What you can do

- Be honest with yourself and your therapists.
- Make a list of those stress factors in your life or situations that you feel contribute to episodes of bulimia. Bulimia is often worse premenstrually, and some of the dietary and supplement advise for PMS may also be relevant (see page 394).
- With your therapist, set goals as to the frequency of bingeing, types of foods you will binge on and the amounts you will consume.
- Do not worry if you do not achieve these goals initially, work towards them; it may take a while.
- Take any supplements prescribed regularly. Supplements of multi-vitamins in particular may be required as well as foods rich in

potassium. These latter are mainly fresh fruits and vegetables, especially bananas and oranges. Fruit juices are another good source.

• Socialise with others. Enjoy yourself in the company of your family and friends, and when you are ready, be prepared to discuss these problems with them.

Complementary therapies

As for Anorexia.

Eczema

This is predominantly an inherited condition, also known as atopic eczema or atopic dermatitis, affecting one to three per cent of the population. It often starts in childhood and is linked to asthma and rhinitis. Itchy skin is the most noticeable feature, with the skin being red, scaly and dry. The distribution varies. It may be widespread, or confined to the bends of the elbows and knees; it may affect just the face and neck, or settle in one or two other areas of the body. People with atopic eczema are more prone to asthma, rhinitis, allergic reactions to drugs and abdominal symptoms due to food allergy.

Who gets it?

Eczema has become increasingly common with estimates showing a doubling or trebling in prevalence in the UK since the Second World War. It seems to be more common in higher social classes with the risk rising with the level of the parents' education. Having one or both parents affected by eczema or other allergies is relevant and additionally eczema has become more common in children from African and Asian families – a perplexing combination of genetic factors. Events in the first years of life and possibly exposure to environmental chemicals seem to be at work in determining who gets it.

What causes it?

Eczema comes about because of a failure to control certain aspects of the immune system. A variety of different white cells which make up much of the immune system are normally busy fighting infections. Nowadays, with many of these controlled, the immune system has less to do and has had to reduce its level of activity. In the patient with eczema this has failed to occur and the white cells themselves, or proteins called antibodies that they produce, target a variety of everyday agents with which we all have contact. In practice it is allergy to these substances, which include housedust mites, foods and bacteria, that can be considered to be the cause of eczema.

It should be noted from the outset that although patients with eczema may have many allergies, and benefit from their identification and avoidance of the relative substance, only a few will subsequently experience complete resolution of their rash and itching.

Possible allergens include:

- *Foods* Cows' milk, cows' cheese, eggs, wheat, corn, yeast (baker's and brewer's), fruits and nuts are all commonly implicated.
- *Infective agents* Bacteria that are frequently present on the skin surface, viruses including *Herpes simplex* (see page 327) and fungi including *Candida albicans* can all play a part in eczema. Relief of symptoms may follow measures to treat these infections or reduce the amount of bacteria on the skin surface.
- *Housedust-mite* This is a common allergen, and seems to be important in some cases of eczema as well as asthma. (For control of housedust mite *see* Hay Fever, page 229.)
- *Others* Pollens and animals may aggravate eczema in the susceptible individual.

What your doctor can do

Your doctor can help in the identification of possible allergens and in the treatment of the skin condition itself.

Allergy tests

Allergy tests come in many guises and all have their limitations:

- Skin prick tests, where a small amount of the suspected culprit agent is placed on the skin which is then scratched, can show a reaction in ten minutes. This is useful in identifying allergies to housedust, pollens and sometimes foods. Many non-eczematous individuals show positive test results.
- Blood tests that measure the level of antibodies against foods and other agents are available. The RAST or radioallergosorbent test can detect a number of quick-acting food allergies. Other tests are being developed to look for delayed allergies to foods but their role is still uncertain. Even if a test shows a number of allergies there is no guarantee that other foods not tested for do not cause problems.

Treatments

- Steroid creams and ointments will, if the dose is high enough, dampen down the irritation and rash. Typically this is the mainstay of treatment for severe eczema and is useful in smaller doses for mild or intermittent eczema.
- Moisturising agents will help with the dryness. Useful for widespread or localised eczema where dry scaly skin is a problem. Several good

ones are available without prescription (E 45 and Unguentum Merck), and may be all that is needed for dry affected hands.

- Treatment for any associated infection. This applies especially to bacterial infection on the skin. Creams that combine antibiotics and steroids, antibiotics by mouth, or antiseptic washes to add to the bath can all be used. Occasionally treatment of thrush, infection with *Candida albicans*, may help eczema.
- Other medicines include powerful drugs to alter the immune system and allergic response. One medicine is worthy of special mention for those with known food allergies. Nalcrom (oral cromoglycate capsules) is a drug that when taken by mouth is not absorbed from the gut but blocks the development of immediate allergy reactions that take place in the gut wall. It has very few side-effects because it is not absorbed, and can therefore allow those with food allergies to respond better to dietary exclusion and consequently be more relaxed with their diet. Nalcrom has to be taken just before meals to be most effective.
- Evening primrose oil can be prescribed by doctors in the UK (as Epogam), and is useful for very dry, widespread eczema. It is best combined with a high polyunsaturated fatty acid diet (see below).

What you can do

- *Change your diet* You could try, with the approval of your doctor, either The Strict Exclusion Diet (see page 466), or The Simple Exclusion Diet (see page 460) for two or three weeks. Cutting out specific foods one at a time is not very successful and is not recommended except for children where exclusion of just cows' milk, eggs, tomatoes and artificial colours is sometimes worth a try. For young children, those with severe eczema, or those with asthma or a history of severe allergic reactions, such diets must only be performed with medical supervision, as the re-introduction of a food after its withdrawal can sometimes lead to a severe allergic reaction.
- *Avoid irritants* Many agents will worsen the eczema even though they are not the cause. Wear rubber gloves, cotton lined if necessary, when in contact with water. Use non-biological washing powders and liquids. Clothes that you wear next to your skin should be made from cotton or silk as they are often less irritating.
- *Take some nutritional supplements* Deficiencies of vitamin B, zinc and EFAs can all effect skin quality. You may need to take supplements for two or three months to see the full effect. They are often usefully combined with supplements of evening primrose oil.
- *Go on holiday and get some sunshine* This is known to help for a number of possible reasons: the rest and relaxation are good for the immune system; a change in diet or the sunshine may help to kill off

some of the surface bacteria, or the warmth and light stimulate the skin's metabolism.

- *Reduce your exposure to housedust mite* After years of suspicion it is now acknowledged that careful avoidance of this allergen can help those with eczema who are known to be sensitive to it. A simple skin prick test will give an indication of this. Measures on housedust mite avoidance are on page 229. In severe cases there may be a case for medical desensitisation to housedust. This is only undertaken at specialist centres.
- *Treat any associated premenstrual syndrome* PMS is associated with a worsening or pre-existing eczema, and some of the dietary and self-help measures for PMS can sometimes benefit any associated eczema.

Complementary therapies

Homeopathy is perhaps the most established complementary therapy for eczema. There are many remedies and their selection depends upon they type of eczema, the patient's response to it and any distinguishing features. Two common remedies are Sulphur and Graphites. These are given as tablets and are usually administered several times per day for a few weeks. More than one remedy may need to be tried before benefit is experienced.

Sheryl's story

Sheryl's partner had been a patient of mine some years ago and when her life-long eczema decided to flare up she decided to seek my advice.

The eczema stretched back to infancy and had required her to use steroids intermittently. She had observed that her eczema was better in the sun and worse after contact with water which seemed to aggravate the itching rather than the rash. A variety of allergy tests in the past had suggested multiple sensitivities to inhalant allergens which caused her some nasal stuffiness.

Simple skin prick allergy tests for foods were performed, but there were no clearcut reactions and we therefore decided to proceed straight away to a strict exclusion diet. There was a good improvement but after a few weeks the diet became very tedious. It took nearly a year of introducing and re-introducing foods before the picture was clear. There seemed to be delayed reactions to dairy products, egg, chicken, fish and we were still uncertain about a variety of other foods.

Blood tests had shown a potential important abnormality. There were very low levels of some of the Omega-6 series – essential fatty acids, especially gamma linolenic acid, the active component found in evening primrose oil.

Her doctor was willing to prescribe this for her, and it produced further improvement in her skin quality, especially lessening the dryness. It became increasingly clear that she had a wide number of food allergies and as her diet was difficult to follow completely she began a course of Nalcrom (oral cromoglycate). This allergy-blocking drug when taken by mouth may help minimise the adverse reactions to foods that may underlie some patients' eczema.

Sheryl was very pleased with the further progress, and her skin was better than it had been for over a decade. Furthermore she was able to deviate from her rather restricted diet without experiencing any severe reactions.

Shortly after this she became pregnant. Calcium supplements were needed to ensure adequate intake of this mineral and she already had been taking supplements of vitamin B and folic acid.

She was asked to be extra vigilant during her pregnancy and whilst breast-feeding as foods to which she is allergic may in some way be transmitted to her baby. Avoidance of common food allergens by mothers with eczema seems to reduce the risk of their off-spring developing eczema as well.

Erectile Dysfunction

Erectile dysfunction is defined as persistent or recurrent inability to attain or maintain an erection sufficient for the completion of sexual activity. This problem becomes increasingly common with age but may be a presenting feature of a number of important, and at times potentially life threatening, diseases. An erection is achieved in the male by the provision of extra blood flow into the blood filled spaces along the shaft of the penis – the cavernous sinuses. For this to occur, blood flow in the penile arteries needs to be good, the relevant nerve reflexes need to be intact and the male needs to be psychologically attuned to having sexual intercourse. This requires the presence of the male sex hormone testosterone.

Who gets it?

Broadly speaking, the causes of erectile dysfunction can be divided into two differing groups. It can be due to a number of physical illnesses listed below, or be psychogenic in origin. The term psychogenic means caused by personal stresses rather than a physical illness. This latter category is more likely to occur in younger individuals – under the age of 40 years, and may well be intermittent and stress-related. It can have a sudden onset at times of acute stress. Despite the problem, those with psychogenic erectile dysfunction may continue to have nocturnal or early morning erections. However, even in those in whom psychological factors are considered important, physical factors must be considered.

Organic or physical causes of erectile dysfunction include:

- Cardiovascular disease including high blood pressure, elevated blood cholesterol, peripheral vascular disease with reduced blood flow to the lower limbs.
- Endocrine disturbance with loss of testosterone production, an underactive thyroid, or excess of the hormone prolactin produced by the pituitary gland. Other symptoms indicative of these problems may or may not be present but fatigue and depression may be features of these endocrine disturbances.
- Neurological disease including multiple sclerosis or any other neurological injury, particularly if bladder function is also affected.
- Smoking, which greatly increases the risk of cardiovascular disease.
- Type II diabetes which, as well as accelerating cardiovascular disease, may also damage the sensitive nerves from the tip of the penis. Good diabetic control is associated with less risk of erectile dysfunction.
- Depression, which in turn can also be due to endocrine disturbance, excess alcohol or nutrition-related problems.
- Excess alcohol, for despite its reputation, it may increase the desire in the short term but usually results in reduced testicular and sexual function in the longer term.
- Due to drug therapy, particularly drugs for the control of blood pressure, anti-depressants and other types of psychiatric medication.
- As a result of bladder or prostate disease.

What your doctor can do

- Examine you to look particularly for cardiovascular, endocrine or neurological disease. This is usually evident from a simple but thorough examination.
- Perform a simple urine test and blood tests for the measurement of testosterone, prolactin and thyroid hormone.
- Perform other investigations if abnormalities appear on examination.
- Ask about depression, personal or marital stress problems.
- Refer you to an appropriate specialist, such as a urologist if urinary or bladder problems are anticipated, or an endocrinologist or cardiovascular disease specialist. Referral to a psychiatrist or Relate counsellor may also be appropriate.
- Review any drug treatment you are receiving in case erectile dysfunction is a side effect of treatment.

- Consider medical treatments to assist erectile function. These include locally administered drugs to improve blood flow to the base of the penis by intra-cavernosal injection (Alprostadil) or via the urethra (Muse), systemic pharmacological treatment with Sildenafil, Viagra, mechanical aids including vacuum constriction and constriction rings and occasionally surgery for the insertion of penile prostheses.

Many physicians may not have the experience or interest to advise appropriately about these treatments and may then pass patients on to specialist clinics.

What you can do

Many patients with erectile dysfunction suffer reduced blood flow to the base of the penis and most of the self-help measures are intended to try and improve these problems. They include:

- Stop smoking. This has both short and long term effects in reducing blood flow. See page 10 for instructions.
- Limit alcohol to a total of two units per day maximum.
- Lose weight if you are overweight. Follow The Simple Weight Loss Diet on page 452.
- Increase physical activity if you are unfit, and do so gradually, particularly if you are not exercising regularly and are overweight.
- Eat healthily with a high intake of fruit and vegetables. If you are a Type II diabetic ensure you follow the standard guidelines for diabetes to produce a glycosylated haemoglobin within the acceptable range.
- Discuss your problems with your partner, if you have not already done so, and try and resolve any difficulties between yourselves, perhaps with the aid of a marital or sexual counsellor.
- Be patient. Unreasonable expectations will not reduce your level of stress or the outcome of treatment.
- Address the stress in your life and work towards a stress free existence. Follow the instructions in the Stress section on page 25.
- Be willing to consider medical treatments as listed above. These are of proven efficacy provided they are selected with care.
- Try taking some nutritional supplements, particularly if you are not eating well and are smoking or drinking heavily. A strong multi-vitamin supplement with good intake of the anti-oxidant vitamins – vitamin C and vitamin E – would be appropriate if you are a heavy smoker and additional daily supplements of vitamin B complex and 30 mg of zinc would be appropriate if you are a heavy drinker.

Eye Problems

For much of our lives our eyes are designed to take care of themselves. They are cleansed by our tears, which naturally contain chemicals that kill bacteria. But our eyes are vulnerable, and at times become the victims of infection or allergy, or may be affected by some other medical condition, like hayfever or seborrhoeic dermatitis.

As we age our eyes change shape. When they change shape from back to front we become short-sighted, and when the change occurs from top to bottom we become long-sighted. Taking care of ourselves generally will also help to preserve the health of our eyes.

Loss of vision

According to iridologists our eyes are a reflection of what is happening inside the body – not something that conventional doctors would agree with. Orthodox medicine acknowledges, though, that hardening of the arteries may be detected in older folk by checking for a pale ring around the iris. Another eye problem that can occur in later life is glaucoma, in which there is an increase of tension within the eyeball as a result of blocked drainage from the eye. Although the symptoms may initially appear like conjunctivitis, with red and bloodshot whites, glaucoma may be a threat to our sight. The tension can be reduced by drugs or the blockage will need to be cleared rapidly, and so it is important to be examined quickly.

Two major causes of loss of vision are cataracts and macular degeneration.

CATARACTS

A cataract is a gradual clouding of the lens of the eye, in which a jelly-like substance grows over the lens of the eye. They are a major cause of blindness all over the world. A number of risk factors for their formation have been identified, some of which are nutritional, and these include:

- age
- diabetes
- sunlight exposure, especially ultra-violet B radiation
- poor diet with poor intakes of vitamin A, in the form of carotene and its relatives which are found in spinach and other dark green vegetables.
- possibly consumption of dairy products with an inability to digest milk sugar or lactose.

- use of steroid drugs and other medicines
- diarrhoea. This is possibly due to loss of nutrients or as a reflection of poor general health.

Free radical damage

Oxygen is the basis of all plant and animal life. It is our most important nutrient, and needed by every cell. In normal biochemical reactions oxygen can become unstable and capable of 'oxidising' neighbouring molecules. As a result, high energy chemical substances called 'free oxidising radicals' (FORs), or more commonly referred to as free radicals, are released in all cells. If they become too numerous, they attack the body and cause damage to the cells and tissues. FORs, when out of control attack the structural proteins, enzymes and cell membranes of the lens of the eye.

The treatment of cataracts usually involves their surgical removal with sometimes replacement of the lens. As yet there is no evidence that they can be prevented (although progress is made by use of nutritional supplements) but this may change with time.

Some protection may be achieved in those taking low dose aspirin or similar analgesic (often used in treating arthritis but also used for the prevention of heart disease). And long-term usage of a vitamin C supplement has also been associated with a reduction in risk, but only after ten or more years.

MACULAR DEGENERATION

The macular is the most sensitive part of the retina, located at the back of the eye, that perceives the majority of fine vision. Healthy function of this part of the eye is necessary for reading, driving, writing and any fine work.

The degeneration of this part of the eye is mainly age related and is a major cause of irreversible blindness among those persons aged 65 years and more. Again, studies have been performed to look at risk factors for the development of age-related macular degeneration. Attention has focused on nutrients. So far we know that the risk of this condition is influenced by:

- smoking, which increases the risk.
- atherosclerosis, or a narrowing of the arteries in the neck, may be an additional risk factor in the elderly.
- a low intake of carotenoids in the diet. Agents like beta-carotene (vegetable vitamin A) that do not have any vitamin function. High concentrations are found in spinach or collard greens.
- low intake of vitamin C from foods, though this effect is small.

In practice what this means is that eating healthily in your formative and middle years may help retard the rate of decay of tissues in later life. Smoking once again seems to accelerate this risk of tissues degenerating.

What your doctor can do

Not much really except refer you to a specialist.

What you can do

- Follow The Very Nutritious Diet (see page 437).
- Ensure that your diet is rich in fresh fruit and vegetables especially spinach, tomatoes, carrots and any dark-green vegetables.
- Consider taking a multi-vitamin containing good levels of selenium, beta-carotene, vitamin C, vitamin E, zinc and the powerful anti-oxidant, superoxide dismutase (SOD). These nutrients are FOR scavengers which, if out of control can damage the retina and micro-circulation in the eye.

Fatigue and Chronic Fatigue Syndrome

Tired when you go to bed, tired when you wake up. Tired at work, tired when you get home. It's a familiar story, and even if you are not a habitual victim of chronic fatigue you probably know someone who is. Indeed this is one of the most common complaints for which we now consult our doctors, and more women suffer than men.

There are, of course, different types of fatigue. Most of us have experienced fatigue after a period of hard and fruitful work, and then hopefully, noticed a return in our energy after a good night's sleep or a relaxing holiday. Some of us, however, suffer from fatigue day in, day out, despite the amount of sleep or rest we have. The causes of this problem vary from the physical to the psychological, and both aspects need to be considered in the majority of those suffering with significant fatigue. This chapter deals with severe fatigue that is troublesome enough to cause the individual to change her lifestyle in some way.

During the last ten years there has been a great deal of research and publicity about severe fatigue, particularly ME (myalgic encephalo-myelitis). This term is now replaced by Chronic Fatigue Syndrome which also replaces other similar terms such as post-infective or post-viral fatigue. Chronic Fatigue Syndrome (CFS) often, but by no means always, follows an acute infectious illness, such as a sore throat, glandular fever or gastro-enteritis.

What causes it?

The interest of doctors in these chronic fatigue syndromes is a landmark in medical thinking, with research being focused on a symptom, for which there are many possible causes, and not a single disease state. There are serious and not so serious causes of fatigue, so it is important to determine into which category an individual falls. Research has shown that up to ten per cent of those with severe fatigue can be found to have some underlying health problem.

Some sufferers may have a physical illness which may not yet be fully developed, some may have recently experienced acute infection, and others may be mainly depressed. The first step must be to eliminate the possibility of any serious underlying cause before progressing to self-help measures.

As a rule of thumb, fatigue which is persistent or prevents you from working and requires you to make drastic changes to your home life and social calendar, should be regarded as possibly being due to a serious cause. This also goes for fatigue that is associated with weight loss, fever, significant pain or any other troublesome symptoms. This should always prompt you to check with your doctor as your first course of action.

Causes of fatigue (not so serious):

- lack of sleep
- stress or overwork
- lack of physical fitness
- poor quality diet.

Causes of fatigue (serious):

- physical illness, e.g. heart, liver or kidney disease
- after viral or other infection, e.g. glandular fever or 'flu
- depression
- rarely, a continuing infection, e.g. tropical.

Wide-ranging surveys have revealed a pattern connecting common non-serious health problems with mild to moderate fatigue which includes muscular aches and pains, bowel problems, headaches, premenstrual syndrome and sleeping difficulties including snoring, and allergies. Addressing these problems can often result in a reduction in the associated fatigue.

When a doctor has to assess a new patient with significant fatigue it is probably best to consider the following four broad groups:

1. It can accompany any acute infectious illness, such as 'flu or a cold. Occasionally, an infection is hidden and this can be the case in some tropical illnesses or parasitic infections. If anyone with fatigue has a fever usually measured at more than 37.5 degrees centigrade, then they should be carefully checked for a possible hidden infection.

2. Fatigue can also follow an infection. After the acute episode has resolved, the individual can be left with fatigue, which instead of resolving in a week or so, drags on for months and even years. This condition is sometimes called 'ME' (myalgic encephalomyelitis). That mouthful simply means inflammation of the muscles and nervous tissue, and there is now evidence that patients with ME can, at times, have evidence of damage or alteration to either the muscles, the nervous system or immune system (the part of our body that fights infection). It seems in some ways that the infection, after causing an acute illness, goes into a slow or hidden phase which can sometimes reappear. This is particularly true for the glandular fever virus, but may also be true of other virus infections.

   The term ME is now commonly replaced with Chronic Fatigue Syndrome (CFS). This is used to describe significant fatigue present for at least three months which typically, but not necessarily, has followed one or more infections. Several of the following features should also be present:
   ○ the fatigue is worse after exercise
   ○ headaches
   ○ forgetfulness or poor concentration
   ○ muscle aches and pains
   ○ recurrent sore throats
   ○ painful enlarged glands in the neck or elsewhere.
   Doctors still disagree about this definition. In practice, if this picture is present, and continuing infection, other underlying illness, drug or alcohol abuse, or severe depression are excluded, then this allows at least a working diagnosis of CFS (or ME).

3. Fatigue can also be caused by a wide variety of physical illnesses, including heart conditions, thyroid disease, arthritis, conditions affecting the immune system or nervous system, kidney problems and so on. These conditions should be suspected in older patients, those who experience weight loss or have other unusual symptoms. They will usually be detected by blood and urine tests, together with x-rays. In order to eliminate the possibility of any underlying sinister problem, it is important that all those suffering with severe fatigue do see their medical practitioner for a check up.

4. Fatigue of varying degree is often caused by nutritional factors. This can either be due to a lack of vitamins or minerals, or sometimes other dietary problems. Though we are often told that the average diet in countries like the United Kingdom, Australia and New Zealand should provide all the vitamins and minerals we need, careful scrutiny of the evidence from both governmental and other sources, doesn't always support this claim. In fact mild nutritional deficiencies are not uncommon, especially among women of childbearing age, the elderly and the ill, and these can affect muscle and brain metabolism and result in loss of energy. This is easily underestimated by the medical profession through lack of knowledge, and may consequently be overlooked.

A relatively recent survey in the UK revealed that up to 20 per cent of adults have a dietary intake below the new minimum recommended by the government's advisers. This applies particularly to the minerals iron, magnesium and potassium, as well as some of the B vitamins. Deficiency of any of these nutrients can cause fatigue. Most are essential to the function of muscles, nerves and the immune system.

There is good evidence that deficiency is particularly common in certain groups. Iron deficiency, for example, causes anaemia in four per cent of adult women of child-bearing age in the UK. This is mainly because of heavy or prolonged periods with a further ten per cent of women of child-bearing age having evidence of low iron stores, and this may explain why fatigue is more common amongst women. Mild fatigue in such women has long been shown to respond to iron supplements, and is a good example of how a mild or severe nutritional deficiency can be a cause of chronic fatigue.

Who may lack nutrients	Deficiency
women with heavy or prolonged periods	zinc and iron
tea- and coffee-drinking vegetarians	iron
those eating junk and fast food	vitamin B and magnesium
those who drink too much alcohol	vitamin B and magnesium
women with premenstrual syndrome	magnesium
those suffering from depression or anxiety	vitamins B and C
those who eat little fruit and vegetables	vitamin C, magnesium and potassium
heavy smokers	vitamin C
those suffering any illness resulting in weight loss	vitamin B and others
the ill and elderly	vitamin B and others
those with poor resistance to infection	zinc, vitamins B and A

Iron deficiency is most likely in women who are having periods, particularly if they are heavy, and in vegetarians or people who don't consume much meat.

Mild deficiency of the B group of vitamins is also quite common, particularly in those who complain of anxiety, depression or mood changes. This may often accompany fatigue. Again, a poor diet, smoking, and drinking too much alcohol, are all significant risk factors for lack of vitamin B.

The mineral magnesium has attracted considerable interest in recent years. This mineral is essential for nerve and muscle function. Intakes in the UK are acknowledged to be borderline or deficient in some 10 per cent or more of adults. In our own surveys of women with PMS we have repeatedly found that over 50 per cent of women with PMS have low magnesium stores.

Go to your doctor if you suffer serious fatigue and . . .

- you have a fever (a temperature of 37.5°C or 99.5°F).
- you are losing weight.
- you have enlarged glands in the neck, armpits or groin.
- you have pains which disturb your sleep or daily activities.
- your facial appearance or colour has changed.
- you have travelled abroad, especially to Asia, the Far East, the Mediterranean, or South, Central or North America.
- you have had contact with animals other than known pets.
- you are troubled by any joint swellings and pains.
- you have bowel problems such as diarrhoea, a change in the colour of your stool or severe abdominal pains.
- you are aged over 50 years.

What your doctor can do

Establish whether there is a serious underlying cause to your symptoms by:

- Taking a history of your symptoms and giving you a thorough physical examination, with routine blood screening, including a full blood count – to look for anaemia or evidence of infection; serum ferritin – to check your iron stores (particularly useful for menstruating women); thyroid function – to assess the status of your thyroid; biochemistry tests to assess kidney and liver function; measurement of blood calcium, sodium and potassium – to assess mineral imbalances.
- Enlightened doctors may care to measure your red cell magnesium level. This is a simple test that can be performed at district hospital level. Reduced red cell magnesium is associated with fatigue, PMS, muscle cramps or fibromyalgia.

- Make some assessment of your nutritional state, and look for evidence of vitamin B deficiency in particular. Lack of vitamin B12 and vitamin B1 can be serious, and fatigue may be one of the earliest symptoms. Moderate deficiencies of several of the B vitamins including vitamin B6 have recently been found in a small group of chronic fatigue syndrome patients. Specialist supplements of vitamin B3 (nicotinamide) are sometimes used.
- Consider referring you to a specialist for further assessment. This is most likely if the fatigue is severe and prolonged, has been accompanied by weight loss, fever or significant foreign travel, or has caused you to make major lifestyle changes as previously discussed.
- Treat depression if this is a major component of your illness, but this should not stop doctors from looking for underlying physical or nutritional causes.
- Refer you to a specialist unit, or a behavioural psychologist, as simple coping techniques have been shown to help speed up the recovery process.

Maureen's story

Maureen was a 47-year-old nurse who lectured in further education. She suffered chronic fatigue and, as a result, her moods were so wildly out of control. She was in the process of disciplinary action at work and finding life generally difficult when she approached the WNAS.

'I had experienced symptoms for nearly 25 years, but they had become markedly worse in the last three years. My doctor had prescribed numerous forms of hormone treatment which seemed to make the symptoms worse. My total exhaustion, irritability, anger and aggression had almost totally alienated me from the world. I was struggling along on the contraceptive pill continuously as my doctor felt my symptoms may improve if we could suppress ovulation.

I had so much time off in the last three years because of exhaustion and my wild moods. I had reached the point where I was afraid to go out of the house. I was so tired that I could not get out of bed in the morning without a friend phoning to command me through the procedure, limb by limb. My doctor had sent me for counselling and had even referred me to a psychiatrist, but I walked out half way through the appointment as I was so angry with his suggestion that I should pull myself together.

I often felt like ending my life. I had upset so many people and had lost most of my friends. At work I was regarded as unreliable, and regarded as an oddity.

Then one day I read about the book, No More PMS! *in* Woman and Home *magazine and decided to read it. To my utter amazement my complete fatigue and mood changes were described almost exactly by other case histories. I made some changes to my diet myself by following the instructions in the book whilst I was waiting for an appointment with the WNAS. After an in-depth consultation I was asked to make considerable changes to my diet. I cut out certain grains, caffeine, and biscuits, which I used to eat day and night. I also took supplements of Optivite and went back to exercising, which I had let slip from my routine.*

At my follow-up appointment, six weeks later, I was able to report that I had been on an even keel with no wild mood swings, and was feeling so energetic that I had taken to early morning walks. I could hardly believe it and nor could my friends and colleagues especially those who had previously had to resuscitate me in the mornings. I came off the pill too, and my headaches also disappeared.

Within three months I had lost half a stone in weight, I was wonderfully stable each day and had regained my energy and enthusiasm for life. I had renewed my friendships, and was promoted to co-ordinator at work within six months. It has now been two years since my treatment with the WNAS. I feel alive again and can't sing their praises enough. I remain healthy and happy, am keeping to the wheat-free, caffeine-free diet and have taken an additional part-time job as a night nursing sister. I am enjoying it immensely.'

What you can do

Many treatments or cures have been put forward, some showing some very high success rates, and there are many self-help measures that can be implemented to help overcome symptoms of fatigue.

- Follow the recommendations for The Very Nutritious Diet on page 437 and the suggested menus for fatigue on page 472.
- Tidy up your diet by concentrating on good sources of magnesium – green leafy vegetables and most wholesome foods – and avoid sugar, sweets, and soft drinks which contain hardly any magnesium at all. Women with PMS often have low levels of magnesium, and it seems that the same is often true of people suffering with fatigue.
- Many other nutrients, if deficient, are known to affect the function of the immune system. These include vitamins A, C, E and the trace element, zinc. A healthy diet and a strong multi-vitamin supplement with 20 to 30 milligrams of zinc should be adequate. Specialised fats

and oils, as found in evening primrose oil and fish oils, have been used to help those with chronic fatigue. In one placebo-controlled trial a supplement of Efamol Marine at 8 capsules daily helped a high proportion of those whose fatigue was post-infective in type. Again this should be combined with eating healthily and possibly a multivitamin preparation.

- In addition to deficiency of certain nutrients, sometimes other dietary problems can cause fatigue. There is evidence in those who have certain types of allergy, that fatigue may be one of the associated symptoms. Intolerance to certain foods seems to be a factor, and this can be suspected if there are symptoms of allergy, including eczema, asthma, nettle rash, migraine headaches and bowel problems including irritable bowel syndrome. In one study, allergy to wheat protein was linked with increased complaints of fatigue, headaches and bowel problems. It is not known how commonly this is a cause of chronic fatigue, but it does seem to be worth considering.

- Symptoms such as anxiety and depression, often accompany fatigue. In fact many physical problems can also cause mental symptoms. Stress, in any form, may also aggravate mental symptoms, and even reduce the ability of the immune system to fight infection. So if you are feeling stressed it is important to find a workable way of overcoming the stressful factors and to spend a little time every day relaxing, see page 29.

- Exercising regularly to the point of breathlessness and losing weight, if you are overweight, can also help mood and stimulate the immune system. You should only exercise regularly if your fatigue is mild and you have no underlying illness.

- Complementary therapies including homeopathy, herbal medicine and acupuncture may be worth considering. One report from Doctors Sheila and Robin Gibson from the Glasgow Homeopathic Hospital concluded that dietary change, nutritional supplements, homeopathy and psychotherapy helped in 70 per cent of participants.

Of course, frantic modern living is likely to contribute to us feeling tired all the time. Many of us devote insufficient time to preparing food or taking adequate exercise or relaxation. Not enough sleep, stress at home or work, lack of exercise and a poor quality diet can all reduce our energy levels. Addressing the problem directly by taking a much-needed holiday, embarking on a regular exercise programme or taking steps to improve your nutritional intake may well be all that is needed to restore your vitality.

Working long hours and not eating wholesome food regularly is likely to make your blood glucose levels fall, which results in symptoms of tiredness. The solution is not merely to suddenly eat more glucose, as the body finds it hard to adjust to the rapid rise and fall that this causes. Rather eat wholesome food little and often. So aim for three good meals, with nutritious between-meal snacks, such as fruit, nuts and raisins, a sandwich with cheese, meat or fish, or rye crackers and peanut butter, which give a more sustained rise in blood sugar.

Some people seem excessively tired and dopey just after a meal. Men seem particularly prone to this phenomenon, which is likely to be worse at lunch time or after a large meal and is aggravated by drinking alcohol. A smaller, lighter lunch, especially one of salad with meat, fish or vegetarian protein, avoiding alcohol and taking a twenty minute walk afterwards will usually prevent this form of transitory tiredness. The alternative is to have a siesta after your midday meal. This is what the Mediterraneans and lions do, and is simply a response to the physiological need to rest while digesting a large meal.

So in less serious cases, excellent results can be gained by making sure you get a little more sleep, cutting your workload a little to combat the associated stress, taking more exercise, improving your diet, and having a holiday if possible.

Fight fatigue
- eat three meals a day, with wholesome snacks in between.
- cut down on sugary foods, refined carbohydrates and chocolate.
- eat three servings of fresh fruit per day.
- eat three portions of fresh vegetables, including a green leafy one, per day.
- eat protein-rich foods at least once a day.
- avoid bran and bran-based cereals and use corn and oat alternatives.
- limit bread to 2–4 slices per day.
- keep alcohol consumption down.
- consume 300–600 ml of milk (^{1}/2–1 pint) per day and 112–225g (4–5 oz) of cheese per week.
- cut down on tea and coffee and try herbal teas and alternative coffees (see page 6).
- enjoy your food.

Complementary therapies
Although most of us prefer not to given a serious diagnosis for our symptoms, when the verdict is 'no apparent underlying cause' it can be immensely frustrating. As well as implementing the advice given in this chapter is would be worth enlisting the help of one or more complementary practitioners.

Acupuncture would regard symptoms of fatigue as a deficiency syndrome. The practitioner would be looking for deficiency of Qi or the life-force in the blood, and will treat the deficiency.

There are numerous homeopathic remedies that are available for the different sorts of fatigue including Apis melifica, useful for aches and pains, Lycopodium clavatum for symptoms of fatigue and inertia, Natrum muriaticum, a remedy for the pale and weak and Pulsatilla, for the frail, pale female with changeable symptoms, and useful for those who do not tolerate stress well. You could try these yourself, or consult a qualified homeopath.

The herbal practitioner also has a lot to offer, and would be worth consulting if symptoms persist. There are many different herbal remedies for fatigue including St John's Wort, vervain, yarrow, echinacea and stinging nettle.

Cranial osteopaths consider that the membranes around the brain and spinal cord can become 'tight' and cause ill-health. Relaxation, massage and a consultation with a cranial osteopath may be very helpful.

See also: References and Recommended reading (*Tired All the Time*).

Fluid Retention

This is also known as idiopathic oedema. 'Oedema' is the medical term for swelling, 'idiopathic' means that the cause is unknown and is just a clever way of doctors disguising their ignorance. Though there are a variety of causes, the commonest is simply the retention of salt and water in the subcutaneous tissues. This shows up particularly in the feet, in the fingers and sometimes in the abdomen. In severe cases the face may be affected.

It is well known that fluid retention is much more common in women and is very often worse in the premenstrual phase. Some studies have shown that it can be associated with fatigue and a tendency to depression, but before deciding that the swelling is simply 'idiopathic', care should be taken to exclude other causes.

What your doctor can do

- Consider the possible causes of swelling including heart failure (see page 233), underactive thyroid (see page 417), kidney failure, swelling due to blocked lymphatic drainage following infection, or possibly due to a familial disorder.
- If simple idiopathic oedema is diagnosed a low-salt diet is recommended, and this should always be the first line of treatment. Careful studies conducted by doctors at Charing Cross Hospital in London clearly demonstrated that a restriction of sodium (salt) leads almost

always to clearance of idiopathic oedema. Our bodies are composed of 70 per cent water, and the reason we retain fluid is because each cell in the body has a mechanism to balance sodium and other minerals. It is primarily sodium that governs the retention of water and it seems that some women are particularly unable to tolerate large amounts of salt in the diet. Our western diet has become laden with salt, with intakes some ten to 50 times our actual requirements.

- Prescribe diuretics if all else fails. This is very much a poor option and a last resort, although it is indeed a common treatment. Low-dose mild diuretics often do not produce lasting benefit as the body adjusts to the effects on their chemistry.

What you can do

- Be vigilant with a low-salt diet (see page 449), as we consume far more salt than we need and most of the sodium salt in our diet comes from hidden sources rather than added salt in cooking or at the table. This will mean doing without crisps, other salted savoury snacks, bacon, sauasages and greatly limiting the intake of bread.
- Avoid wheat if you also suffer with abdominal bloating. This might indicate a food sensitivity. When the body perceives a food as 'toxic' it may accumulate fluid in the cells.
- Fluid restriction is not required although it is inadvisable to drink very large amounts. Watch out for some mineral waters which actually contain significant amounts of sodium, and choose those rich in calcium and magnesium if possible.
- Lose weight if you need to.
- Restrict your alcohol intake to no more than two units per day.
- Follow the The Very Nutritious Diet (see page 437). High intakes of magnesium and potassium will help the body get the balance of sodium right.
- Take supplements of magnesium and multi-vitamins (see Premenstrual Syndrome, page 394, for further advice).
- Ginkgo biloba has been used in the treatment of oedema due to its ability to improve circulation, particularly to the extremities. Ginkgo should not be taken if you have been prescribed anti-coagulant medication or you are pregnant.
- Put your feet up. Lying down aids clearance of fluid from the legs and also the body's ability to pass it out in the urine.
- Have a cup of coffee? This has modest diuretic effects. Perhaps a cup of coffee first thing in the morning, whilst putting your feet up for a couple of hours to read the newspaper, may help you to offload some of the fluid that has accumulated overnight.

Complementary therapies

Most herbal remedies have diuretic properties, so see a qualified herbalist for advice.

A homeopathic remedy, Agis mel, is traditionally used to treat this sort of problem. These avenues are worth exploring but will not replace the need for a low-salt diet. Manual lymphatic drainage is a useful therapy in conjunction with dietary modification, but you must consult a professionally trained practitioner.

Alison's story

Alison was a 38-year-old welfare worker with two children who suffered severe water retention which made her life a misery. She felt swollen and tired for two weeks each month which was severely disrupting her life.

'For two weeks before my period each month, with unrelenting regularity, my body would begin to swell. Within days, my middle swelled up so much that I looked at least five months pregnant. My waist would increase by inches and my face puffed up. My eyelids felt tight and my breasts sore because of the swelling. I could hardly fit into my bra, and even walking felt uncomfortable.

Every month I'd be so bloated, I felt like a pudding and everything was an effort. I was lethargic and lacking in energy. My doctor prescribed progesterone suppositories which made me feel even more bloated. When I returned to ask for further help he told me I needed to see a psychiatrist. I felt insulted as I knew that my symptoms were not psychological. I went off and tried to help myself with vitamin B6 and evening primrose oil. They did help a bit, but not significantly. My doctor's reaction had put me off trying to get help, so I struggled on for another couple of years.

My husband read an article in the newspaper relating to the work of the WNAS in which one of the patients reported symptoms similar to mine. I wrote off immediately to ask for help. The detailed questionnaire and diet diary arrived shortly after and I set about completing it. The WNAS worked out a programme for me that involved cutting out chocolate bars, which I used to crave, and bread, tea and coffee had to go too. Instead I was asked to concentrate on fresh foods. Every day I had to eat lots of vegetables, salad and fruit. I drank herbal tea and fruit juice, and small amounts of decaffeinated coffee. As well as the fresh foods, I had to take vitamins and minerals to help speed up my recovery and to exercise regularly.

I had a constant headache for the first week and felt sluggish. Once the first two weeks were over I felt smashing. Within two *months I was really feeling slim and positive. The bloating disappeared and my breasts were no longer tender.*

Six years on now I'm still full of energy, my skin looks smooth, my nails no longer split and break, and I no longer have cravings for food. I am two stones slimmer now without dieting, I'm more confident and can honestly say that I feel like a different person, I'm really amazed.'

See also: Standard references.

Food Craving

Just as cars need regular petrol and oil, so our bodies have specific nutritional requirements in order to keep them running efficiently. Too little 'nutritional fuel' results in us running out of steam and having difficulty maintaining our bodyweight. Equally, too much food and drink can leave us feeling wiped out, both physically and mentally. Craving food, particularly chocolate, is very common, and affects approximately three-quarters of all women in the UK to some degree, with 60 per cent feeling that chocolate was a problem for them. It is not uncommon for women to get into a routine of eating in excess of six bars of chocolate each day, sometimes whole packets of fun-size bars, followed by biscuits, cakes and sweets. A little of what you fancy does you good, but excessive consumption does little for our self-esteem, or our waistlines.

What causes it

The brain and nervous system require a constant supply of good nutrients in order to function normally. Eating nutritious food little and often would probably provide all that was needed, and indeed is the way we were designed to sustain ourselves. Many of us are not shopping regularly for fresh food or spending time in the kitchen preparing proper meals. We often rely on pre-prepared meals and fast food in order to satisfy our hunger, without realising that these do not fulfil our need for nutrients. Then, little by little, we reach for these sweet foods in order to give us a boost, which they undoubtedly do, but it is short lived. A biochemical merry-go-round develops, which becomes less and less under our control as time progresses. The progress and results of this are listed below.

- When we haven't eaten for a while or consumed much nutritious food our blood sugar levels drop.
- The brain, which requires glucose in order function normally, sends out a red alert asking for more glucose, ideally in the form of nutritious

food. Unfortunately as we are not educated about nutrition, we often supply the body with refined sugar in the form of a sweet processed snack, or chocolate, which is largely composed of refined sugar, which doesn't contain any vitamins or minerals whatsoever, but does demand good nutrients in order to be metabolised.

- The result of eating the refined sugar snack is that the blood sugar levels shoot up rapidly, flooding the blood with sugar.
- The brain then sends another message to say that there is too much sugar in the blood, which triggers the release of the hormone insulin, whose function it is to drive the sugar back into the cells. It does this so efficiently that the blood sugar levels then goes back to low again, and the whole cycle begins again as a result.

The trick is knowing how to break this cycle, which often develops into a real addiction, and just like alcohol, drugs or smoking, involves a period of withdrawal.

LOW BLOOD SUGAR

Low blood sugar levels usually follow some traumatic event in a woman's life, or alternatively can occur gradually due to poor nutritional intake. Very often women feel low after pregnancy and periods of breast-feeding, when the nutrient demands placed on our bodies are greater than at other times in our lives. Following a broken relationship, we often become vulnerable, so we shun normal meals in favour of comfort eating. Equally, when life becomes stressful, whether with financial pressures, dissatisfaction at work or loneliness, we often find our way to the chocolate counter. It is not simply lack of will that stops us taking control, but real biochemical needs that develop as a result of poor dietary management over a period of time. There is nothing wrong with enjoying food and eating modest amounts of chocolate after a proper meal, but when the cravings take control of you it is time to do something about it.

The WNAS have undertaken several surveys on low blood sugar and food cravings, and some fascinating factors were revealed:

- Women, it seems, suffer more commonly than men, probably because of our hormone cycle, and because the nutritional demands that are placed on their bodies vary throughout the stages of their lives.
- From a sample of 1,000 patients, we initially discovered that just under 80 per cent suffered with cravings for sweet food in their premenstrual phase, in the days before their period was due.
- A further survey of 500 women of all ages showed that 78 per cent admitted wanting to eat less chocolate, and 60 per cent claimed it was a problem for them.

- Weight gain, poor skin quality, fatigue and flagging self-esteem were the commonest resulting problems experienced.
- The most recent survey we undertook on 295 women also revealed this and the following :
  - 74 per cent crave sweet food.
  - Sweet food consumption was related to age and occupation.
  - Most felt worse after eating sweet food, with fatigue being the worst complaint.
  - Women who consume lots of sweet food tend to drink more coffee, smoke more cigarettes and eat a less healthy diet.
  - Retired people, housewives and unskilled workers consume far more sweet food than managers and directors.
  - Chocolate and cakes were the most popularly craved foods. Severe sufferers burning their way through at least £15 per week in order to satisfy their cravings.

HYPOGLYCAEMIA

There are three main types of hypoglycaemia. The most common type is that caused when an insulin-dependent diabetic either injects too much insulin or fails to eat soon enough, or to eat an adequate amount of food after an insulin injection. The effect of an excess of insulin is to lower the blood glucose to levels that can cause a marked reaction.

Hypoglycaemia can also occur as a result of certain diseases. Very rarely, a tumour of the pancreas may cause secretions of insulin and profound hypoglycaemia, particularly if the person goes without food for several hours. Additionally it can accompany disorders such as liver disease, especially alcoholic liver disease, over- or under-activity of the thyroid gland, as a side-effect of some drugs, after operations that change the emptying pattern of the stomach and after alcoholic binges.

More severe forms of low blood sugar, often referred to as reactive hypoglycaemia, can be measured and dealt with medically, and indeed persistent symptoms should be medically investigated. Reactive hypo-glycaeamia is the term used to describe a fall in blood sugar following a rise brought about by eating a meal with a high content of starch or refined carbohydrates, sucrose or glucose. There has been much debate over the significance of reactive hypoglycaemia. It is probably much less common than was at first thought. The exact nature of the chemical signals involved has not yet been worked out, but it probably involves changes in carbohydrate and protein metabolism in the brain.

Low blood sugar can cause profound changes in mental function as well as physical ability and our mood. Some of the associated symptoms are:

- irritability
- faintness
- dizziness
- weakness

- hunger
- nausea
- headache
- fatigue

- palpitations
- sweating
- apprehension
- anxiety

What your doctor can do

It is fair to say that food craving as opposed to low blood sugar is not really recognised as a syndrome, and because of lack of education about nutrition, it is not something that most doctors would be equipped to deal with. Your doctor can:

- measure your fasting blood sugar levels.
- investigate for any other underlying medical problem like diabetes.
- assess your dietary habits to see whether you have an eating disorder.

Gail's story

Gail was a 36-year-old working mother with two young children who had been suffering with uncontrollable premenstrual bingeing since she finished breast-feeding her youngest child.

'I've always been a vegetarian – very health conscious and sporty. Not the type you'd think would suffer PMS. But all that changed after I had my second baby.

When my periods returned, they returned with a vengeance. I suddenly found myself craving bars of chocolate and junk food. At first it was just one or two bars of chocolate a week but, within months, my craving for chocolate was insatiable and I was eating only junk food.

I'd raid the house for anything chocolatey and if I couldn't find anything, my poor husband would have to go and get me my 'fix'. I'd eat five or six bars in one sitting and still fancy more, even though I didn't really like the taste of it. I'd even raid the children's chocolate box. This went on for 21 days out of my 28 day cycle. I put on so much weight, and experienced feelings of violence and aggression which were vented at my family for no reason.

I visited my GP and was told that my symptoms were psycho-somatic. I felt guilty and sure I should be able to control my cravings. During my one clear week each month I'd tell myself that next time it would be different. But, of course, a week later I was that madwoman all over again – cramming my face with chocolate and hating myself for it.

Thank heavens I read about the work that the WNAS were doing. Their programme helped me to withdraw from chocolate and caffeine. The first couple of weeks were awful. I had headaches and suffered terrible withdrawal symptoms. But I had been warned to expect this and so persisted with the programme. Within a few months I was completely back to normal. I had no cravings and began losing weight. All my premenstrual symptoms were gone. It's been five years now and I've never looked back. Personally and professionally, thanks to a resurgence of self-belief and awareness brought about by the WNAS programme, life is wonderful. For the past three years I have studied incessantly to increase my knowledge of financial services, and practice as a financial advisor. I have since been adopted as a partner – all thanks to the WNAS.'

What you can do

A report produced by The Committee on Dietary Reference Values recommends that we cut down our non-milk extrinsic sugars by 50 per cent – this includes any foods or drinks containing sugar. It is not necessarily an ideal recommendation, as it really depends on how much you were eating in the first place. However, it does present an achievable goal that should bring about substantial improvements in both dental and general health.

The COMA (Committee on Medical Aspects of Food) Report on Dietary Sugars and Human Disease recommended improved food labelling – if we are to cut down we need to know precisely how much sugar is in each packet of food we buy. The same report recommended that medical students should be learning about human nutrition as an integral part of their course.

- *Avoid obesity* Obesity is associated with poor blood sugar control and at its worst can sometimes precede a diabetic state. The message is to keep your body weight in the normal range for your height and bone structure.
- *Reduce intake of alcohol* Alcohol can cause liver damage, which can lead to significant hypoglycaemia. Replacing a meal with two or three gin and tonics, for example, can cause a profound rise and subsequent fall in blood glucose levels, producing all the symptoms of hypo-glycaemia.
- *Stop smoking* Smoking can increase the release of insulin and glucagon, another hormone which causes a rise in blood glucose, which is also released by the pancreas. Smoking is a powerful appetite suppressant in the short term. If a balanced meal is not consumed, blood glucose levels will inevitably fall.
- *Cut down on tea and coffee* If these are consumed in large amounts, they can also cause an increase in the release of insulin. Large amounts of sugar consumed in tea or coffee can contribute to an unstable blood glucose level.

- *Eat regularly* Irregular eating can lead to swings in blood glucose levels. This is particularly significant for insulin-dependent diabetics. Missing a meal or fasting will cause blood glucose levels to fall to the lower end of the normal range in susceptible individuals.
- *Take exercise* This is the one factor that can improve the control of blood sugar, as well as having many other health benefits. Exercise increases the sensitivity of the body's response to insulin, leading to smoother control of blood sugar levels. Ideally you should be doing at least four sessions of exercise per week to the point of breathlessness.

Useful tips

- Consume nutritious food little and often to keep blood sugar levels constant. Eat breakfast, lunch and dinner each day, with a wholesome mid-morning and mid-afternoon snack to keep the blood sugar levels constant.
- It is very important not to skip meals, as this will only serve to make matters worse. If your day starts with just a cup of tea or coffee and no breakfast, by mid morning energy levels tend to crash and symptoms occur which include cravings for sweet foods. It is the body's way of informing you that the blood sugar levels are low. Having a lunch time drink, and several cigarettes instead of a meal is about the best way of producing swings in blood sugar levels.
- Concentrate on eating foods with a low glycaemic index – those which are converted into sugar at a slow to medium rate. Foods include wholegrain rice, pulses and most fresh fruit and vegetables. *See* the section on Diabetes (page 165) for further information.
- Eat fresh homecooked foods wherever possible.
- Eat foods that are intrinsically sweet like dried fruit, fresh fruit, nuts and seeds.
- Relax whilst you are eating and enjoy your food.
- Plan your meals and snacks in advance.
- Take wholesome snacks out with you so that you don't get caught short.
- Always shop for food *after* you have eaten.
- Concentrate on a diet rich in chromium, magnesium and vitamins B and C. Although we need a constant supply of all the important nutrients, three specific groups of nutrients have been shown to be needed to maintain normal blood sugar control. B vitamins are also necessary for optimum function of the brain and the nervous system, as is magnesium, which is also necessary for normal hormone function, and incidentally, is the most common nutritional deficiency amongst women of childbearing age. Chromium is a curious mineral of which we have only tiny amounts at birth, and these gradually lessen as the years go by. Chromium, like magnesium and B vitamins can be sourced

in food, but we have to know where to look for it, so this calls for a little study of the Nutritional Content of Food lists on page 483.

- At the WNAS we recommend nutritional supplements of vitamin B, magnesium and chromium in the form of a preparation called Normoglycaemia, which acts as a short-term nutritional prop to regulate blood sugar levels.
- Take regular physical exercise, five sessions per week to the point of breathlessness.
- Use the menus for Sugar Craving on page 476 as a guide.

See also: Obesity, Alcohol, What's wrong with present-day diet and lifestyle?, Nutrition is the key to health, Recommended reading (*Beat Sugar Craving*), References, A very nutritious diet and the Menu for sugar craving.

Gallstones

Gallstones are formed in the gall bladder, whose function it is to collect and concentrate a dark green fluid produced by the liver called bile. This fluid aids the digestive process, especially that of fats, and contains cholesterol, other fats, calcium and pigments derived from the breakdown of blood cells. Gallstones form slowly, usually over many years, when the concentration of cholesterol, calcium and other chemicals normally found in the bile is so great that they can no longer remain in solution. Often the presence of a small amount of bacteria acts as the focus for the onset of gallstone formation. There may be just one stone or many small stones. Often the stones are 'silent' – being present, but without any symptoms. Their presence, however, may cause pain or other symptoms relating to digestion and liver.

What are the symptoms?

The pain caused by gallstones is often severe, episodic and can last up to two hours. The sufferer is likely to be doubled up by pain, which is usually, though not always, located in the upper right-hand side part of the abdomen. Typically the episode passes off after a few hours. Minor episodes may occur, and can be associated with a feeling of sickness, or alternatively an aversion to large or fatty meals which may indeed trigger the attacks. Sometimes infection also develops in the gall bladder in which case there may be a fever, the pain is more prolonged and the sufferer is visibly unwell. If the gallstone moves and blocks the passage of bile from the liver to the bowel then the person becomes jaundiced and the stools become pale.

So much for the full-blown picture. We now know that gallstones are in fact very common and may cause milder intermittent symptoms of abdominal discomfort, nausea and aversion to fats. In this situation the picture is similar to that of irritable bowel syndrome or of a peptic ulcer. The treatments for these three common conditions are very different, so doctors as well as the sufferer need some understanding of what is going on.

Who gets them?

They are rare in children, but do develop if there is a blood condition that leads to an increase in the breakdown pigments from haemoglobin. This can run in some families. Recent surveys reveal that the prevalence of gallstones, detected by ultrasound examination (like that used to look at unborn babies) rises steeply with age especially after the age of 40 and especially in women. Figures of between ten and 20 per cent in the middle-aged and the elderly are not uncommon. Studies show that gallstones are an example of a 'Western diet' – overconsumption of refined foods, low fibre and an insufficient intake of fresh fruit and vegetables.

What causes them?

- Being female, as women carry approximately twice the risk of men.
- Getting older.
- Being overweight, especially if the fat is distributed around the abdomen rather than the hips. Obese teenagers are especially at risk, as are those who gain weight later in life.
- Fluctuating weight. Feasting then dieting may cause changes to the chemistry of the bile that promotes gallstone formation.
- A diet high in sugar and low-fibre carbohydrates, e.g. potatoes, and low in fresh fruit and vegetables.
- Lack of alcohol! Just one drink per day seems to offer reasonable protection.
- The oral contraceptive pill can cause a slight increase.
- Severe constipation in women is associated.
- Some diseases of the liver and bowel are associated.
- A high level of fats called triglycerides in the blood. This is associated with being overweight, being diabetic, or consuming a lot of alcohol or sugar.

What your doctor can do

- *Ignore them* Gallstones that are found coincidentally, and cause no or very few symptoms, require no treatment. Gallstones are a phenomenon that many of us will acquire if we live long enough. However we may not all live long enough for them to be a problem.

- *Remove them with an operation* This is necessary for most of us if they start to cause problems like severe pain, infection or jaundice. The operation may be needed as an emergency, or more usually is tackled when any acute episode is over. During the operation the gall bladder and the stone or stones are removed, and special attention has to be paid to make sure that all the stones present are found.
- *Dissolve them using chemical treatments* Preparations of acids with cholesterol-dissolving properties are a possible treatment for some with stones made mainly from cholesterol. This technique is useful when the stones do not contain a lot of calcium and are contained within a relatively healthy gall bladder.
- *Destroy them using high energy sound waves* This is technically known as extracorporeal shock-wave lithotripsy. With the abdomen immersed in water, high-energy wound waves can be focused upon the gallstones when they shatter. Combining this with chemical means leads to a 90 per cent success rate in selected patients.

What you can do

If you need an operation have it. Then select those pieces of the following advice that may be relevant to you. If your gallstones are not really a problem, and there is no need for definitive treatment, the following advice may reduce the risk of their becoming worse. Increasing numbers of people will fall into this category. These measures may also be helpful if your gallstones are being dissolved by chemical means.

- Lose weight if you need to (see The Simple Weight-Loss Diet page 452).
- Alternatively follow The Very Nutritious Diet or The Vegetarian Diet (see pages 437 and 455).
- Allow yourself one alcoholic drink per day.
- Don't let yourself become constipated (see page 136).
- Take a supplement of magnesium. The WNAS recommend magnesium amino acid chelate for its ability to relax the smooth muscles of the gut to promote healthy bowel function.
- Don't miss meals. Eat regularly and always have breakfast.
- Supplements of vitamin C, 1g per day, might help by encouraging the breakdown of cholesterol.
- Gallstones are easier to prevent than to treat so ensure that you are following a healthy diet from the outset!

Complementary therapies

Traditional naturopathic texts refer to the treatment of gallstones using the juice of six lemons and 300 ml (half a pint) of olive oil. A small number of our patients have apparently used this treatment after an overnight fast. According to their testimony they have subsequently passed a number of small stones and been relieved of their gall-bladder pain. This is a potentially dangerous treatment for most patients with gallstones especially those with large or multiple stones. If any reader of this book has successfully passed stones in this way we would be grateful if they would contact us. Photographic evidence or a suitable affidavit would be required! This truly is a kill or cure treatment.

Genital Herpes

In the 1980s there was a 90 per cent increase in the incidence of genital herpes in North America, and a similar increase occurred in the United Kingdom. The term herpes is derived from the Greek word *herpein*, meaning 'to creep', and it was first described by Hippocrates. Genital herpes is a disease that is spread through sexual contact, and may be passed to new partners without either party being aware of the risk. It cannot be cured, it may cause cancer, and it may be passed on to newborn babies who either die or become severely brain damaged. When compared to genital herpes, syphilis and gonorrhoea appear to be relatively mild diseases.

The virus that causes genital herpes is the herpes simplex virus type 2 (HSV-2). This is one of a family of five herpes viruses that cause a wide range of human ills, including chickenpox, shingles, infectious mononucleosis (glandular fever), and birth defects such as mental retardation. Research suggests that HSV-2 is a complicated virus, with over 100,000 different strains or varieties of its basic structure. HSV-1, the virus that causes cold sores can also cause genital herpes as well . As people 'swap' mucous membranes during sexual intercourse, it is likely that either of these types of virus may be present in genital herpes.

What are the symptoms?

Genital herpes affects the vulva, perineum, buttocks, cervix, the vagina, thigh or anal area, and sores can erupt in any of these areas.

Any combinations of the following symptoms may occur:

- Itching
- Fever
- General malaise
- Burning
- Painful urination
- Swollen lymph glands
- Blisters
- Immobility
- Painful bowel movements
- Open sores
- Headaches

When genital herpes repeats itself, as it does, particularly in the first year following the primary attack, some of these symptoms may recur. The attack usually begins when a person experiences an itchy tingling sensation over a reddened area of the skin, which is followed hours or days later by a single blister, or cluster of highly infectious fluid-filled sores that will erupt in one to two days, and then crust over after three or four days. These sores usually appear on the cervix, in the vagina and in the urethra, and in men the sores are generally on the penile shaft.

The primary outbreak may involve intense pain for as long as three weeks, but subsequent outbreaks tend to be less and less severe as time passes, and in some cases they are almost unnoticeable.

What causes it?

The virus can be passed to a woman in any of the following ways:

- sexual intercourse with an infected partner with active sores.
- sexual caresses from a partner with herpetic whitlows, sores on the fingers.
- oral sex with a partner who has a herpes sore on the mouth.

It can also be triggered by internal stimulation of the latent virus which has been hiding in the body, by any of the following:

- emotional stress
- over-exertion
- sunburn
- fever
- ultraviolet light
- onset of a period
- anxiety or depression over the illness
- persistent vaginal discharge
- chafing
- impaired immune system which may be caused by some of the above and by a lack of essential nutrients.

What your doctor can do

- Prescribe Acyclovir, the only effective anti-viral agent. It can be given as a cream for those suffering their first attack, but this does not help recurrent episodes. In tablet form it is not always well absorbed. A dose of 200 mg five times per day for five days can be used to treat repeated attacks, but to be of any use it needs to be taken as soon as symptoms begin, often before there is definitive evidence of the infection. This means your doctor giving you a prescription to carry around with you in the event of a further attack. Long-term use of Acyclovir

to prevent attacks is sometimes used. The dose is 200 mg per day. This is only rarely required.
- Assess you for the presence of other genital infection especially candida.
- Assess and treat your partner.

What you can do

- Report early when you have symptoms.
- Use symptomatic treatment to control the discomfort, which includes painkillers, e.g. aspirin or paracetamol, especially if there are generalised 'flu-like symptoms, and local applications of iodine ointment (messy but effective), ice packs, or used tea bags (an old folk remedy).
- Refrain from sexual intercourse – just in case you wondered.
- Wear underpants in bed at night to minimise the risk of spread to other parts of the body, e.g. the hands and eyes.
- Wash your hands thoroughly every time you go to the toilet.
- Try supplements of Lysine. Lysine is an amino acid found in foods and can replace the chemically related amino acid arginine which is needed by the virus to replicate itself. Supplements of lysine have been used in the treatment of oral herpes with some benefit. Not all studies have been positive. The dose is 500 mg three times per day. Some advise taking it with vitamin C, 1g three times per day.
- Follow a diet rich in lysine and low in an opposing amino acid arginine. This means avoiding nuts, chocolate, carob, oats, wholewheat and soya beans. You can eat more of fish, chicken, meats, milk, cheese, mung beans and other beans but not soya.
- Try supplements of multi-vitamins and zinc in the longer term as a means of improving resistance to infection. Zinc applied topically as zinc sulphate can give immediate benefit, but treatment given in its early stages is more effective. Also follow The Very Nutritious Diet (see page 437).
- Oral consumption and topical application of vitamin C can increase the rate of healing of herpes. It is most effective when treatment is administered in its early stages.
- B-complex helps combat the virus and helps to keep it from spreading. It also works synergistically with the amino-acid lysine to prevent further outbreaks.
- Tea tree oil is a powerful natural antiseptic and is best applied during an outbreak. Use it neat or dilute in distilled water or cold-pressed vegetable oil. Avoid contact with the eyes.
- Liquorice root inhibits both the growth and cell damage caused by the virus. *Do not take* for more than seven consecutive days or if pregnant. AVOID it completely if your suffer with high blood pressure.
- Applying black walnut or goldenseal extract to the affected area may help. See a qualified medical herbalist for more specific advice.

- Garlic in capsule form has natural antibiotic properties and has also potent immune boosting properties.
- Avoid those factors that seem to precipitate an attack.
- Do not get pregnant until this problem is sorted out. You should probably see a venereologist if your genital herpes is recurrent, and you and your partner are planning a pregnancy. It is possible for a woman with genital herpes to bear a normal healthy child, if medical screening procedures are methodically followed prior to delivery. If the screening shows that the infection has become active near or during labour, the baby can be protected by being delivered by caesarean section.

Complementary therapies

Anything that helps to strengthen the immune system may help to increase your rate of healing. The main four therapies – cranial osteopathy, acupuncture, herbal medicine and homeopathy are all geared to do this in their own way. It is a matter of preference which combination of therapies you try.

Julie's story

Julie is a 36-year-old mother of three who works as a receptionist at a Family Planning Clinic. She had suffered with herpes for thirteen years and although she and her doctor tried all sorts of medication nothing really kept the herpes at bay.

'I have been suffering with herpes for so long and they have been much worse for the last couple of years. I remember two years ago we went on a family holiday in the sun and my whole top lip swelled up. It really ruined the holiday. I also had boils on my chin to accompany the herpes which made me feel like nothing on earth. Last year we went on holiday – there wasn't even any sunshine – but I still had an attack. In fact, when I think about it I have had herpes every couple of weeks for years and it seems to last for about ten days each time so I have been rarely free of an ugly cold sore on my lips.

My doctor had prescribed all sorts of products. We have tried antiseptic and I have even tried anti-biotics but nothing seemed to help. In fact, some of the products for herpes seemed to make the sores spread.

I approached the WNAS for some help with my premenstrual syndrome, after reading their book on PMS, No More PMS, three months ago. Not only is my PMS relatively non-existent now but I haven't had an outbreak of herpes or boils since I began. I can't really believe it and I am thrilled to bits. We are off to Cornwall this year and I am looking forward to a normal family holiday.'

See also: References.

Haemorrhoids

Women are particularly prone to haemorrhoids, or 'piles' as they are commonly known, which are varicose veins that form inside the rectum. Sometimes after childbirth or following an episode of constipation, because of the straining and pressure in the area, they become external, and resemble a small bunch of grapes. They can vary from being mildly uncomfortable to extremely painful, and they often bleed, as their thin walls may be ruptured by a passing motion.

Our veins contain valves, which prevent blood flowing backwards. When the vessels are healthy and strong, this system works well. However, when the valves themselves become weak and inefficient, blood flows backwards and pools at certain points making the vessel wall swell out into a varicose vein.

What are the symptoms?

- Pressure and a feeling that 'everything is falling out' of your rectum.
- Soreness, irritation and sometimes sharp pains in the rectum.
- Itchiness around the anus.
- Small amounts of fresh red blood in the stools.

What causes them?

- The constant pressure of carrying a baby during pregnancy can precipitate haemorrhoids in a woman who has not previously been a sufferer.
- Straining on the toilet when constipated can weaken the vessel walls in the area.
- Lack of adequate nutrition – for example we know that vitamin C and bioflavanoids are necessary for the health of the walls of our blood vessels.
- Lifting heavy goods on a regular basis.
- Bouts of coughing.

What your doctor can do

- Examine your back passage to determine whether haemorrhoids are present, or whether there is likely to be any other physical problem, like a tear or a growth.
- Prescribe some soothing cream, suppositories or topical anaesthetic to help relieve the pain, if it is severe.
- Supply you with an anal dilator to manually replace external haemorrhoids after a motion.

- An enlightened doctor will tell you to increase your consumption of fruit and vegetable fibre, but not necessarily cereal fibre, which can sometimes make constipation worse.
- Give you, or refer you for, a course of injections, which over a period of three months cause the haemorrhoids to shrink.
- In severe cases, refer you for surgical removal of the haemorrhoids. This is a particularly painful operation, and there is no guarantee that the haemorrhoids won't re-form, unless you tackle the underlying cause.

What you can do

- Keep your motions very soft by eating a good diet. Follow the recommendations for The Very Nutritious Diet on page 437 or, if you think you may have food sensitivities, follow the recommendations for The Simple Exclusion Diet on page 460.
- Take supplements of magnesium at night to keep the motions soft, and two tablespoons of organic linseeds with your morning cereal to make the motions smooth, rather than dry and lumpy. The magnesium needs to be taken to gut tolerance level (see Constipation, page 136). This will prevent you from straining, which stresses the haemorrhoids further.
- Drink plenty of fruit juice, water and herbal tea.
- After each motion, gently bathe your tail end, and use some soothing herbal cream, either from the health-food shop or ask your herbal practitioner to make up a prescription for you.
- If you have external haemorrhoids, take care to manually replace them with an anal dilator greased with herbal cream.
- During an acute episode, keep your feet up when you can, until the pain and soreness has diminished.
- Make up a small bag of frozen peas and sit on it for 10 minutes. This should be repeated throughout the day when symptoms flare up, and will help to reduce the swelling and inflammation in the area.
- Take warm baths or showers rather than hot baths, as the intense heat may encourage even more blood into the area.
- Take regular exercise, including exercises for your pelvic floor and your tail end. Draw your muscles in as if you are trying to stop the flow of urine mid-cycle. Hold it for the count of ten, and then slowly release. You can repeat this exercise at convenient moments during the day.

Complementary therapies

Acupuncture, homeopathy, herbal medicine and cranial osteopathy all have something to offer in their own way. Improving the flow of fluid around the body will help to unblock the areas of stagnation. Additionally acupuncture may also be able to help strengthen the walls of the vessels.

See also: Standard references.

Hair Loss

There are different patterns of hair loss in women and men. In men there is often a receding hair line which is due to the action of the male hormone testosterone. Women may occasionally experience this pattern, but more usually have either generalised diffuse hair loss or alopecia areata.

Alopecia areata involves discrete patches of hair loss that are completely bald. It is common in young adults, and often recovers spontaneously. Treatment sometimes involves injection of steroids and always patience. There seems to be little that the patient can do to speed up the natural turn of events. Diffuse hair loss is exactly what it says it is, with generalised thinning and loss of hair from the top of the head. Generalised, often mild, scalp hair loss can also accompany any disease of the scalp such as psoriasis and eczema.

Research has shown that a large proportion of women reporting hair loss had low ferritin levels. The main reason for this is due to the loss of blood during menstruation, which is just enough to cause a gradual depletion of iron stores, particularly in women who suffer with heavy periods or eat little or no red meat.

What your doctor can do

He can investigate the cause by checking for:

- an underactive thyroid gland or other hormonal disturbance.
- a pregnancy.
- a fever or any severe illness.
- a side-effect of drugs.
- iron deficiency, or a mild lack of iron, might follow blood donation.

What you can do

- Eat The Very Nutritious Diet (page 437).
- Take a supplement of iron if you are anaemic or if the haemoglobin level is normal but at the lower end (11.0 to 12.5 mg/dl). A small supplement such as one tablet of Ferrous Sulphate taken daily with fruit juice for six months is safe and should correct any mild deficiency. You will need to take it for six months though as recovery is slow.
- Vitamin C works synergistically with iron, enhancing its absorption. Take a supplement of at least 1000 mg a day, and ensure that you drink a glass of orange juice when taking your iron supplement.
- Avoid tea as it contains tannin. This binds with iron, therefore inhibiting its absorption.
- Supplements of zinc and multi-vitamins might be helpful. Again they will need to be taken for several months.

Complementary therapies

Watch out for some unusual shampoos. Local applications are unlikely to make much difference and sensitisation can occur. For advice see a qualified trichologist (see your local Yellow Pages).

Halitosis

Bad breath, or halitosis as it is medically known, is detected in most cases by someone other than the sufferer themselves. It is not a very social topic of conversation, and even dentists, who are responsible for keeping us orally fit, are sometimes embarrassed about mentioning it to a patient. In the UK only four out of ten of us visit the dentist regularly, and some 15 per cent of regulars have moderate to severe gum disease, which is thought to cause some 60 per cent of bad breath.

The mere thought that our breath may be unsavoury does little for our self-confidence, and is likely to make us feel introverted and nervous. If you think you may be a sufferer check it out with your partner or a close friend, and ask them to be absolutely honest. A bad taste in your mouth doesn't always translate to a bad smell, and it is difficult to smell your own breath. If you do suffer, you need to know so that you can deal with it without delay.

What causes it?

- The most serious cause is an infection of the gums, where the bone supporting the teeth is eaten away after plaque (bacteria in the mouth) has been allowed to stagnate in the pockets of gum surrounding the teeth. Plaque becomes rotten and smelly as it ages, which is what causes the odour.

   The milder form of gum disease is known as gingivitis, which means inflammation of the gums, and a more advanced form, which involves bone resorption, is called periodontitis or periodontosis. Not all gum infections cause bad breath though. It usually has to be an acute flare up or advanced gum disease before it affects the nostrils of others. Acute ulcerative gingivitis, or trench mouth as it more commonly known, will make the breath smell foul, and should be treated quickly.
- Stomach disorders such as hiatus hernia can create an oral odour.
- Infections of the tonsils and respiratory tract may also make the mouth smell.
- Hormonal changes, particularly a rise in the level of the hormone progesterone, can cause gums to be swollen, resulting in a bad taste and sometimes a bad smell. This is why symptoms are sometimes worse before a period or during pregnancy.

- A dry mouth, which can arise from stress or other illnesses, or simply as a result of too much exertion and not enough fluid, often causes bad breath.
- Food allergies often cause a reflux, food returning to the mouth after it has been digested, which is smelly.
- Crash diets affect the flow of saliva, and this is the body's natural mouth wash, flushing away odour-producing bacteria. Some drugs like sleeping pills can also dry the mouth. Constipation can be associated with halitosis (see page 136).

What your doctor can do

- Check to see whether you have a hiatus hernia, an upper respiratory tract infection, like infected tonsils, or constipation. If so, these should be treated and the problem will resolve by itself.
- If you are on medication, check to see whether you are suffering a dry mouth as a side-effect.

What your dentist can do

- Check for the presence of any form of gum disease, and if so treat it, see page 326. Gingivitis can be eliminated by careful tooth-brushing and flossing between the teeth, over a period of weeks or months. More severe forms of gum disease, where pockets of calculus (old, hard stagnated plaque) have developed between the gum and the tooth, may involve dental intervention. The pockets can be cleaned out by the dentist or the hygienist, and in severe cases where bone loss has occurred, but substantial bone still exists, the bones can be remodelled. Once the mouth has been cleaned up, your breath will undoubtedly feel fresher.
- Diagnose AUG – acute ulcerative gingivitis – or trench mouth, (see page 326) which needs urgent treatment with metronidazole, a special form of antibiotic.

Julia's story

Julia was a 36-year-old part-time sales assistant with two children. She had developed halitosis (bad breath) which made her feel extremely self-conscious.

'With hindsight I think my problem started years ago when my two children were small. Our eldest child had open-heart surgery as a toddler and I knew that he would need a further operation when he reached his teens. We had concerns about the little one at school plus my mouth and throat had become dry, which I presumed was

directly related to the anxiety. My husband eventually confirmed my worst fears, that my breath was very smelly, particularly in the two weeks before my period. I had a foul sour taste in my mouth and when I ran my tongue across my teeth I was aware of an equally unpleasant smell.

My first thought at the time was that I must have a dental problem. I was very embarrassed when I consulted my dentist, and extremely dismayed when he could find nothing wrong with my teeth, and only minor inflammation on the gums which I corrected with improved brushing. I read that halitosis can be caused by a number of illnesses, like lung disease and gastric ailments like hiatus hernia. But my doctor confirmed that there was nothing wrong with me in these departments.

I began to wonder if my problem had something to do with the food I was eating, so I made a point of avoiding all the acknowledged obnoxious smelling foods like onions, garlic and blue cheese. I brushed my teeth several times each day, flossed between them, gargled with mouthwash and chewed and sucked fresh-breath sweets and gum. Nothing worked and I became so embarrassed about the problem that I made sure I stood well away from people when I spoke to them. I even got into the habit of covering my mouth with my hand when having a conversation.

I felt very humiliated and self-conscious. I was used to being such a lively and outgoing person, it's hard not to be inhibited when you are trying to keep your mouth firmly shut. Most people are too polite to comment, but I knew they could smell my bad breath, which was so distressing. What didn't make sense was that the smell was worse for two weeks before my period, and seemed to improve after my period had begun. I had been having other premenstrual problems for many years which eventually lead me to the solution to my bad breath.

I read an article in a magazine about premenstrual syndrome, and not dreaming that my breath problem could be connected, I wrote for information. When I received the questionnaire from the WNAS I was stunned to see that bad breath was one of the premenstrual symptoms they asked about. I came to discover that life events and stress can upset the brain chemistry which influences our hormones. It turned out that I had an allergy to wheat, which seemed to cause a chemical reaction in my body, particularly before my period. Once I tidied up my diet and avoided wheat the bad breath cleared up completely. The only problem was that I had cravings for pasties in the two weeks before my period, and each time I indulged I'd feel the bad breath taste welling in my mouth. Once I tuned in to my body I realised that the pasties and other *foods containing wheat affected my gut too. This explained why my breath was worse premenstrually.*

It's ten years since I kissed my bad breath goodbye. Occasionally I get the cravings for a pastie, and if I do indulge I feel that old familiar taste return. I managed to overcome the other premenstrual symptoms too and feel totally in control. It's wonderful to be able to smile and chat without having to be self-conscious.'

What you can do

- Follow The Good Oral Hygiene Plan on page 332.
- Omit from your diet any foods that you are aware upset your tummy, and of course avoid the known smelly foods like garlic and onions.
- Use an anti-bacterial mouth wash before brushing your teeth which helps to decrease the plaque levels, and thus reduce the smell.
- Coffee and cigarettes can dry your mouth, so it's best to cut these down, or better still, cut them out altogether.
- Ninety per cent of adults in the UK have gum disease and many suffer with halitosis or bad breath! Unlike toothbrushes and mouthwashes, dental floss can reach the plaque bacteria, decaying food and toxins, hidden beneath the gum line, which cause bad breath, gum disease and can lead to tooth loss. The WNAS recommends Glide floss which should be used daily in conjunction with tooth brushing by anyone who is keen to adopt a thorough, comfortable and effective oral hygiene routine.

See also: Allergies, Constipation, Influenza, recurrent coughs, colds and sore throats, The simple exclusion diet, References and Recommended reading.

Hay Fever and Allergic Rhinitis

Nasal irritation, discharge, sneezing and blockage are all the hallmarks of rhinitis which literally means 'inflammation of the nose'. This can occur at fixed times of the year, being related most frequently to pollens and is known as hay fever. Non-seasonal rhinitis may occur separately, or as well, and is often related to housedust mite allergy, but there are other possible causes. The symptoms of nasal irritation may be accompanied by throat itching, irritation in the ears, conjunctivitis with red watery eyes, and in more severe cases, asthma (see page 89).

The basic mechanism involved is that cells, called mast cells, present in the nose and lungs are stimulated by an allergen (a substance to which the individual is allergic), and subsequently release a variety of powerful irritating chemicals, including histamine. These chemicals produce the symptoms of rhinitis, and in particular stimulate the production of mucus, possibly in an attempt to 'wash away' the triggering allergen as though it were a serious threat to health. The mast cell contains, on its surface, specific antibodies of a type called IgE that interacts with specific antigens. Other chemicals and cells found in the lining of the nose determine the degree to which the body produces this sensitising IgE antibody.

Who gets it?

Something like 10–15 per cent of the UK population suffer. There appears to have been a substantial rise in consultations for these problems over the last 40 years.

Air pollution, especially in cities, may have led to this rise in prevalence despite, in some situations, a fall in the seasonal pollen count. Pollutants such as sulphur dioxide may damage the lining of the nose. The magnitude of exposure to housedust mite or animals as a youngster may be a determining factor. In occupational allergies, cigarette smoking again seems to increase the chance of developing such allergic reactions.

There is some association with other allergic conditions such as eczema and asthma and there is therefore probably a genetic component in determining who is likely to suffer.

What causes it?

It will be useful to separate seasonal and non-seasonal allergies:

Seasonal allergies

- Tree pollens are present in the spring from early April onward to late May in the UK. Sensitivity is common, and symptoms start at these times before the grass pollen season is underway.
- Grass pollen is abundant from mid-May to early August, with the earlier times being more relevant to the warmer southern areas. Pollen counts rise in warm dry conditions and in the evening, as the air cools, pollen counts at ground level reach a maximum.
- Weed pollens follow grass, and are around from July to September in the UK.
- Sensitivity to mould is again not uncommon. There are many varieties present from June until the autumn. Moulds are Mother Nature's garbagemen, breaking down vegetable matter, and releasing millions of invisible spores. Depending upon the variety, this can occur in either warm summer weather following rain, or after a heavy dew. In the house, damp dark places, especially cellars, attract moulds. In the garden, compost heaps, piles of grass cuttings and the soil are all places where some moulds proliferate.

Non-seasonal allergies

- Housedust mites are the commonest perennial allergen. They are abundant in most homes and live on shed human skin scales, thriving in the warm, moderately moist conditions that are the norm in most centrally-heated modern homes. Carpets, bedding materials and furnishings are the major preferred residences for these common allergens. Dustmite counts tend to peak in the spring and autumn, and their level is greatly influenced by the type of materials found in the home, and cleaning habits.
- Animals, especially domestic pets, are again another common source of allergic material. This is often from the saliva of cats which is passed on to their hair but can also be present in the air and mixed in with housedust. Dog, rabbit, and horse hair as well as feathers are other possibilities. Sensitivity to an animal's urine can also develop in farm and laboratory workers.
- Cockroaches in semi-tropical climes and now some inner-city buildings are again a potential source of allergic rhinitis.
- Occupational exposure to animal products, chemicals, flour, yeast, enzymes in biological washing powders and in flour improvers, and rubber are all possibilities.
- Foods are a possibility though this is an uncertain area. From adult and child experience it would seem that sensitivity to artificial colours, dairy products and oranges are especially likely. Only repeated withdrawal and challenge will determine the issue.
- Sulphur dioxide is worth a special mention. This is a chemical pollutant found in the air, especially in relation to inner cities and industrial areas. Some are particularly sensitive to it as it readily irritates the lining of the nose and lungs. Small amounts of this and related chemicals called sulphites are used as a preservative in foods and beverages (E 220–227). It is a surprisingly common additive in wine, especially cheap acidic white wine and in some this tipple will aggravate symptoms of rhinitis and asthma. Concentrated squashes are another possible source.

What your doctor can do

- Help identify the allergen from your history, from skin prick tests or, occasionally, blood allergy tests.
- Advise about allergen avoidance (see opposite).
- Offer drug treatment with steroid nasal sprays, antihistamine tablets and nasal sprays, and a nasal spray of sodium cromoglycate which blocks the allergen's interaction with IgE and the activation of the mast cell.
- Rarely desensitisation is used for isolated grass-pollen sensitivity.

What you can do

Avoiding the allergen is a central part of treatment for most sufferers:

- It may be difficult to completely avoid seasonal allergens. Staying indoors with windows and doors closed during times of high grass pollen count is for many a thing of the past because of effective drug treatments. For some, going to the seaside and sitting on the beach with an on-shore wind blowing, is a way to reduce one's exposure to pollen.
- If mould sensitivity is a problem, make sure that you are not being exposed to mould in the house. Watch out for damp patches with dark discoloration of wallpaper, and treat such patches with an antifungal paint. If there is a lot of damp, then a builder may need to be consulted. Treat any dry, as well as wet rot, that affects wooden structures. It may be advisable to remove houseplants which encourage mould growth.
- Measures to reduce exposure to housedust mite can be highly effective though this can take two or more months before the full benefit is experienced. The following measures are recommended in approximate order of importance and cost:
  - Use a modern powerful vacuum cleaner with an efficient filtration system once or twice weekly in the bedroom and main living areas.
  - Vacuum the carpets, furniture and the mattress and pillows.
  - Clean sheets and duvet covers weekly on a hot wash.
  - Renew pillows, opting for a synthetic and not feather filling.
  - Use a synthetic filled duvet rather than wool blankets and sheets.
  - Put the pillow and duvet out into bright sunshine on a dry day for several hours each week or month when possible. This helps to kill off dustmites.
  - You can also wash pillows and duvets from time to time. Putting pillows into the freezer for 24 hours and then into a tumble drier for 30 minutes will help curtail the mite's activities.
  - Keep the temperature and humidity in the bedroom low.
  - Minimise the use of soft furnishings, cuddly toys and carpets in the bedroom.
  - Buy a new mattress.
  - Use specialised occlusive corners for the mattress and pillows. This is worth considering if symptoms persist despite simple measures, or if mite sensitivity is a factor in asthma which is severe enough to require regular treatment with substantial amounts of steroids.
- In the case of animal sensitivity, remove the animal from bedrooms and main living areas. Many children with asthma, without obvious animal sensitivity, are well advised not to have cats or dogs as pets in case they develop a sensitivity.

- In the case of exposure to a possible allergen at work, expert advice may be needed, particularly in the case of asthma that is severe enough to affect the quality of life.
- If food sensitivity really is suspected then try The Simple Exclusion Diet on page 460 (*only* with medical supervision if you have asthma).
- Try limiting exposure to sulphites in foods and beverages (this latter will include some beers and many acidic tasting wines).
- Exercise might help! A run or 40 minutes' aerobics is a pretty good way of clearing your nasal passages. Regular exercise over several weeks might reduce the overall degree of sensitivity of the lining of the nose.
- Avoid drugs that might worsen nasal congestion. Sensitivity to aspirin is a not infrequent problem. Be suspicious of this if there are also nasal polyps, a personal history of asthma, or a family history of aspirin intolerance. Paracetamol is usually a safe alternative. Those who are very sensitive may need expert advice, and may benefit from a specialised diet low in fruits, vegetables and other foods containing salicylates.
- Vitamin C, 1g twice daily, has a moderate antihistamine effect. It's simple, cheap and free from side-effects.
- Supplements of vitamin B or multi-vitamins might help. Vitamin B6, pyridoxine, is needed by the body for the breakdown of histamine.
- The bioflavonoid quercetin stabilises the membranes of the histamine-releasing cells which triggers allergic symptoms.

Headaches

The type of headache ranges from a classic migraine to an eyestrain headache, hunger headache to a sinus headache. However, for the purpose of this chapter we are going to examine tension headaches, which are familiar to practically everyone, being the most common human complaint. At least 80 per cent of the population suffer with tension headaches at some point, and they are essentially due to contractions of the muscles of the scalp, neck and face. It is primarily an adult problem, with women affected three times as often as men. About half of those afflicted will have headaches that are severe and disabling, and it is thought that between 10–20 per cent will consult a doctor about their headaches, as a primary symptom. Unlike migraine, which occurs periodically, the tension headache is often a daily occurrence. It usually gets worse as the day goes by, and it is not associated with visual disturbance.

What are the symptoms?

The symptoms of a tension headache usually consist of an aching or squeezing discomfort on both sides of the crown, temples and forehead. The description most often used to illustrate the headaches is 'It feels like a tight band around my head, like a skull cap' or 'as if a clamp or vice was squeezing my head'. Others feel as if their head is about to 'burst or explode', and they stress that there is a feeling of pressure as well as pain.

The neck is often involved, and so too, sometimes are the nose and jaw. The headaches may only last for a few hours, but can last for days, weeks and even months.

What causes them?

Tension headaches are frequently associated with spasm of the muscles of the scalp, neck or shoulders. Anxiety and depression are other emotional associates. A somewhat different view is that of cranial osteopathy which believes that tension headaches often come about because of stress to the fascia, the connective tissue structure under the skin . This can apparently be the result of physical, mental or emotional trauma.

The cause is usually a combination of overwork, stress, lack of exercise or an emotional crisis of some sort which causes the muscles to go into spasm. Whilst headaches may stand alone as a problem, they may also be a manifestation of various general medical diseases, or problems affecting the nervous system or the head. The risk of headaches being due to a serious condition increases after the age of 65 years of age. Other possibilities include bleeding or leakage from blood vessels at the base of the brain, and only very rarely a brain tumour.

What your doctor can do

- Examine you physically, and take a history of the problem, which is important for three reasons: firstly, to eliminate the possibility of the symptoms being anything other than a tension headache; secondly, to locate the source of the headache, such as the neck, which may have been forgotten; and thirdly, to put your mind at rest. Anxiety about an underlying brain haemorrhage or something will only serve to make the headaches worse.
- Once the cause is located, it may be that drugs are unnecessary. However, analgesics, and even sedatives, tranquillisers and other tension-relieving drugs are sometimes used. If drugs are used they should only be limited to short courses.
- Refer you to a neurologist if there is any cause for concern.

What you can do

- Eat a good diet. Follow the recommendations for The Very Nutritious Diet on page 437.
- Avoid excessive amounts of tea, coffee and alcohol.
- Identify any food allergies or sensitivities. Dairy products and caffeine have been implicated in the onset of headaches. However, caution is needed when cutting these foods out of the diet, because withdrawal symptoms can manifest, which can actually worsen headaches and induce feelings of nausea. The best advice is gradually to cut out the offending foods over a period of weeks.
- Avoid foods containing tyramine, which include chocolate, bananas, cheese, citrus fruit, peanut butter, pork, smoked fish, wine and products containing yeast. Tyramine can cause blood pressure to rise, resulting in a dull headache.
- Never miss a meal, as low blood sugar can often precipitate a headache.
- Talk through any problems you face, and aim to get a workable solution underway.
- Learn to manage your time, so that you have time for regular relaxation, (see page 29).
- Try to reorganise yourself so that you can avoid further stressful situations recurring (see page 25).
- Take regular exercise, preferably in the fresh air and sunlight when available, see (page 32).
- Massage your own scalp, forehead, temples and ears regularly, or treat yourself to a regular massage. Use some of the gentler and more relaxing aromatherapy oils like lavender, melissa or geranium.
- Take daily supplements of strong multi-vitamins and minerals, with a strong B complex. Add an extra supplement of magnesium, in the region of 300 mg per day, as magnesium acts as a muscle relaxant. It may take two or three months before it is fully effective.
- When you feel the stress is getting the better of you, try going for a walk or doing some deep breathing.
- Try chewing some ginger, either root or crystallised, as this old remedy can often reverse the process of a headache if caught in time.
- Always seek and treat the cause of the headache, rather than the symptom, as long-term reliance on painkillers can switch of the brain's natural ability to fight the headache.

Complementary therapies

Cranial osteopathy is the first choice of treatment, and may sort out the underlying physical cause of your headaches. Other therapies like herbal medicine, homeopathy and acupuncture all have something to offer.

See also: References.

Heart Failure

At its simplest, it is a failure of the pumping action of the heart. For a variety of reasons the heart may not be able to pump enough blood forwards around through the lungs and around the body. The heart has two sides: the right side pumps blood to the lungs where oxygen is collected and carbon dioxide released; the refreshed blood returns from the lungs to the left side of the heart from whence it is pumped around the body. This requires a greater degree of force and consequently the left side of the heart is bigger than the right side. Blood is prevented from flowing back in the wrong direction by a series of valves and chambers in both sides of the heart.

What are the symptoms?

- shortness of breath, especially with any activity, or at night when lying down
- fatigue
- ankle swelling
- cough
- irregular breathing pattern when asleep
- poor appetite
- sometimes, loss of weight

Who gets it?

The elderly are the largest group at risk, and heart failure is now one of the commonest reasons for admission to hospital throughout the developed world.

What causes it?

Often there is more than one cause. The main ones are:

- high blood pressure
- ischaemic heart disease
- disorders of the heart muscle or the heart valves
- alcoholism
- nutritional deficiencies
- rarely, infectious anaemia

What your doctor can do

- Assess the cause and severity. This often requires specialist referral for blood tests, x-rays, ECG (electro-cardiogram – an electrical heart tracing) and ultrasound examination of the heart which can look at the function of the heart muscle and valves.

- Treat the failure with diuretics or water pills, digitalis (a very old-fashioned but effective drug derived from foxglove), and drugs that help to open up blood vessels and reduce the pressure under which the heart works. These latter drugs, called ACE Inhibitors, have greatly improved the outlook for many with heart failure and need to be prescribed more frequently. Occasionally treatment with beta blocker drugs.
- Advise about the need for supplements of potassium which may be deficient or in excess as a result of drug treatment.

What you can do

- Rest in bed with your feet up. This helps in the removal of excess fluid in acute episodes of heart failure. It is most useful to do this in the morning after the first dose of any diuretic or water pill.
- Follow The Low-Salt Diet (see page 449) as salt in the diet contributes to a build-up of water in the body and creates more work for the heart to do.
- Limit your intake of fluid to 2.5 litres per day.
- Make sure the diet is adequate in essential nutrients, especially protein, vitamin B, potassium and magnesium.
- Spread meals out during the day, as eating little and often is a good rule for you to follow.
- Limit alcohol to seven units per week.
- Avoid all alcohol. It is actually a poison and damages the heart muscle.
- Take supplements of multi-vitamins and magnesium, with your doctors approval as these may well make a difference if you are not eating very well.
- Weigh yourself regularly, as rapid weight loss or weight gain may signify deterioration in heart function.
- Exercise. Amazingly, very careful graded exercise is appropriate for those with mild to moderate heart failure once any acute episode is over. In fact this can lead to considerable improvement and actually helps correct the underlying weakness of the heart muscle in a way not achieved by drug therapy. Again specialist advice from your doctor is needed.

See also: Standard references.

HIGH BLOOD PRESSURE

The blood in our body circulates around due to the pumping action of the heart which causes the blood leaving the heart in the arteries to be at a higher pressure than that which is returning to the heart in the veins. When the heart contracts, the pressure rises to reach a peak called the systolic pressure, and between contractions the pressure falls to what is termed the diastolic pressure.

When you have your blood pressure measured, both these levels are recorded and are expressed as the systolic value over the diastolic value. They are measured as millimetres of mercury which are written as 'mm Hg'. Elevation of either can be associated with an increased risk of a stroke and other disorders of the circulation. The clear association of a raised blood pressure with stroke risk, and the now established benefit of reducing blood pressure, means that doctors commonly measure blood pressure during routine examinations and patient visits.

Blood pressure values vary considerably from one person to another and from country to country. Furthermore our own blood pressure shows a substantial variation during the course of the day rising with stress, physical pain, exercise and sexual intercourse. There is usually a modest rise with age in most urban populations and much of this age-related rise has been attributed to the relatively high intakes of sodium salt found in the diet of developed communities.

Definitions of high blood pressure vary. In the USA and now in most other developed countries, many experts accept that if the blood pressure is consistently greater than 140/90 mm Hg, then this is worthy of a diagnosis of hypertension, and more importantly a signal to do something about it. For most adults a rise in either the diastolic or systolic readings above these values is associated with an increased risk of premature death. Values up to 159/99 are considered to be mild hypertension and may be improved by non-drug approaches. Hypertension with blood pressure values above 160/100 almost always needs drug treatment and, especially if there is evidence of damage to blood vessels, the kidney or heart. If not tackled vigorously, it is associated with greatly increased risk of early death usually from a stroke, kidney damage or a heart attack. The risk of all three rises as blood pressure rises, and there is also an increase in the furring up of arteries in the legs which leads to peripheral vascular disease. These conditions are dealt with elsewhere in this book. The optimal goal of treatment particularly in young people and diabetics is to lower systolic pressure to 140 or less and diastolic to 85 or less.

The mechanisms behind these diseases are damage to the walls of the arteries that are subjected to this increase in pressure. The artery wall becomes thickened, the lining damaged and more prone to the deposition of cholesterol, particularly if the blood level is elevated. The risk of blood pressure to health is thus greatly magnified if the person is overweight, smokes cigarettes, drinks excessively, has an elevated blood cholesterol, or eats a diet low in fresh fruit and vegetables.

The symptoms of a high blood pressure are few and far between. Usually with a mildly elevated pressure there are none, and the diagnosis is made by chance at routine examination. Headaches, giddiness, recurrent nose bleeds, a sensation of fullness in the head are all possible symptoms, but equally have many other causes. Dangerously high blood pressure can cause these as well as visual disturbance, symptoms relating to nerve damage, and even epilepsy or loss of consciousness. Symptoms relating to another condition causing the high blood pressure may also be present.

Who gets it?

The prevalence of high blood pressure obviously depends on the criteria set for its diagnosis. In the USA 33 per cent of white men and 38 per cent of black men in the age range eighteen to 74 years have a blood pressure above 140/90. The rise in systolic blood pressure with age means that the risk of high blood pressure is greater in the older population. Generally high blood pressure is more common in women compared with men, mainly from the age of 50 onward. In the UK the rates of high blood pressure in whites, Asians and blacks are similar. Urban populations tend to have higher pressures than those from rural communities. If Australian aborigines return from an urban to a rural existence there can be a substantial fall in blood pressure as well as reduction in other heart disease risk factors such as obesity and altered blood-fat levels. Reductions in salt and alcohol intake are top of the list of necessary changes.

What causes it?

The causes of high blood pressure have been one of the most hotly contested topics for the last 30 years. There are usually many minor contributing factors which produce a noticeable effect. This has important implications for treatment. Causes can be divided into three main categories:

- genetic
- environmental (e.g. diet)
- disease (e.g. hormonal disorders).

Genetic factors

These would seem to account for about 30 per cent of the variation in blood pressure, and are less important than environmental factors. The genetic mechanism may involve other factors such as weight, hormonal changes and a propensity to retain sodium. The effect of these is in turn capable of being reversed by appropriate dietary changes.

Environmental factors

There are many environmental factors considered on page 239 under the section 'What You Can Do', which interact with each other, and there is potentially substantial benefit in addressing most of them in every person with high blood pressure.

Two environmental factors that should be mentioned at this point are the effect of oestrogen and environmental poisons.

- The oral contraceptive pill and hormone replacement therapy (HRT) can cause a rise in blood pressure in a small percentage of users. This is in the region of 1–2 per cent of users only, but necessitates the doctor to monitor blood pressure levels when prescribing these or similar hormonal treatments.
- Steroid drugs and occasionally other medicines cause an elevation of blood pressure and require an alteration of the dose or change of treatment.
- Rarely, a raised blood pressure is due to past exposure to lead or possibly cadmium. These are two toxic minerals that can damage the kidneys and as a consequence cause high blood pressure as well as other health problems. A history of working with these minerals, no matter how long before should make one suspicious.

Disease factors

These are relevant to probably less than 10 per cent of newly diagnosed patients, and are for the most part outside the scope of this book. Brief details only will be given about these possible causes. Blood pressure can be raised in a wide variety of conditions including:

- kidney disease
- an underactive or overactive thyroid gland
- excessive production of adrenaline, cortisone and related substances
- structural abnormalities of the main artery leaving the heart, and occasionally a metabolic disorder.

Many of these conditions are rare but their importance is that their management may be very different from 'ordinary' high blood pressure and in some instances a cure can be genuinely achieved. Such conditions should be suspected if:

- there is a very high blood pressure, especially if it is not easily controlled by standard means.
- there is a family history of these rare causes or hormonal disorders.
- there is a personal history of kidney or urinary problems.
- there are persistent or severe headaches, palpitations or sweating and in all young people with a very high blood pressure.

Careful physical examination, blood tests, urine tests and a chest x-ray will detect the majority of them, and consequently all patients with high blood pressure should be carefully assessed by their doctor before beginning treatment.

What your doctor can do

- Assess your blood pressure by measuring it on three separate occasions. You should be sitting or lying down, relaxed and with no restrictive clothing on the upper part of the arm.
- Assess any possible damage that may have developed as a result of an elevated blood pressure. Enlargement and weakening of the heart, damage to the kidneys and changes to the blood vessels at the back of the eye are all possible, though now much less common due to the benefits of good treatment.
- Assess the possible causes, especially the presence of underlying medical conditions even if they are rare. The nature of any associated symptoms, examination, and results of simple blood and urine tests usually serve as a guide to these possibilities.
- Assess associated risk factors. An elevated blood pressure by itself may have relatively little health implication for the individual. Add one or more of the following and that can change dramatically: high alcohol intake, cigarette smoking, obesity, an elevated blood cholesterol, a poor diet and lack of exercise. These should all be discussed as appropriate by your doctor and the necessary advice given.
- Treat your blood pressure with drugs. There are many different types of drugs, and within each type of drug a variety to choose from. Commonly used drug types are:
  - *Diuretics* Now usually given as a very low dose, and are very useful in the elderly. They have the added bonus of possibly reducing calcium losses from the skeleton.
  - *Beta-Blockers* These act by blocking the action of adrenaline. They are more suited to young and middle-aged patients, especially if they suffer from coronary artery disease.
  - *Calcium antagonists* This family of drugs is useful for those with coronary artery disease. Some may cause ankle swelling as a side effect.
  - *Angiotensin Converting Enzyme Inhibitors* These act by counteracting one of the hormonal mechanisms that underlie high blood pressure. They are particularly suited to those who have a weakened heart, and diabetics. Chronic dry cough is a common side-effect.
  - *Alpha-Blockers* Another type of drug that also acts against adrenaline. It may be particularly suited to blacks and diabetics.

- Monitor your progress, which is vital. Regular frequent checks at the start of therapy are needed, and when control is achieved these can reduce to once- or twice-yearly checks. Those with a very high blood pressure, heart disease or diabetes will need more careful monitoring with regular urine and occasional blood tests and x-rays.

What you can do

Once upon a time there was nothing for the patient to do except to have faith in their doctor and the treatment. That has changed. In fact it is probably fair to say that today the patient's efforts are considered as important as the doctor's. You can choose whether or not to address the environmental factors that so often play a part in high blood pressure, and the doctor should direct you to the most important areas to address, and work out how to combine them with appropriate drug therapy.

To explain it all a little further, there are a collection of factors relating to our day-to-day existence that determine our blood pressure. These probably interact with any genetic predisposition for the blood pressure to rise.

For example, blood pressure levels, both systolic and diastolic, rise with age in virtually all communities around the world. The rise is quite substantial in some, but does not develop in those communities where there is a very low intake of salt. It seems likely that this environmental factor, salt intake over many years, will influence blood pressure, especially in those who are predisposed to respond this way.

Another important factor is the age of the person, and how long these environmental factors have been at play. Initially blood pressure readings may fluctuate considerably with high levels being recorded intermittently. This is termed 'labile hypertension'. Eventually this usually leads to an established raised blood pressure, though it may take many years. If you set about tackling some of the environmental factors in the early stages it is likely that you will achieve substantial results, whereas in an older person with persistently elevated blood pressure, drug treatment is more likely to be needed in order to achieve satisfactory control.

The British Hypertension Society issued guidelines in the year 2000 that all hypertensive and borderline hypotensive should be advised about self-help non-drug approaches. The most important areas that may need to be tackled, and can be tackled by you, are:

- *Weight* Obesity is a major determinant of blood pressure, which also influences blood cholesterol, heart disease and stroke risk. Weight reduction is often all that is needed to control mildly elevated blood pressure that is newly found in an overweight person. Follow The Simple Weight-Loss Diet (see page 452).

- *Alcohol* Consuming anything other than very modest amounts of alcohol can raise blood pressure. This can happen temporarily the day after an evening's socialising, but in regular heavy drinkers the elevation in blood pressure can be very substantial. In one study of young heavy-drinking Australian men, the drop in blood pressure after several week's abstinence was better than the improvement achieved by use of standard drug therapy. Modest consumption of alcohol may protect against heart disease, so a reasonably conservative guide for those with a raised blood pressure would be seven units per week for women and ten for men which is half the safe amount recommended by The British Hypertension Society.
- *Salt* As we have already mentioned, salt seems to be an important determinant of a community's blood pressure. For individuals, modest salt restriction, reducing sodium intake from the current average of around 150 millimols per day to half this value, can produce a small fall in blood pressure of usually no more than five to ten points in either systolic or diastolic. Very severe salt restriction can be more effective, but such diets are very difficult to follow in the long term. It is rare that this measure alone is enough to control raised blood pressure. However it would seem unwise not to advise those with an elevated blood pressure to not make some restriction of their salt intake. See The Low-Salt Diet on page 449.

These three factors are the most important and should really be considered by all those with established or labile hypertension. The remaining factors are worth considering, particularly as they may be relatively easily corrected by making simple dietary changes and because these same changes may bring other important health benefits.

- *Potassium* Increasing the balance of this mineral, which broadly speaking is the antagonist of sodium, also helps to lower blood pressure. The effect is small and it is no longer considered advisable to use supplements of potassium too freely as they can easily cause stomach irritation. A high dietary intake of fresh fruit and vegetables which are the main sources of this mineral will normally suffice. This is sound advice for almost all of us, as high fruit intakes are associated with a reduced risk of having a stroke. The British Hypertension Society recommend a total of seven portions of fruit and vegetables daily.
- *Magnesium* The sister of potassium. Poor or barely adequate intakes are common certainly in adults in the UK, and losses can also occur as a side-effect of some diuretics (water pills) used in the treatment of high blood pressure. One Scandinavian study showed that supplements can help lower blood pressure levels slightly in women but not all similar studies have shown this small effect. Magnesium supplements can help

improve the balance of potassium. Consider trying a daily supplement of 200–300 mg. It should not be taken without medical advice by those with kidney problems.

- *Calcium* The big brother of magnesium, at least so far as the bones are concerned. It too may have an effect of mildly lowering blood pressure. This is small and of uncertain value until the results of further current trials are published. To its advantage it is simple, cheap and safe, and of course mostly worth considering for older people who may also need to minimise their risk of developing osteoporosis. An effective dose is not clear, but probably between 500 and 1000 mg per day.
- *Fats and oils* Cutting down on saturated fats, which come mainly from animal sources, and increasing the intake of polyunsaturates, can also help lower blood pressure slightly. There does seem to be some particular effect by fish oils, particularly the Omega-3 essential fatty acids.
- *Avoiding liquorice* The black chewy sweetmeat of our childhood, prepared from the root of a Mediterranean and Asian plant, has one interesting side effect: it encourages the retention of salt by the body which can lead to a rise in blood pressure, so avoid it.
- *Exercise* There are many reasons for doing it, and yes, you can add controlling high blood pressure to the list. Experts recommend a daily jog or brisk walk or any other pleasurable and easy-to-do regular exercise of your choice. Some 40 minutes three times per week is a good goal. The British Hypertension Society recommend walking briskly for 20 minutes each day. Exercise lowers blood cholesterol and is also associated with lowered risk of heart disease, stroke and osteoporosis. So what are you waiting for!
- *Stress avoidance* This is now broadly accepted as being effective. Relaxation exercises and even meditation have been successful in controlling blood pressure. Do it the simple cheap way and fit it in with your lifestyle and daily schedule. Try relaxing very fully at home (see page 29 and page 242).

Finally for those who have followed the self-help advice carefully and achieved a normal blood pressure your doctor could then reduce or even stop your daily treatment. In one British study 22 per cent of well controlled hypertensives were able to remain off medication but they should all be followed up regularly.

Everyone with high blood pressure should be careful about their weight, should not drink excessively, should limit salt intake and follow the general recommendations for The Very Nutritious Diet (see page 437) with an emphasis on a good daily intake of fresh fruit and vegetables and exercise. There is a great deal you can do to influence your blood pressure.

Complementary therapies

Relaxation therapies, acupuncture and herbalism are all possibilities to be considered. Whichever of these you choose, make sure that your blood pressure is monitored by your medical adviser. Alternatively you can, with his approval, buy a blood pressure machine called a sphygmomanometer and record it yourself at home. If you want to do this then you should keep a careful record of the readings you obtain and check these results with your doctor who should oversee the whole activity. A very high blood pressure is a danger and the consequences of it remaining untreated or under-treated are substantial.

Kathy's story

The reason Mrs Hadley wanted to see us was because of her long standing rheumatoid arthritis which had begun 30 years ago and had required her to take low dose steroids for the last ten years. Weight gain had become inevitable and had probably contributed to the recent deteriorations in her arthritis. However, this did not prove her main problem.

She was overweight at 83 kilos (13 stone) and many joints, especially those of her hands and knees, had been severely damaged by the arthritis. Her blood pressure was very high, recorded at 250/140, and her weight was increased to 84.5 kilos (13 stone 6 pounds). There were changes in the blood vessels at the back of her eye indicating that this elevation in blood pressure was not just a one-off. Routine blood and urine tests were fortunately satisfactory.

She was immediately put on a weight-reducing low-salt diet together with a beta-blocking drug. Within two weeks her weight was down to 81.75 kilos and her blood pressure had fallen to 185/104. The headaches that she had barely mentioned at her first appointment had cleared up and she felt a lot better in herself.

Over the next three months her weight finally came down to 80 kilos and blood pressure 160/100. She was eventually prescribed a lower dose beta blocker with a small amount of diuretic, continued to follow her reduced calorie, low-salt diet and took supplements of calcium and magnesium together with multi-vitamins. If left untreated, this very high blood pressure would almost certainly have brought substantial consequences.

See also: Standard references.

Hysterectomy

The term 'hysterectomy' originates from the Greek words *hystera* meaning uterus, and *ektome*, meaning to cut out. The earliest hysterectomies on record were performed 1,600 years ago in Greece, and despite the high death rate, this method of treatment continued. The procedure involves the removal of all or part of the female reproductive organs. When the ovaries are removed (oopherectomy) as well as the uterus, the procedure is referred to as a full or radical hysterectomy, and when the uterus alone is removed, it is known as a partial hysterectomy.

It is one of the most common operations performed on women these days, surpassed only by caesarian section. It is offered, mainly for the control of heavy bleeding, to 50 per cent of women in the USA, 22–34 per cent of Australian women, and 20–25 per cent of women in Britain. Despite these large percentages, there are many unanswered questions about how appropriate it is to perform a full or radical hysterectomy on many of the chosen women, and the effects that this operation then has on long-term health and life expectancy.

Although there are times when a hysterectomy may be a life-saver, as in the case of uterine or ovarian cancer, in our experience there is substantial evidence that it is often performed unnecessarily, without giving the patient sufficient information to make an informed decision. In the case of heavy bleeding, where the ovaries are healthy and there is no history of ovarian cancer in the family, it may not be necessary to remove the ovaries as well as the uterus. A full or radical hysterectomy will prematurely rob you of your supply of oestrogen, which plays a key role in keeping your body youthful (see Menopause on page 298). And yet, many uneducated women are told that it is better to have the ovaries removed at the time of surgery in order to avoid further trouble later. Let us now test this premise.

Apart from obvious fertility, some women associate their uterus with femininity, and feel that its presence makes them more sexually appealing to their partner. This may be particularly relevant in societies where the ability to reproduce is a highly respected function. At the WNAS we have encountered numerous patients who went into hospital believing that they were having relatively minor surgery, and woke up to find that they had lost both their uterus and their ovaries. Surely we are all entitled to fully informed consent, no matter what the operation. In the case of a radical hysterectomy, the consequences may be great, and it is impossible to turn back the clock. All too often we hear of gynaecologists who suggest a radical hysterectomy after childbirth, assuming that as no further children are desired there is little point in retaining the reproductive organs. This is still occasionally recommended for the treatment of PMS, which is totally unacceptable.

The advantages of hysterectomy

- no more periods
- an end to heavy bleeding and period pain
- no further risk of pregnancy
- no need to use contraception
- elimination of the threat of cancer of any of the reproductive organs
- no further need for cervical smears
- no more gynaecological operations needed

The disadvantages of hysterectomy

- an earlier menopause, with increased risks of the bone-thinning disease osteoporosis, and heart disease. The risks of this latter are reduced by taking HRT, but not all women will tolerate this
- little further protection by oestrogen from ageing
- surgery and an anaesthetic required
- possible complications, either at the time of the operation or afterwards
- time needed to convalesce after the operation
- help needed at home during the recovery period
- the prospect of needing to take HRT in the long term, without first demonstrating that it suits you
- lack of fertility
- possible reduced sexual satisfaction for you or your partner, and less comfortable sex (the vaginal tissues dry as a result of the falling levels of oestrogen)

The reasons for an hysterectomy

The most common reasons for performing an hysterectomy are heavy periods or fibroids (lumps of fibrous tissue that grow inside the uterus).

- *Heavy bleeding* When periods become heavy, especially if there is flooding or associated anaemia, your doctor may suggest hormone therapy treatment with tranexamic acid, which affects blood clotting, or an hysterectomy.
- *Fibroids* Usually, with careful surgery, these can be removed, and the uterus left intact.
- *Prolapse* Where the uterus has dropped down in the pelvic cavity, but this can usually be repaired.
- *Endometriosis* Where the lining of the uterus grows outside the uterus, around other organs. This can often be improved by non-surgical means (see page 363).
- *Pelvic Inflammatory Disease* This includes all manner of infections and pelvic pain, which should be treated with drugs, antibiotics and natural means (see page 366), with an hysterectomy being the last resort.

- *Cancer* It goes without saying that a hysterectomy should be performed quickly in any life-threatening situation. Cancer of the uterus, ovaries and cervix are major killers, which means there is no room for hesitation.

A study performed by the Australian Institute of Health and Welfare of the estimated 30,000 hysterectomies performed in Australia each year demonstrated that:

- fibroids accounted for 22 per cent of the hysterectomies
- heavy menstrual bleeding for 18 per cent
- prolapse 7–21 per cent, depending on the type of hospital and State
- endometriosis and adenomyosis (endometriosis growing within the thick wall of the uterus) 6–23 per cent
- cancer 1–12 per cent
- pelvic inflammatory disease 2–8 per cent, with a number of other reasons given for the remaining hysterectomies.

Types of hysterectomy

- *Total hysterectomy* The removal of the uterus, the cervix and the supporting ligaments, leaving the fallopian tubes and ovaries intact.
- *Partial hysterectomy* The removal of the upper two-thirds of the uterus only, leaving everything else intact.
- *Total hysterectomy with salpingo-oophorectomy* The removal of the uterus with the cervix and supporting ligaments, together with one or both sets of ovaries and fallopian tubes.
- *Radical hysterectomy* The removal of the uterus, cervix, supporting ligaments, both ovaries and fallopian tubes, as well as lymph nodes in the area, and the upper portion of the vagina. In women with cancer that may have infiltrated other areas, there may be little choice but to choose this option. For others there may be some flexibility.

Surgical alternatives to hysterectomy

Various techniques have been developed in the last few years to destroy the endometrium, the lining of the uterus, rather than removing the uterus itself. These methods, in principle, are usually performed through the vagina, possibly under local anaesthetic. They are far less invasive and traumatic, and the recovery time is a fraction of that for a hysterectomy. They are useful tools for women who suffer heavy bleeding that is resistant to drug therapy, or where there are side-effects to the drugs, and for women who are intolerant to general anaesthetic, or for whom anaesthetic may be life threatening (the obese, for example). However, they are not thought to be so suitable for women with large fibroids, endometriosis or a retroverted uterus (tilted backwards).

The methods use lasers, an electrically heated rollerball, and more recently a thermal technique, which involves passing hot water through the uterus, and are collectively known as 'endometrial ablation and re-section'. We already know that they are not risk-free procedures, but the risks seem to be lower than for hysterectomy. They can cause infection, bleeding, damage to other organs, vessels or fluid overload. The worst scenario is that two women in every 10,000 die as a result of these proce-dures, compared with between two to six women out of every 10,000 that have a hysterectomy.

It is acknowledged that doctors performing these techniques need to be experienced, previously performing between ten and 80 operations, so as not to cause damage or perforate the uterus itself. Having said that, there are many satisfied customers. Periods may continue after surgery, but they are usually light. The stay in hospital is likely to be only one night, and women are often back at work within two weeks. Those with fibroids may need the procedure repeated in the future, and some even resort to an hysterectomy eventually.

What your doctor and consultant can do

- Give you an honest appraisal of what is physically wrong with you. So if you have fibroids, for example, you want to know how large they are and whether they could be removed without taking the uterus with them. It is possible to remove very large fibroids with skilled surgery, leaving the uterus intact.
- Give you a rundown of the treatment options available, before consid-ering an hysterectomy.
- Assure you that, if the removal of your uterus seems necessary, the ovaries will remain, unless they are diseased. Leaving even part of an ovary puts you at an advantage.
- Have a respectful attitude towards your reproductive organs.

What you can do

- Read widely on the subject of hysterectomy (see Recommended read-ing on page 490).
- Take your time making a decision, and discuss the pros and cons with your partner.
- Follow the recommendations relating to your problem in this book for three or four months to see whether there is any improvement before agreeing to surgery.
- If you do have surgery, and cancer has not been diagnosed, explore the alternatives to hysterectomy with your surgeon, and put your views and requests relating to your ovaries in writing to the consultant before the operation.

Complementary therapies

Many of the complementary therapies have a great deal to offer in helping with period problems. Herbal therapy would be top of our list. Vitex agnus castus has been shown in one early study to reduce heavy bleeding in 60 per cent of the patients included. There are other herbs and homeopathic remedies that may be useful, and acupuncture is worth a try. Follow the recommendations for your specific problem by referring to the appropriate chapter.

Indigestion

One of the main functions of the stomach is to produce acid of a strength great enough to dissolve metal! Dangerous stuff, but only if not confined to a healthy stomach. Leading into the stomach is the oesophagus which carries swallowed food from the mouth down through the chest, pierces the diaphragm and, via a muscular valve-like mechanism, joins the top of the stomach. This muscular valve is intended to keep the contents of the stomach in the stomach and prevent them from washing back up into the oesophagus. But if this happens, this acid reflux (as it is known) will irritate the delicate lining of the oesophagus, causing pain and spasm. It can even trigger chest problems and asthma (see page 93).

A common factor with indigestion in middle-aged and older people is a hiatus hernia. This is when a small portion of the stomach passes up through the diaphragm. The protective valve-like mechanism is lost, and indigestion results.

What are the symptoms?

Typical symptoms include burning discomfort at the top of the abdomen and the lower part of the chest, which is often worse shortly after eating if bending or lying down. There may also be a desire to belch wind and a loss of appetite when it becomes difficult to swallow. It raises the possibility of scarring of the lower end of the oesophagus as a result of long-standing acid reflux, or even of a cancerous growth causing a partial blockage.

What causes it?

There are a number of factors that can lead to acid reflux with or without a hiatus hernia. They all have the potential to relax the muscular valve mechanism, stimulate an excessive amount of acid from the stomach or damage the protective covering of mucus that lines the lower end of the oesophagus. They include:

- smoking
- alcohol
- being overweight
- tea and coffee
- fatty foods
- possibly other foods to which there is an intolerance.
- stress

What your doctor can do

- Assess the severity of your symptoms.
- Investigate those with swallowing difficulties or who fail to respond to drug treatment.
- Prescribe one of three types of medicines:
  - Alkaline medicines based on magnesium or aluminium to neutralise the acid. These are suitable for mild symptoms.
  - Drugs that stop acid production. These can be very effective, especially Losec.
  - Drugs to help the muscles of the stomach to pass its contents out of the stomach.
- Rarely refer patients for surgical correction of a hiatus hernia. This once common operation is now hardly needed as drug therapy has become so effective.

What you can do

- Stop smoking. Tobacco increases stomach acidity and releases the muscular valve at the lower end of the oesophagus.
- Lose weight.
- Eat slowly. Chew your food well too.
- Avoid very fatty foods. Follow the recommendations for The Very Nutritious Diet (see page 437).
- Don't eat late at night. If you do, when you go to bed your stomach will still contain a significant amount of food and acid when you are lying down in bed.
- Prop the head of your bed up. Place books under the top legs. A pair of telephone directories will do the job nicely. This reduces the flow of acids upwards from the stomach.
- Avoid spicy food. This may be best, although, despite its reputation it only rarely causes problems.
- Reduce tea and coffee consumption. Use alternatives (see page 6).
- Peppermint tea has been traditionally consumed after a rich meal or to treat heartburn.
- Ginger in the form of tea, root or crystallised, is a natural carminative traditionally used to treat morning sickness, nausea, motion sickness and indigestion.
- Avoid foods that commonly cause digestive problems. These include

wheat, especially in wholemeal bread, bran, and wholegrain breakfast cereals, eggs, dairy products, citrus fruit and foods containing yeast. You could try The Simple Exclusion Diet (see page 460) if all else fails.

Complementary therapies

Acupuncture, homeopathy and herbalism may all have something to offer.

Ingrid's story

Ingrid was a 53-year-old licensee who had two grown up children. At the time she began taking HRT, to address her menopause symptoms, she developed a mystery gum disease and rather severe gastritis.

'I hadn't had any problems with my gums or my digestion before I started taking HRT and for the first two and a half years didn't link the two. My gum problems came on gradually and eventually became extremely painful. They felt very irritated, almost as if the gums were too big for the spaces between my teeth and no matter how much I cleaned them or rinsed them with mouthwash the symptoms persisted. The gastric reflux also began about the time I started taking HRT but my doctor insisted that neither of these conditions were related to the medication.

I eventually went off to see my dentist who said there was nothing wrong with my teeth. I simply had gingivitis, inflammation of the gums. He gave me a series of mouthwashes and dental paste to use which masked the problem for a while but did not seem to get to the root cause. I saw the dental hygienist every two months. She agreed there was a problem but also could not put her finger on what was causing the problem. I felt so miserable, in constant pain, it really wore me down.

I read about the natural approach to the menopause in the Daily Express and did not waste any time contacting the WNAS for some help and advice. I felt certain inside that the HRT was not really helping my gums, plus I was still experiencing menopausal symptoms despite taking it.

The WNAS programme involved making dietary changes and taking supplements aimed at helping my menopausal symptoms, plus also extra vitamin C to help with my gums. During the first month I noticed that the gum problem was easing and that the reflux was calming down. Before I could not eat a meal without feeling bloated, nauseous and experiencing heartburn. The worst side effect of the reflux was breathlessness where I felt I could not fill my lungs easily and panicked. My doctor's explanation was that *the acid from the gastric reflux was tipping into my lungs. However, it got to the point where I was vomiting after eating and drinking which made me feel awful and obviously restricted my social life.*

Now, six months later, I am happy to report that my gums are healthy, the gastric reflux has gone and I don't experience any sickness or even feel sick after eating or drinking. I can almost eat everything. Occasionally I get an acid feeling after overdoing it but that really is rare now. I feel so much happier and the quality of my life has improved beyond belief. I'm grateful for every symptom-free day.'

Infertility

Although many women manage to conceive without any difficulty, approximately one in six couples experience problems. There are many underlying causes, which include the woman's age, the man's sperm count, and an assortment of other factors. About one in ten couples take more than a year to conceive, and one in 20 take more than two years.

There is no need to rush to be investigated if you are under 35, unless you have been trying to conceive for over two years. If you are over 35, having had regular sexual intercourse for a year, and experiencing a disturbed menstrual cycle, it would be acceptable to be investigated without further delay.

Infertility is best regarded as a problem of the couple, rather than the individual, and nutritional causes will often overlap, resulting in self-help measures being much the same for both. To fully understand the causes, it is best to separate them into female and male.

Causes of female infertility

By the time a woman is born, all the eggs that her ovaries will hold have already been produced! Several million eggs are in place initially, but only about 400 of them will reach maturity. The supply is influenced by smoking, even before birth, and daughters of women who smoked during pregnancy have fewer eggs, have more difficulty conceiving, and may reach the menopause earlier than the offspring of non-smokers.

The monthly release of an egg from the ovary is known as ovulation, and occurs at approximately mid-cycle with menstruation coming fourteen days later. Ovulation does not always occur with every cycle, but when an egg is released from the ovary it is picked up by the finger-shaped projections at the end of the fallopian tubes and then passes along towards the womb.

Failure of ovulation

A guide to whether or not an egg is being produced each month is whether the periods are regular, between twenty-five and thirty-five days. Ovulation can be checked for by measuring the blood level of the female sex hormone progesterone seven days before the next period is due. Usually this is day 21 of a 28 day cycle, but can be day twenty-eight in a 35 day cycle.

A rise in early morning body temperature of 0.5°C should also be observed in the few days after ovulation, but this is less reliable than measuring the progesterone level. Often day 21 progesterone level is checked in two or three cycles in couples with fertility problems, especially if there is some uncertainty about ovulation.

Failing to ovulate can be due to:

- Hormonal problems, including an early menopause.
- An under- or over-active thyroid gland.
- Disturbance of the pituitary gland, especially an excess of the hormone prolactin in the blood, can inhibit ovulation. Often the first clues that this is the case are the presence of a milky white discharge from the nipples, known as galactorrhoea, and infrequent periods. However, only one-quarter of those with galactorrhoea will have a high prolactin level, and this then requires further investigation.
- Nutritional deficiencies. Even changing your diet can affect ovulation. Following a 1,000 calorie weight-loss diet for six weeks may suppress normal ovulation. The World Health Organisation survey of infertility found that recent weight loss or gain was a mild risk factor for infertility.
- Any chronic illness, especially if there is weight loss.
- Stress, which can be a powerful factor.
- Excessive physical activity and an inadequate calorie intake, resulting in loss of weight, can prevent ovulation taking place each month. When the body is not well nourished perhaps this is Mother Nature's way of preventing a pregnancy.

Blockage of the fallopian tubes

This is very often due to past infection, most commonly by an organism called chlamydia. It is usually acquired following sexual intercourse, particularly in those who have had multiple partners, and causes lower abdominal or pelvic pain, a vaginal discharge, painful periods and sometimes a fever.

The reporting of infection with chlamydia more than doubled in the UK between 1976 and 1986, and damage to fallopian tubes is now the commonest cause of infertility in many developing countries because of the high prevalence of pelvic inflammatory disease (PID), an acute illness which requires treatment with antibiotics (see page 366).

To confirm the diagnosis a more detailed assessment by laparoscopy, examination of the pelvic organs with a telescopic instrument passed into the abdominal cavity, and x-rays of the fallopian tubes may be performed. Blocked or damaged tubes can be corrected by surgery, but assisted fertilisation is often the simplest way to achieving pregnancy.

Endometriosis

This condition, in which the cells from the lining of the womb grow outside the uterus, such as around the ovaries or adjacent to the outer walls of the womb, can cause infertility. Difficulty conceiving, very painful periods and abdominal distension are common problems of endometriosis. Diagnosis is often made after investigative surgery, a laparoscopy, to examine the pelvic organs. Unfortunately treatment is not very successful.

Polycystic Ovarian Disease

Up to 20 per cent of the normal female population suffer with cysts on the ovaries which cause a shift in the balance of sex hormones resulting in:

- irregular and infrequent periods
- excessive hair growth
- reduced fertility
- often, but not always, obesity.

Contraception

Users of the oral contraceptive pill may experience delayed fertility, as it sometimes takes several months to re-establish a normal menstrual cycle after being on the pill. Users of intra-uterine devices have a slight increased risk of PID (pelvic inflammatory disease) resulting in reduced fertility.

Abortion

A history of abortion does not seem to reduce the future chance of conceiving, according to recent research.

Medical drugs

Many drugs can interfere with a woman's fertility. This is almost always reversible and can follow use of:

- anti-cancer agents.
- hormone preparations, as may be used to treat period pains or premenstrual problems.
- drugs such as used in the treatment of schizophrenia and depression.
- drugs such as metoclopramide and domperidone used in the treatment of nausea.

- the drugs reserpine and methyldopa used in the treatment of high blood pressure, all of which can increase the level of the pituitary hormone prolactin.

Medical conditions

Diabetes and thyroid disease can cause infertility in women, but only if they are not well controlled.

Social poisons

Many, though not all, studies show slightly reduced fertility rates in those women who drink or smoke. Coffee consumption has also been studied, and there is a possible slight adverse effect on fertility. The same may be true of the consumption of soft drinks that have a high sugar content and contain colourings and additives. There are many other possible explanations as those consuming these social substances often have a poorer nutrient intake.

Recreational drugs, including marijuana, may reduce the chances of fertility, and are likely to have a substantial effect on pregnancy outcome.

Exposure to environmental chemicals

This has been shown in studies, especially in the work-place, to reduce fertility. Those who work with textile and leather dyes, lead, mercury, benzene, petroleum and related chemicals, and possibly other chemicals used in the plastics industry, are most likely to be at risk. Additionally, female dentists, anaesthetists and assistants, have been reported as having delayed conception, possibly due to their exposure to the anaesthetic gas, nitrous oxide.

Nutritional deficiencies

It is widely accepted that in developing countries a significant degree of malnutrition, resulting in severe weight loss, is likely to stop women menstruating and could result in her being infertile. Surprisingly little work has been done however to determine whether *mild* nutritional deficiencies contribute to infertility in women from developed countries. Several small reports have documented the association of deficiencies of iron (without anaemia), vitamin B12 and vitamin B3 being associated with reduced fertility.

Other causes

In rare cases, infertility may be associated with:

- structural deformities of the uterus or vagina which may be a barrier to fertility, or prevent successful implantation of the fertilised ovum.
- genetic problems which cause some women to fail to menstruate at all.

- antibodies to sperm or allergic reactions to it! Some women suffer from these, but treatment with assisted conception can get round this problem.

Despite careful assessment of both partners, no cause for infertility is found in some 20 per cent of couples. If spontaneous pregnancy has not occurred within three years, then some form of treatment is deemed appropriate.

What your doctor can do

This depends on the discovered cause of infertility.

- He could treat failure of ovulation either by correcting any underlying hormonal abnormality, or by inducing ovulation through short courses of agents that encourage the ovary to release an egg. These measures might be aided by attention to diet and lifestyle which we will come to shortly.
- He could arrange for Tubal Disease – blocked or damage to the fallopian tubes – to be treated by surgery to repair the damaged tube(s), or by assisted conception. Tubal repair surgery is actually not very effective as it is difficult to repair damage to the delicate tube lining, but it is useful for reversal of sterilisation procedures. Newer specialised techniques – trying to remove scar tissue from inside the fallopian tube by passing an ultrafine tube via the uterus – may be more successful.
- He could also advise you on Assisted Reproduction Techniques (ART). Women with unexplained infertility of more than three years' duration, and those with ovulation problems that have not responded to more simple measures, may be advised to choose this method. It can also help where the male partner has very few sperm or when the woman has no eggs and is willing to use donated eggs.

These techniques involve collection of a woman's eggs, often after treatment with hormonal agents, collection of sperm and their careful preparation. This is followed by either *in-vitro* fertilisation (IVF) or test-tube fertilisation with placement of the embryo in the womb, or placement of both the prepared eggs and sperm in the fallopian tubes (gamete intrafallopian transfer or GIFT), or some of the newer techniques being piloted. In some circumstances it may be appropriate to use donor eggs from (usually) younger women together with the partner's sperm.

Causes of male infertility

Sperm are produced in the testes by specialised cells, and slowly mature over four months. During orgasm they are ejected from the part of the testis called the seminiferous tubules, mix with fluid from the prostate gland and other tissues, and are released into the outside world. Millions are produced, even though only one is required to fertilise an egg. The number and quality of sperm as well as the health of the prostate gland are all important in deciding how fertile any one male is.

Sperm production takes place most efficiently at a temperature of 33°C (91.4°F), and thus the testicles are *outside* the body, which has a temperature of 37°C (98.6°F). A normal ejaculate should:

- be greater than 2ml (or millilitres)
- contain at least 20 million sperm per ml
- have 30 per cent or more with a normal shape
- have 50 per cent actively mobile (it is quite normal for some 50 per cent of sperm of be 'duds').

Assessment of male infertility requires asking many questions about diet and lifestyle, a physical examination and examination of a sample of sperm. Quite often a sperm sample can be collected by using a post-coital test, which will also determine how it responds to the cervical mucus.

Absent or deformed testicles

Sometimes testes may have failed to descend from their original position high up in the scrotum or lower part of the abdomen. Newborn and infant boys are routinely checked to make sure the testes are descended. Small testes may be due to past injury, illness or sometimes developmental problems. Enlargement is most commonly due to a varicocele – enlargement of the veins around the testis – and this is present in 10 per cent of the normal population. This can raise the temperature of the testes, and contribute to a poor sperm count. Surgical treatment is often necessary.

Blockage of the vas deferens

A blockage of the duct leading from the testicles to the base of the bladder will result in a very low sperm count or no sperm in the ejaculate. Previous vasectomy is an obvious cause, and can be reversed by surgery. Sometimes the sperm-carrying ducts are distorted as they reach the area of the prostate gland. Consequently some or all of the ejaculate does not reach the outside world directly, but passes into the bladder. Sperm are detected in the urine that is passed after intercourse. This commonly happens after surgery on the prostate gland.

Excessive heat

The sort of heat which may be encountered by steel workers and bakers can be associated with a reduced sperm count. Severe obesity and tight underwear and trousers may play a part too.

Damage to the testicles

The chromosomal material in the sperm itself, or the motility of the sperm, can be damaged by:

- infection, especially sexually transmitted disease like chlamydia or non-specific urethritis (NSU)
- infection with mumps during adolescence or early adult life
- drugs as used for cancer and colitis or Crohn's disease
- radiation treatment
- exposure to environmental pollutants – lead, cadmium, mercury, pesticides, herbicides and other chemicals that have effects similar to the female sex hormone, oestrogen
- cancer of the testicle.

Chronic illnesses

Diabetes, cystic fibrosis, chronic disease of the nervous system, any chronic infection or unexplained fever, an underactive thyroid gland, disease of the pituitary gland and kidney disease can all affect sperm count. Sperm counts also fall in men who are paralysed by a spinal injury.

Social poisons

Alcohol and cigarette smoking are the most important, but marijuana and other recreational drugs can also affect the quality and quantity of sperm.

Lack of essential nutrients

Some nutrients seem to be particularly important to sperm production, and these include zinc, vitamins B and C. One experiment in healthy volunteers presenting mild zinc deficiency showed a dramatic reduction in sperm quantity and quality, and testosterone (male sex hormone) production, which took nearly a year to fully correct.

Stress

This might also be a factor in reducing a man's sperm count.

The modern world

A group of Danish doctors in 1992 published an important review of the fall in sperm count that seems to have taken place over the last fifty years. Looking at 61 papers detailing the results in nearly 15,000 men, there appears to have been a 40 per cent decline in sperm concentration and a 20 per cent decline in seminal volume over this time. Combined with the known increase in testicular cancer and developmental abnormalities of the genitals in new-born boys, this strongly suggests an environmental cause, probably due to pollution.

Smoking, alcohol and lack of some essential nutrients may also be factors. The escalating use of the oral contraceptive pill and hormone replacement therapy, traces of which can find their way into the general environment, should give us all something to be concerned about. Increased use of plastics and related chemicals, the pesticide DDT and the chemical PCBs used as insulators for electrical cables prior to 1970, have also been suggested as factors, because of their mild oestrogen-like effects. Decline in reproductive capacity could also be interpreted as an indication that the planet is becoming too crowded, and is Mother Nature's answer to the problem.

What your doctor can do

This does of course depend upon the cause, but unfortunately most of the treatments tried are not very successful. Self-help measures may be more effective at improving sperm count and function than are drug therapies.

- A wide variety of drugs and hormonal treatments, including steroids, have all been tried with either no benefit or uncertain benefit being recorded. Steroids can be useful in those men whose infertility is due to antibodies that attack their own sperm. Hormonal treatments are helpful only for the small percentage of men with true hormone deficiency.
- Surgery is useful if blockage of the ducts from the testicles is causing a low sperm count. Enlargement of the veins of the testicles, a varicocele, can be treated by surgery if there is a low sperm count, when infertility has been present for two or more years, and if there is no associated hormonal disturbance.
- Antibiotics are necessary to treat any infection of the testicles or prostate gland. Treatment for several months may be required.
- He could advise on Assisted Reproduction Techniques (ART), as on page 254. Test-tube fertilisation or *in-vitro* fertilisation (IVF) are often the best hope for many couples where a low sperm count is the main barrier to conception. Such techniques involve the collection of the partner's sperm, treatment with an agent that improve its function, bringing together the sperm and egg – sometimes by actually injecting healthy sperm into the egg – and return of the fertilised egg into the womb. In this way pregnancy can be achieved when there is a very low sperm count.

If there is no sperm, then donor sperm will have to be used, and the donor can be chosen to have similar physical characteristics to those of the male partner.

What you can do

Whilst none of what follows may be as important as the hormonal and surgical techniques that have revolutionised female infertility treatment in particular, they all have their importance. It seems foolish not to take simple common-sense measures to improve health before embarking upon costly assisted reproduction techniques. Remember that most of the advice that follows will take three to six months before it has a detectable effect upon body chemistry and therefore a subsequent influence upon your reproductive ability.

Certain nutrients seem to play a crucial part in the way ovaries respond to pituitary hormones (magnesium and possibly the EFAs), and in influencing female sex hormone metabolism in general (vitamin B, essential fatty acids and possibly magnesium and zinc). Severe deficiencies of these nutrients are rare except in women with very poor diets, or who are seriously ill or alcoholic. However there is now substantial evidence that mild undetected deficiencies are quite common, and they may have a modest effect upon the regularity of your menstrual cycle and ovulation.

What you both can do

- Cut down on alcohol and cigarettes. Ideally, you should both stop. Cigarette smoking in women is associated with reduced fertility and means a lower success rate in those undergoing assisted reproduction techniques.
- Eat a healthy diet with plenty of fresh fruit and vegetables. The high content of vitamins A, C and E act as anti-oxidants that help limit the adverse effects of many environmental pollutants. Ensure a good intake of protein-rich foods of either animal or vegetable origin. These are particularly important for men as they are good sources of zinc, which seems to play such a crucial role in sperm production and function.
- If you are very overweight then lose weight, and if underweight try to gain weight, but always by eating healthy nutritious foods. Rapid weight change, gain or loss, is usually undesirable, especially in women.
- If you are on long-term drug therapy ask your doctor or specialist to review your need for medication. The goal is the minimum effective dose for a drug or drugs, with the least risk of side-effects. In men, drug therapy for mental problems or Crohn's disease could be reducing sperm count.
- If you have any chronic illness that is not being adequately treated at present, then check with your doctor.
- Limit exposure to environmental chemicals. Take especial care if your work involves handling heavy metals, pesticides or industrial chemicals.

For women

- Follow the preconception programme on page 386.
- Limit consumption of tea and coffee to a total of four cups per day. More might have a small adverse effect on the chance of conceiving.
- Do not consume more than three cans of soft drink, low calorie or normal type, per week. This is about 1 litre (1³/4pints) in volume.
- Consider taking nutritional supplements, depending upon your health circumstances. Expert advice is often desirable and if you are receiving infertility treatment then you should always check with your specialist about these before commencing.
- Iron may be needed by those who:
  - have heavy periods
  - are poorly fed, such as vegetarians who are also tea drinkers
  - have symptoms of iron deficiency, e.g. recurrent mouth ulcers or a sore tongue
  - have flattened or up-turned nails
  - have poor hair growth.
- Folic acid should be taken by all women who are trying to or who might conceive. The dose is 400 mcg per day. Those women who have had a previous pregnancy complicated by a neural tube defect will need to take 4 mg per day.
- Vitamin B Complex could be needed by those who:
  - eat poorly
  - consume more than an average of two units of alcohol daily
  - suffer from significant anxiety or depression
  - have any illness that has caused recent weight loss
  - have recurrent mouth ulcers or a sore tongue.
- Vitamin B12 may be needed by vegans. All women wishing to become pregnant should be taking folic acid, and as a wise precaution all vegans should also take a vitamin B12 supplement. A mild deficiency of vitamin B12 could be made worse by taking folic acid, resulting in damage to the nervous system and numbness in the hands or feet. An appropriate dose of vitamin B12 is 5 mcg per day.
- Zinc is necessary for optimal functioning of the reproductive organs.
- Magnesium might be useful for those who are deficient, and have trouble ovulating regularly. Early symptoms that could indicate a lack of this essential mineral are:
  - premenstrual syndrome – physical or mental symptoms
  - muscle pains or cramps
  - fatigue.

An appropriate dose is 300 milligrams per day. Once pregnant, your need for these supplements may well change. Again check with your GP or specialist.

For men

- Avoid use of jockey-style underwear and underwear made from synthetic materials. Cotton boxer shorts will help keep the testicles at the right temperature.
- If your sperm is low, then rather than 'saving it all up for one good go' it would seem better to have more frequent intercourse, especially around mid-cycle. The optimum frequency of intercourse to maintain a good sperm count is two or three times a week.
- Do not have excessively hot baths or showers. Limit the time you spend in a sauna. Avoid exposure to excessively hot environments, at work for instance.
- Take nutritional supplements of Vitamin C (about 500 mg) and a good quality multi-vitamins. These can all help improve sperm count, especially if you have low levels of vitamin C. Vitamin C prevents the sperm from clumping, making them more motile. These moderate doses can be safely taken in the long term, but the positive effects are likely to take three or six months at least to be felt. Supplements of other nutrients may be needed if you have deficiencies or other health problems.
- Zinc is fundamental for reproductive health and enhances sperm production.
- Deficiency of the mineral selenium has been linked to a low sperm count.
- The amino acid L-arginine plays an important role in increasing sperm count and sperm motility.
- Manganese maintains sex hormone production.

Remember that all of these factors are likely to take some time to show results. Whilst getting yourselves into better condition, you will both need a little patience. If you haven't managed to conceive after two years of regular sexual intercourse you will need to see your doctor with a view to organising some specialist investigations. Most doctors do not initiate any treatment until after three years, though this can be less in older couples.

Complementary therapies

Whilst complementary therapies cannot be relied upon to solve the problem of infertility, it may be worthwhile having some acupuncture from an experience practitioner or consulting a cranial osteopath in order to free any blocked energy.

Carole's story

Carole was a 33-year-old who was experiencing problems with infertility at the time when she approached us.

'I had been investigated for infertility in the mid 1980s as we were trying for a baby for three years without any success. The doctors did not think I was ovulating, although there was no concrete evidence, and eventually I managed to fall pregnant. We were hoping to have several children in quick succession but after a further two years without any success we began investigations again. Our GP referred us to a consultant who confirmed that I was not ovulating. My periods were very irregular at the time and I was put on Clomiphene for three months and then a double dose for a further six months. However the tests didn't change – even after the treatment I was still not ovulating.

By this time I had developed very severe premenstrual tension. I think the strian of trying to conceive had got to me. My behaviour was utterly uncharacteristic and I experienced all manner of symptoms ranging from migraine to mood swings, bloating and irritability, from which I seemed to have no respite. When I was not knocked out by migraines or an upset stomach I was prone to violent mood swings and at one point tried to attack my husband. I regularly wept for no apparent reason. I felt so ill I was never in the mood for sex, which affected both our marriage and our plans to conceive. My husband actually phoned The Samaritans at one point because I was so emotionally out of control. He had asked me why I was unhappy and I replied 'I'm not unhappy, I was just ill'. Of course it was difficult for him to understand.

My doctor said I was causing the symptoms because I wanted to have a baby so much, so eventually I decided I ought to go and see a psychiatrist. At about that time a close friend of mine read an article about the work of the WNAS and suggested I bought a book called No More PMS! which I did. I put myself on the diet straight away and contacted the WNAS for some help.

As a fifteen-coffees-a-day woman and a Diet Coke addict, I was advised to cut these out and also to initially stop eating wheat and other grains, except rice and corn, and I also gave up cheese. I was told to exercise and take nutritional supplements. For the first time for as long as I could remember I had two normal regular cycles with no PMS. A week later the migraines stopped. Inside two months my erratic moods had abated. A regular cycle had been re-established which I hadn't had for years, and my libido was restored. I felt so well that I decided to relax the diet and then had a dreadful month with a 50-day cycle.

When I went back to the clinic and went over my charts it seemed that the wheat that I had recently been eating had aggravated the situation. I was asked to cut it out again and after having some tests I was given some extra zinc and magnesium as well as my other *supplements. I am delighted to say that I fell pregnant the next month and had a very smooth pregnancy and a lovely baby daughter.*

I have to stick to the diet which I sometimes find difficult, as wheat, chocolate and dairy products all seem to affect me in different ways. I have since added a herbal preparation to my supplements as it seems to help to normalise my cycle. My husband was both relieved and delighted that not only was I able to overcome my symptoms but also that I was able to conceive without difficulty for the first time in years.'

See also: Standard references and Recommended reading (*Healthy Parents, Healthy Baby*).

Influenza, Recurrent Coughs, Colds and Sore Throats

Hardly anybody needs to be told but for those few who might never have suffered, the common cold is a short-lived infective illness due to one of several easily transmitted viruses. Symptoms include nasal stuffiness with the production of profuse watery catarrh. A fever, which is not usually great, may be present too. Severity varies from person to person and depends also upon changes in the virus that allows it to bypass the immune system's defence mechanisms. In most people the illness lasts a few days and rarely more than a week.

Influenza is a viral infection that typically occurs as a widespread outbreak. It is caused by several strains of the influenza virus known as A, B or C. Typical features are headache, muscle aches which can be severe, a fever, sore throat, cough and nasal catarrh. The illness lasts from two to seven days unless secondary infection with bacteria develops, causing bronchitis, pneumonia or sinus infection.

Sore throats are most often due to viral infections which may cause inflammation of the conjunctiva (red eyes), or a cough due to a chest infection. Occasionally, though, they are due to bacterial infection that may need antibiotic treatment. Many of us will experience around four to six such infections each year though half of these may be so mild as to pass virtually unnoticed.

With simple viral infections, provided they are uncomplicated, there should be little constitutional disturbance, unlike influenza. Some people seem prone to these viral infections, especially in the elderly or those with poor resistance to infection.

Who gets them?

We all do, especially young children. Influenza is more common in the winter months. As the virus can spontaneously make subtle changes to itself, thus evading the immune defences caused by previous infections, we are all prone to infection every few years especially with new strains. Immunisation is effective, though not completely so, and is offered yearly to those with heart, lung or kidney disease, the elderly, diabetics, those with poor resistance to infection, and some health-care workers.

Colds and sore throats are common throughout the year, though slightly more so in the winter months. Incubation following initial contact with these viruses is one to six days.

What your doctor can do

- For all viral illnesses affecting the upper airways there is little treatment. Prevention by immunisation is only effective for influenza, and it is only appropriate for those groups already detailed.
- Aspirin may help with the fever and pain of these infections but actually increases the shedding of common cold viruses. A drug called amantidine is effective for reducing the severity of influenza caused by type A infections, but only if given before the illness starts so it can be used early on in some outbreaks.
- Antibiotics are needed if an infection with a bacterium follows causing a cough or nasal discharge with yellow or green mucus.

What you can do

- Ignore it if symptoms are mild.
- Since there is no real cure for the common cold, the best remedy is to prevent getting a cold in the first place by boosting your immune system.
- Take supplements of vitamin C (1 g three times per day) although the evidence in favour is small.
- Suck zinc lozenges three times a day – these have been shown to reduce the duration of a sore throat. The high concentration of zinc in the throat may be harmful to the virus, and the zinc that is absorbed can act as an immune stimulant.
- Vitamin A is useful as it helps heal the inflamed mucous membranes and strengthens the immune system.

- Take the herb echinacea which is renowned for its potent immune-enhancing properties. It works more effectively if taken only at the onset of a cold or when feeling low. If it is taken on an ongoing basis the body's own immune mechanism might become compromised. Echinacea can be taken in tablet form or as a liquid tincture.
- Have a steam inhalation. These are old fashioned but effective at reducing the duration of symptoms especially if there is nasal stuffiness. The steam needs to be as hot as possible. Pour freshly boiled water into a large bowl which is securely placed on a table. Sit at the table and place a large towel over your head and breathe in deeply through the nose. Do this for ten minutes three times a day. Such inhalations are particularly useful if there is a lot of sticky phlegm on the chest or nasal catarrh that is difficult to clear. You can add some eucalyptus or menthol preparations to it if you like.
- It may be worth going on a mild fast for two or three days. Drinking plenty of clear liquids and eating mainly fruit could help, as strict fasting can stimulate immune activity. Furthermore, if there is a degree of nasal sensitivity to a food (most commonly, dairy products) then avoiding this could benefit some. For those who have more than two upper respiratory tract infections each year, especially if this has led to taking antibiotics then the following may be helpful:
  - Eat The Very Nutritious Diet (see page 437).
  - Don't smoke, and drink very little.
- Take supplements of a moderately strong multi-vitamin, zinc 15–20 mg, and vitamin A, 4,000 IU per day. If deficient, the latter can make it easier for bacteria to adhere to the lining of the airways. The first two were taken in a trial of healthy elderly regularly over one whole year and were shown to approximately halve their rate of these infections and subsequent use of antibiotics.

Pamela's story

Pamela had had a full and busy life and now, at the age of 75, she was troubled by persistent fatigue. In fact she had felt fatigue for about 30 years, then when she was still bringing up three children she had a severe viral pneumonia and had felt that her energy levels had never been the same since. She had managed through her middle years but now, as an elderly lady her reduced energy level meant that she spent most of her time at home indoors and rarely enjoyed the walks and gardening that she had managed in the past. She seemed predisposed to recurrent minor infections, coughs, colds and sore throats that never missed their opportunity to punctuate her winter months. Fortunately, she rarely required antibiotics. She had lost a few pounds in weight but there were no other features to think that there was anything more sinister. Indeed she had been very thoroughly assessed by a local physician a few months earlier and all routine tests were satisfactory. She had occasionally been found to have a low white cell count in the past, perhaps indicating her reduced resistance to infection. However she herself had tried taking a variety of nutritional supplements with no clear cut benefits.

She found it difficult to keep her weight much above 51 kilos (8 stone), she also found it difficult to eat large or rich meals which caused her to experience abdominal bloating and discomfort.

Nutritional investigations had shown a surprisingly low level of retinol (vitamin A), 136 mgs per litre (200–650). The level for zinc was also very reduced at 7.6 mmols per litre (11.5–20) and a number of other essential nutrients were also reduced. Low levels of zinc and vitamin A are quite strongly linked with poor resistance to infection and repeated upper respiratory tract infections which were clearly part of Pamela's problem. Perhaps her poor digestion lay behind it.

She began supplements of strong multi-vitamins and zinc and was advised to take some digestive enzymes with her meal. It actually took about six months before her nutrient levels came up, and as they did she gained a few pounds in weight, her energy level improved and she began to experience fewer coughs and colds. There was significant improvement in her levels for zinc and vitamin A.

All the patients are predisposed to mild to moderate nutritional deficiencies which may significantly impair their resistance to infection. For many in this situation it would seem a good policy to take moderately strong multi-vitamin and zinc preparations.

In Pamela's case it is not known how long she really had the deficiencies.

Insomnia

Anyone who has ever suffered from disturbed sleep will tell you that sleep is a vital part of our life, probably taken for granted by those who have never experienced problems. Whatever the reason for the insomnia, be it anxiety, bereavement or simply jetlag, it leaves us feeling washed out, with our vitality crushed. We feel unrefreshed, irritable and listless, and as we are not as alert, we are more prone to making mistakes.

The main features of insomnia are difficulty falling asleep, an inability to stay asleep, or waking in the early hours and not being able to get back to sleep. Sufferers usually feel frustrated because they feel they should be asleep, and they invariably feel tired and washed out the next day.

Insufficient sleep may have serious repercussions in people of all ages. In children it may cause growth retardation, it can affect the academic performance of adolescents, cause under-achievement in the workplace and contribute significantly to the cause of accidents.

- Nearly four out of ten individuals do not get a regular night's sleep which affects their alertness.
- One-third of adults experience difficulty falling asleep or remaining asleep.
- Approximately 60 per cent of the elderly suffer from disorders that disrupt sleep, like snoring or sleep apnoea, where breathing ceases temporarily.
- Sufferers are often more tired during the day, not sufficiently alert to even drive a car. Road traffic accidents, for example, have been associated with sleepiness in 27 per cent of cases, and in one study accounts for 83 per cent of the deaths on the road, even more than deaths from alcohol-related accidents.

What causes it?

There are a variety of underlying factors that disrupt our sleep pattern:

- It is thought that in 50 per cent of complaints of insomnia there is underlying anxiety or depression. Stress, tension, grief or fear can all keep us awake.
- Caffeine, found in tea, coffee, chocolate and cola-based drinks, can stimulate us to the point of insomnia.
- Some drugs may produce side-effects which include insomnia, or may induce disturbing dreams which cause us to wake during the night.
- Withdrawal symptoms when coming off certain drugs.
- Alcohol in excess will also produce insomnia.
- Any painful condition e.g. arthritis.
- Any condition that causes you to break your sleep e.g. cystitis or diarrhoea when you need to go to the toilet.
- Day-time napping can prevent us having a sound night's sleep.
- A cold bedroom, especially for the elderly, could be enough to keep them awake at night.
- Shift work, which involves working some nights and not others is likely to severely disrupt your sleep pattern. We regularly see nurses and air hostesses with problems that relate to their poor sleeping routine, as the menstrual cycle is disturbed by the lack of routine.

What your doctor can do

- The first step is to exclude the possibility of any underlying cause, especially if there is pain. He should do a physical examination and routine blood screening to check for thyroid problems, diabetes, low iron stores, infection or other serious problems.

- Check to see whether anxiety or depression is keeping you awake.
- Give you instructions about 'sleep hygiene' – going to bed at a regular time, not napping during the day, making sure your room is warm enough, that your bedcovers are comfortable, and that there is no external noise to disturb you.
- Reassure you that your problem is likely to be short-lived.
- Prescribe sleeping pills in the very short term to break the pattern of insomnia and re-train you to sleep through the night.
- If you are depressed, he may prescribe antidepressants, and in severe cases refer you to a psychiatrist for further investigation and treatment.

What you can do

- Pinpoint the reason for your insomnia, either by visiting your doctor if you feel it may be a symptom of a medical condition, or by discussing your problems with your partner or a close friend.
- Take concerted steps to sort out the problem to alleviate your worry or anxiety. The problem may take some time to resolve, so you will need some intermediate measures to get you through.
- Eat well. Follow the instructions for The Very Nutritious Diet on page 437. Never miss a meal, and eat wholesome snacks between meals, especially in your premenstrual week if you are menstruating, as your calorie requirements are increased by up to 500 calories per day.
- Never go to bed on a full stomach: eat earlier on in the evening allowing sufficient time for your food to digest. This is more important for older patients or those with digestive troubles.
- Take plenty of exercise during the week, at least four or five sessions, out in the fresh air when possible.
- Learn how to relax your body and mind by practising daily one of the relaxation techniques (see page 29). You can use these techniques before going to bed (or in the night to help you get back to sleep).
- Eliminate the stimulant caffeine from your diet completely, and use alternatives (see page 7). Cut down gradually or you will get a withdrawal headache.
- Cut down on cigarettes if you smoke, or give up completely, as nicotine can act as a stimulant.
- Keep your alcohol consumption to a minimum, especially at night. Many people are under the misconception that alcohol is a hypnotic; it does induce sleep, but as it metabolises it acts as a stimulant.
- In the evening try eating bananas, figs, dates, yogurt or a milky drink. These foods are high in the amino-acid tryptophan which promotes sleep. Eating a grapefruit at bedtime may also help.

- Avoid bacon, cheese, chocolate, and red wine. These foods contain tyramine which increases the release of noradrenaline – a brain stimulant.
- Take a supplement of 5HTP, the precursor to the amino acid tryptophan, which in turn is converted into the neurotransmitter serotonin. 5HTP is much closer to serotonin than tryptophan and it is not dependent on a transport system for entry into the brain.
- Co-factor nutrients that assist the conversion of tryptophan into serotonin should be supplemented for maximum benefit. A B-complex together with the mineral magnesium ensure its conversion to serotonin.
- Protein should be avoided when taking 5HTP because the amino acids in the food competes with tryptophan for transport into the central nervous system. Eat a small carbohydrate snack alongside taking the supplement.
- Take a supplement of magnesium, preferably as amino acid chelate which is better absorbed. Magnesium works by relaxing the central nervous system and promoting uninterrupted sleeping patterns.
- Herbal preparations like valerian have been used for centuries for the natural treatment of insomnia. Several studies have confirmed valerian's ability to improve sleep quality and alleviate insomnia.
- Passion flower is also a good adjunct which has been widely used in traditional folk medicine for its natural sedative and analgesic properties.
- Make sure that you have a quiet, warm and comfortable environment in which to sleep. Having a good mattress with clean bedding might well help.
- Train yourself to go to bed at a regular time each night, before midnight, but not too early.
- Don't watch any scary films or upsetting television programmes before going to bed.
- When in bed, don't think about the day's activities, try to concentrate on something pleasant, and consciously relax your muscles.
- Cuddle up to your partner if you have one. The warmth of another person can help you get to sleep.
- An orgasm will often induce sleep – so this may be one problem that your partner will be only too keen to help you solve!
- Set your alarm for a regular time, unless you are a shift worker, as this will help you re-establish a routine.

When you wake in the night

- Instead of lying awake worrying, get up, make yourself a warm drink and read, watch a video or practice some relaxation technique, before returning to bed. This often does the trick and takes the frustration out of the situation.

- Go back to bed when you feel sleepy. Practice relaxing your muscles again and getting your mind to wander to a favourite location (see page 31).
- If you are still awake 10 minutes later, get up again, go to another room, do some more reading or relaxing.

Try not to worry or get too frustrated about not being able to sleep, as it is much more tiring than just being awake!

Complementary therapies

They are tremendously valuable in the treatment of insomnia that does not have an underlying physical cause. Acupuncture is very effective, but it requires a course of treatment to gradually ease you back into a proper sleep pattern. Herbal preparations and homeopathic remedies are useful tools, but you would be advised to seek professional help, as there will more than likely be other related problems that need addressing, too. It would be worth visiting a cranial osteopath to see whether there are any lesions that need attention, and having a massage before bed, with some relaxing aromatherpy oils like lavender, geranium or melissa, which will help to induce sleep. A useful homeopathic remedy is Coffea 6X, taking two before you go to bed.

Angela's story

Angela was a 56-year-old teacher with two children. Despite being desperately tired she was unable to sleep. Her health had been so badly affected that she had retired from her job.

'For eleven years, prior to the menopause, I had heavy periods, headaches and moodswings. My last period was in November 1993. Since then I had suffered with hot flushes, my libido had disappeared, and my vagina was dry. My doctor prescribed HRT which I took for five months, but the side-effects were so severe that I had to stop taking it. I was unable to sleep at all and experienced terrible panic attacks, plus my curly hair went straight and unmanageable.

Not being able to sleep seemed to be affecting my brain. I couldn't retain anything in my mind, and was anxious about everything. I usually play bowls but did not have the energy or the confidence to go to games. I have a super husband and lovely grandchildren, but I couldn't be bothered with them either. I felt really cheated as I knew I was missing out on life, but I just wanted to be left alone to doze in the afternoon.

A friend recommended that I go to the WNAS clinic, which in desperation I did. I was asked to get my doctor to measure my serum ferritin levels, which is a test to detect low iron stores. Plus I was given a programme which consisted of making dietary changes, relaxation, supplements and exercise.

My doctor did find that my serum ferritin was very low, and as a result I was put on a course of iron pills. I followed the programme closely and within a month felt that my symptoms were calming down. I began to sleep for parts of the night, my flushes were calming down and I didn't feel quite so tired. The next couple of months were hampered a little because I developed diarrhoea. We eventually discovered that I was reacting to the vitamin E and ginseng which were designed to help with the flushes, and when I stopped taking them my bowel settled down.

I continued to make gradual progress through the year. I avoid wheat and coffee completely, even decaffeinated which seems to upset me. I feel that I am now back to my old self and have been able to cope well with two family crises that have occurred. I am able to sleep through whole blissful nights again, my social life is restored and so is my sense of humour, and as an added bonus my libido is back. My husband is relieved and we are both very grateful to our friend who suggested we visit the WNAS.'

See also: What's wrong with the present-day diet and lifestyle?, Alcohol, Cystitis, Diarrhoea and Arthritis if applicable, The very nutritious diet, References and Recommended reading.

Irritable Bowel Syndrome (IBS)

Irritable bowel syndrome is the modern name for a condition that was formerly known as spastic colon. It is the most common functional gastrointestinal disorder, and is present in up to 20 per cent of the general population in the UK, yet its diagnosis by simple means remains a dilemma. This, however is not a true figure, as many sufferers decide that their bloating is not a real problem, and therefore do not seek professional advice. If they were all to decide to consult their doctor or a consultant, this would place an impossible burden upon medical care facilities in the UK. IBS accounts for almost 50 per cent of outpatients seen by British gastroenterologists each week. The other costs of IBS are mainly in lost quality of life and the effect it has on social life and family health.

The occurrence of IBS almost exclusively in civilised nations, places it in the class of so called 'civilised diseases', stemming from its main causes which are dietary and lifestyle. A typical western diet, consisting largely of refined and adulterated food, over-consumption of one or two staple foods and hurried meals are just a few of the underlying causes of IBS. Epidemiologists often refer to IBS as an acquired disease to which food and environmental factors are the most likely contributing factors. If so, they are largely avoidable, yet the medical profession's first response is not prevention but medication.

For a diagnosis of irritable bowel syndrome to be made, a patient must have no underlying sinister symptoms, but be suffering with either constipation or diarrhoea or both, and abdominal pain and/or bloating and wind.

According to a large UK study published in 1965, a 'normal' bowel habit was considered to be anything from passing motions three times per day to three times per week. At the time 99 per cent of the population survey fell within these limits. It was also discovered that despite this many people still complained of diarrhoea or urgency, or constipation with stools difficult to pass. A further American survey some twenty years later revealed that 94 per cent had a stool frequency of between three times a day and three times per week. However, further questioning about a variety of bowel symptoms revealed that a total of 17 per cent had symptoms indicative of bowel dysfunction.

Surveys on precisely how common IBS is, vary from between 10 to 25 per cent. The most recent UK survey conducted on 2,000 adults from the Southampton area found that a total of 24 per cent of women and 19 per cent of men reported symptoms consistent with IBS. Many people who are troubled by it do not consult their general practitioner but muddle on alone. One wonders how the medical facilities would cope if everyone with IBS turned up for help!

What are the symptoms?

- constipation – opening the bowels infrequently, or hard stools
- diarrhoea – loose rather than just frequent stools
- alternating diarrhoea and constipation
- abdominal discomfort or pain
- abdominal bloating
- excessive wind
- mucus or slime in the stool
- nausea and loss of appetite
- indigestion

It is usual with IBS that patients will suffer with either diarrhoea or constipation, or a combination of the two, together with abdominal bloating and some discomfort or pain. These are the most common and typical symptoms.

What causes it?

- *Age* Many people develop IBS symptoms in young to middle age, although approximately 12 per cent of those with IBS did experience symptoms during their childhood.
- *Operations* It has been observed that approximately 10 per cent of women are more likely to suffer symptoms of IBS following an operation like a hysterectomy or surgery on the ovaries. These operations can leave internal scar tissue which is thought to be connected in some way to the onset of symptoms.
- *Radiotherapy* When the abdomen has been targeted by radiotherapy, scarring can occur which may then once again produce symptoms of IBS.
- *Gynaecological problems* The female reproductive organs have a very close relationship with the bowels. The womb, or uterus, is next to the end of the colon and a significant amount of the small bowel sits loosely coiled on top of the uterus. Many conditions relating to the uterus can release powerful chemicals which also influence the gut. A study by Dr Prior and colleagues on a sample of 200 women found that many of them noticed improvements in their bowel functions following a hysterectomy. Twenty-two per cent of his sample had IBS before surgery, and two-thirds reported improvement in their symptoms following the operation.
- *Gastrointestinal infection* Most of us have experienced a severe tummy upset whilst on holiday or after eating a take-away meal. Sudden onset of diarrhoea, sometimes accompanied by pain and fever, can either be caused by bacteria or by a virus. Usually it doesn't last for more than a few days, but sometimes the gut never seems to feel the same again, and symptoms of IBS develop.
- *Other bowel conditions* Older people sometimes develop a condition called diverticulosis of the colon, when the weak walls of the colon begin to bulge, and this can sometimes cause symptoms of IBS as well. A lack of fibre may lie behind both conditions. Patients suffering with ulcerative colitis, a severe inflammation of the gut which causes diarrhoea and bleeding, may also experience symptoms of IBS, even when the colitis is controlled by drugs.
- *Drugs* Some pain-killing drugs can cause symptoms of IBS, either shortly after they are taken, or several months later. Antibiotics, certainly if taken in the long-term, can cause diarrhoea as a side-effect which may set up IBS-type symptoms in some. This seems to be due to

a build up of *Candida albicans*, the organism responsible for thrush. This is often self-limiting and passes off, but for some it persists. Sometimes supplements of iron or multi-vitamins and minerals containing iron can irritate the gut also and produce symptoms of IBS.

- *Stress* There is now plenty of evidence to show that stress can worsen symptoms of IBS. The stress factors affect the muscles in the gut and can cause them to go into spasm, rendering the bowel inefficient, and causing pain. Chronic sufferers of IBS sometimes suffer with anxiety and depression as their symptoms remain unresolved, which produces a vicious circle.

- *A change of diet* Food intolerances sometimes develop after a period of eating substantial quantities of the same food, or when new foods which are hard to digest are introduced. Further information on this subject can be found in the information on Food Allergies (see page 58).

- *Nothing* Strangely, it seems that symptoms of IBS occur out of the blue with no single precipitating factor. Perhaps a subtle combination of circumstances may be the underlying cause or perhaps there may be genetic factors at play.

What your doctor can do

Twenty years ago, it used to be fashionable in medical circles to investigate patients complaining with symptoms of IBS, with a view to diagnosing a stomach or duodenal ulcer, gall stones, digestive problems or problems with the colon, or large bowel, particularly diverticulosis. IBS was a diagnosis made by the doctor when nothing else could be found. This meant that patients were often subjected to numerous tests including blood tests and x-rays, that were unnecessary. This was frustrating for patient and doctor alike.

Times have fortunately changed. It has become recognised that IBS is often the diagnosis for young to middle-aged patients, with abdominal pain or disturbance of bowel function. There are no tests to verify the diagnosis of IBS, it is often made on a balance of probabilities. It is important to be screened by your doctor to eliminate the possibility of any sinister underlying cause to your symptoms.

What you can do

- Follow an exclusion diet outlined in the Menu for Irritable Bowel Syndrome on page 472. An exclusion diet involves avoiding all commonly allergenic foods for a set period of time, then reintroducing them one by one. The most frequently implicated foods are wheat, dairy, eggs and citrus foods.

- Take a probiotic supplement which provide a standardised dose of the healthy bacteria *Lactobacillus acidophillus* and bifido bacteria. Eating live yoghurt might also be helpful, but supplements ensure a more precise dose. Most probiotics require refrigeration, but some do not have special storage requirements.
- If you are constipated add 1–2 tbsp of organic golden linseeds to your wheat-free breakfast cereal daily. They can be crushed and soaked in water or milk (soya or rice 'milk') for maximum efficiency. Crushing and soaking them reduces the risk of any associated discomfort such as bloating. Refer to the chapter on constipation for more information.
- Take supplements of magnesium amino acid chelate to improve bowel function if your are constipated. Magnesium works by relaxing the smooth muscles of the gut. The WNAS recommend taking it 'to gut tolerance' which means that too much can result in loose stools. Monitor and adjust your dose accordingly.
- Aloe vera is a good adjunct to a specific dietary and supplement programme. Aloe vera is used primarily to heal the digestive tract. Be aware of cheap inferior brands on the market, and choose one from a reputable manufacturer. Aloe vera is available in liquid or gel form.
- Take some digestive enzymes. These function to mimic the natural enzymes secreted by the pancreas and stomach. Sometimes these are lacking in patients with IBS, especially those who suffer with chronic bloating and a feeling of fullness soon after eating, even small quantities. They shouldn't be taken in the long term as the body might lose its ability to produce these enzymes naturally.
- Charcoal tablets are quite a good standby for the immediate relief of bloating and discomfort. However do not take daily or at the same time as nutritional supplements because the charcoal can actually inhibit the absorption of nutrients.

Complementary therapies

Creative visualisation is a wonderfully simple and most enjoyable method of relaxation, that requires little or no training. It is perfect for those who haven't had the time to learn how to practice yoga or meditation. We advise patients to lie flat on the floor, with a cushion beneath the head. Bend your knees and place your feet flat on the floor, so that you are in what is called 'The Alexander position' after the founder of the Alexander Technique. Next, close your eyes, take some slow steady breaths, and consciously relax your face, your fingers and your toes. When you feel comfortable, whilst still breathing slowly and steadily, you simply visualise any fantasy you fancy, from a world cruise to a good night out! The trick is to keep your mind on the trip in question. It seems to be an acquired skill, and one that you may have to work at. If you have a very busy mind, you may need to have a pen and paper handy at first, in order to download your thoughts. You need to do this for fifteen or twenty minutes per day, and then gently come back to reality, rolling over on to your side prior to standing. Some patients feel so relaxed doing their creative visualisation, that they fall asleep!

Sinister symptoms

It is essential for you to become familiar with some of the possible sinister underlying symptoms, which may produce IBS-type symptoms, but are not IBS, and their treatment is quite different. Here is a check-list of further symptoms for you to examine:

1. **Have you recently developed symptoms which are severe?** In this case it is always best to have a medical examination.
2. **Do you have severe abdominal pain?** For example, can it wake you from sleep? Does it cause you to stop what you are doing? Does it put you off eating?
3. **Have you lost weight because of your bowel symptoms?** Losing any more than a few pounds in weight should not be regarded as IBS.
4. **Do you regularly pass more than four stools per day?** Diarrhoea from any cause can contribute to a loss of essential nutrients, even if there is no weight loss.
5. **Have you passed blood in the stool or passed dark coloured stools?** Loss of blood from the bowel requires investigation because it may not always be due to IBS.
6. **Have you had a fever with your bowel symptoms?** Infection in the bowel from parasites or other causes should be considered. Some parasitic infections can be found in the UK without travelling abroad.
7. **Have you had any abdominal operations including an appendectomy?** Past operations can leave behind strands of tissue called adhesions that can interfere with normal bowel function. If your bowel symptoms followed an operation you should return to your doctor.
8. **Are you aged fifty years or more?** This increases the risk of symptoms being due to bowel cancer or a polyp (a small growth inside the bowel) which may become cancerous. Again you should check with your doctor if you have not already done so.
9. **Did your mother, father, sister or brother develop cancer of the bowel under the age of fifty?** If so, you should also check with your doctor. Sometimes this type of problem can run in families affecting relatively young or middle-aged members. Early detection of those at risk is now possible with a marked improvement in outlook for them.

10. **Do you have any vaginal discharge, pain on intercourse or pain very low down in the abdomen?** Infection of the fallopian tubes is particularly common in young women with these symptoms, which can sometimes aggravate, or be confused with IBS.
11. **Are your periods painful, heavy or irregular?** A number of gynaecological problems may cloud the picture at times. Fibroid growths of the womb, cysts on the ovaries, and sometimes hormonal problems should all be considered if you have any of the above.

Once the diagnosis of IBS is made, what is on offer from your doctor will depend whether you are suffering with diarrhoea, constipation or a combination of both. For further details of what your doctor can do, and what measures you can implement yourself, you will now need to refer to the chapters on Constipation (page 136), Diarrhoea (page 174) and Abdominal Bloating (page 45).

The good news is that symptoms of IBS are both treatable and curable. We have written a book called *No More IBS!*, which is based on our success treating this condition at the WNAS. If you require personal advice you will find details of our clinics and help-line services on page 511.

Belinda's story

Belinda was a single 32-year-old who had been suffering with severe bowel problems for two years prior to approaching the WNAS. She was very distressed as both her work and social life were affected.

'Looking back I realise that my symptoms began at about the time that my relationship ended with my boyfriend. We had been together for two years, and I found it very difficult to cope with the break-up. I began to have severe episodes of bloating and constipation every day, with extreme abdominal pain. I even found it difficult to sit down at work. Each day by the evening I was in so much pain, I could only go to bed and wait for the pain to subside. I felt awfully drained and lost quite a bit of weight, which I could ill afford to do.

I was referred to the hospital for tests, including a small bowel enema, ultrasound and x-rays, and in November 1992 I was diagnosed as having IBS, and told to go on a high-fibre diet. The hospital doctor told me there was no known cure, and when I asked in desperation what I could do as I was still in constant pain, and with a redundant wardrobe, due to the swelling, he said I would have to buy bigger clothes. I was very shocked and angry by his unsympathetic response.

So a vicious circle began. I took painkillers, which brought on severe constipation and distress, which could only be relieved by laxatives. My doctor prescribed Colpermin, to make eating easier, but this only brought me out in a rash and the list of possible side-effects was quite alarming.

In May 1993 I went along to the WNAS clinic at the suggestion of a friend who had been treated successfully by them. I must admit feeling sceptical when I went along for my first appointment, as I couldn't imagine that diet alone would be the solution to this severe problem. I was put on to a basic diet, asked to keep daily symptom charts and seen fortnightly for a review. While I did have some good days, I still had more bad days. After three months and very little change I was on the verge of giving up, when I was told that in addition to excluding the foods we had so far, I should also leave out rice, corn, potatoes and bananas. It was also suggested that I take linseeds with my cereals and extra magnesium at night to relieve the constipation. To my utter amazement, my symptoms calmed down. The constipation was no longer a problem and the pain and bloating subsided.

I am happy to live on a restricted diet as I have traded the foods that upset me for my health. I am making great progress at work and have found a wonderful new boyfriend. I am very grateful as I now look forward to each day.'

See also: Stress, exercise and relaxation, The simple exclusion diet, The strict exclusion diet, References and Recommended reading.

Ischaemic Heart Disease

This is a disease in which there is a narrowing and eventually blockage of the blood vessels that supply the heart muscles. These vessels, which are called the coronary arteries, carry a very substantial flow of blood and oxygen to the ever-active heart muscle. The narrowing is due to the slow development of what is termed a plaque. This is made up of fatty deposits, and fibrous tissue which develops in response to the fat deposit. The internal diameter of the blood vessel is reduced and even a small plaque can halve the flow of blood through one of the several coronary arteries. This process of arterial narrowing and hardening is called atherosclerosis, and the same process takes place in other major arteries, leading to strokes and poor circulation to the legs.

Very often the slowed blood that is attempting to flow through the coronary arteries is sticky, and a clot easily forms and adheres to the surface of the plaque. This leads to a complete blockage of a major coronary artery, which in turn leads to the most important manifestation of ischaemic heart disease, a heart attack or acute myocardial infarction (literally heart muscle that is stuffed with old blood). Needless to say that the heart muscle previously supplied by the now occluded artery will die, and the patient will at the very least be left with a weakened heart.

The next most important consequence of ischaemic heart disease is angina. The narrowing of a coronary artery does not always lead to blockage. The artery may have an adequate blood supply for the needs of the muscle it supplies provided that the heart is not working too hard. But when walking briskly, walking uphill or running, the supply of oxygen may be inadequate. The level of certain chemicals rises in the heart muscle which leads to pain usually felt as a 'tight' pain in the centre of the chest, which may also pass into the left arm, up into the neck or through into the back. The pain is often sufficiently severe to cause the sufferer to stop whatever they are doing and rest, which in many cases is enough for the pain to ease. The whole episode may only last a few minutes but recur every time the person tries to exert themselves.

Unfortunately not all ischaemic heart disease presents in this way. Sometimes the first event is also the last. Sudden unexpected death in a young to middle-aged man is very often due to this condition. Then there is no opportunity to undertake some of the medical and preventative measures that are proving successful in this condition.

Ischaemic heart disease can also cause palpitations with changes in the rhythm of the heartbeat, and also heart failure. This latter may be as a consequence of several heart attacks, or develop slowly and silently in older patients. The diagnosis of coronary artery disease is usually made as a result of one of these clinical pictures with confirmation from an ECG, blood tests, specialist x-rays of the coronary arteries called an angiogram, or other specialist assessments. Very often the assessment of ischaemic heart disease, especially in a young person, will involve an assessment of the main risk factors as well.

Who gets it?

Atherosclerosis, the process of narrowing and hardening of the main arteries, and the development of ischaemic heart disease, are common. In England and Wales 22 per cent of all female deaths, and 30 per cent of male deaths, are due to ischaemic heart disease. In most developed countries around the world, death from disease of the coronary arteries rose substantially in the latter half of this century. This rise peaked and has fallen since the 1960s in the United States and is now falling in western Europe. The rise is still continuing in eastern Europe. An appreciation of the risk factors, changes to reduce them where possible, and better medical treatment probably lie behind these falls.

The main risk factors that determine who is likely to develop ischaemic heart disease are:

- age, the risk rising from age 40 to mid-70s then falling.
- being male.
- race (greater risk in those from South Asia).
- dietary factors:
  - eating too much and being very overweight
  - too much saturated (animal) fat
  - too little fruit and vegetables
  - not enough high-fibre grain products
  - possibly poor intake of vitamins B, C, E, and the minerals magnesium and chromium
  - not consuming certain 'protective' foods and beverages such as oily fish, small amounts of wine, certain nuts (walnuts, almonds and pecans).
- body shape with excess weight being deposited around the abdomen rather than on the hips (being an 'apple' instead of a 'pear').
- family history (coronary heart disease in a first-degree relative under the age of 55).
- cigarette smoking.
- personality type. The aggressive, striving ambitious deadline-driven 'type A' personality as it is known, is more prone than the relaxed sort who could barely care if the deadline is met or not.
- stressful situations at work and at home such as the death of a spouse.
- lack of physical exercise.
- soft water (within the UK, being in an area where the water is soft thus low in natural calcium and magnesium).
- diabetes mellitus.
- high blood cholesterol (over 5.2 mol/L).
- high blood pressure.
- an early menopause and loss of the 'protective action' of oestrogen.
- an excess level of blood-clotting factors.
- an increase in the level of the amino acid homocysteine in the blood not only recently but at any time from youth onwards.
- poor growth in the first year of life, especially if the birth weight was low.

Many of these risk factors interact. For example the level of cholesterol in the blood is in turn influenced by genetic factors, diet, smoking and exercise. Also not all these risk factors are as important as each other. A very high cholesterol, above 9.0 mmol/L, is a major risk factor, especially if combined with smoking. A slightly elevated blood pressure in a woman with no other major risk factors hardly adds to her risk of ischaemic heart disease. Once there is evidence of actual ischaemic heart disease (e.g. an actual myocardial infarction, angina when physically active or an abnormal ECG) the need for aggressive therapy with diet and drugs greatly increases. Young patients (under the age of 40) will rarely need treatment for an elevated blood cholesterol unless it is very high or they are carrying several other major risk factors. For them simple, cheap, safe, non-toxic measures will suffice (a very healthy diet, exercise and possibly supplements of vitamin E 200+ IU per day) until they are older when the higher risk may then justify a more vigorous diet and cholesterol-lowering drugs.

What causes it?

The cause of ischaemic heart disease has been the subject of intense research both of populations and in the laboratory. This has led to the identification of the above risk factors, an understanding of their interaction, and how they lead to actual narrowing of a coronary artery. A full discussion of how these risk factors actually cause heart disease is beyond the scope of this book. What is important is to understand how some of the main risk factors work together and the potential for prevention of this major killer. Obviously there are some risk factors that cannot be changed. Age, sex and race are not under our control.

Fats and cholesterol

There is a strong connection between the amount and type of fat in the diet, and the risk of ischaemic heart disease. Historically attention has focused upon blood cholesterol. This is influenced by two factors. About one-third of the cholesterol in the blood is derived from the cholesterol that we eat. The remainder is made in the liver, and the amount made is determined by genetic and dietary factors. We use cholesterol to make all kinds of necessary body chemicals such as vitamin D, oestrogen, testosterone and for the structure of some cells. A high cholesterol level in a form that is easily deposited to make an atheromatous plaque is dangerous. This high-risk cholesterol is called LDL, and the beneficial protective form is called HDL. These cholesterol sub-fractions can be measured from a blood sample taken usually after an overnight fast.

High intakes of saturated animal fats add to the risk of heart disease probably because such a diet will increase the production of cholesterol in the LDL form by the liver and may cause other blood changes, encouraging the depositing of that cholesterol on to the inner wall of the artery. Other fats do not have this effect, such as the oleic acid found in olive oil and rape seed oil and of the polyunsaturated fatty acids derived from a variety of plant and fish oils. These oils may actually shift the balance toward the good HDL cholesterol. The degree of protection that these 'healthy oils' provide is debated, and of interest not only to the general public and doctors, but also to farmers and politicians. The majority of expert recommendations recognise a need for the 'average' consumer to reduce their total fat intake by cutting down on saturated animal fats, maintaining a modest intake of the polyunsaturates and to making little change to the consumption of oleic acid. Arguments will continue to rage about the role that these different fats play in heart disease.

Many of the risk factors also influence this balance between the good HDL and the bad LDL cholesterol. Stopping smoking, correction of obesity and regular physical exercise may have a marked effect, reducing the total cholesterol and raising the proportion of the good type. In patients with furring up of their coronary arteries or of those arteries in the legs, meticulous attention to diet and use of drugs to lower cholesterol has been shown to reverse the process of atherosclerosis. If other relevant risk factors are tackled, then the prospects for sufferers will look better still. Do not forget that the type of advice given to someone who has had a heart attack and has a high blood cholesterol level may be quite different to that given to a healthy middle-aged woman or man with low to average risk factors.

Broadly speaking the recommendations for healthy eating take into account the main dietary risk factors for ischaemic heart disease. Their implementation will hopefully lead to the prevention of heart disease in the general population who have yet to have a heart attack. This is termed primary prevention. Our recommendations for The Very Nutritious Diet on page 437 are appropriate for the majority of those who wish to delay the development of ischaemic heart disease. We say 'delay' rather than 'prevent' as this problem may be inevitable for many. Remember age is a major risk factor and for those aged 80 years and more, a heart attack could be viewed as a relatively attractive way of ending one's days.

It is now recognised that increased levels of homocysteine are implicated in the risk of heart disease. Homocysteine is a suphur-containing amino acid produced from the breakdown of another amino acid called methionine. Homocysteine levels in the body rise if there is a relative deficiency of folic acid and to a lesser degree, vitamins B6 and B12. An elevated level of this amino acid increases the risk of athero-sclerosis, where the arteries become blocked, leading to both heart attacks and also strokes. Elevated homocysteine levels are also linked to raised levels of LDL cholesterol which causes blocked arteries. A diet rich in folic acid, from green leafy vegetables and fortified cereals, is recommended, together with a reduced intake of saturated fats from meat and full fat dairy products.

Some other dietary factors have also been shown to protect against heart disease:

- *Garlic* The active ingredient of which is allicin, and which gives it its characteristic smell, has been demonstrated to reduce blood cholesterol, lower blood pressure and have a positive effect on blood clotting which are all risk factors in heart disease. Garlic can be incorporated into the daily diet, but for some the taste can be overpowering, so it is more convenient and pleasant to take it in supplement form.

- *Phytoestrogens* It was discovered that soy protein lowers cholesterol levels almost by accident. In the late 1960's researchers set out to find out whether soy could be a palatable alternative protein to meat, and in doing so they noticed a marked reduction in cholesterol levels in the soya consumers. Almost a decade later soya was once again put under the microscope by Dr Sirtori at the University of Milan. He discovered that soy protein lowered cholesterol levels by an average of 14 per cent within two weeks, and by 21 per cent at the end of the three weeks. Since that time, much more research has been undertaken to look at the effects of soya on cholesterol levels. An analysis of 40 published studies was undertaken by Dr Kenneth Carrol at the University of Western Ontario. His conclusion was that 34 of the studies did produce a drop in LDL cholesterol levels in particular, by 15 per cent or more. Other more recent studies have shown that as well as reducing the level of LDL, soya has been successful in raising levels of HDL, the desirable cholesterol. Even genetically raised cholesterol levels have been seen to drop by 26 per cent in a four week Italian study, published in 1991.

    Another interesting study, conducted by Dr John Eden from Sydney, Australia, showed that menopausal women on Novogen Red Clover supplements, containing 40 mg of isoflavones per tablet, showed an 18 per cent increase, on average, in HDL cholesterol. Furthermore, trials using Rimostil, Novogen's newest isoflavone dietary supplement showed a significant improvement in the lipid profile in healthy post-menopausal women. HDL cholesterol levels increased by up to 28 per cent while apolipoprotein B decreased by 10 per cent after six months. The increase in HDL cholesterol potentially represents an approximate 40 per cent reduction in the risk of cardiovascular death in women.

    A recent study by Professor Kenneth Setchell, reported at the 3rd International Symposium on the Role of Soy in Preventing and Treating Chronic Disease in Washington DC confirmed that it is possible to raise HDL, the good cholesterol, whilst lowering LDL, the bad cholesterol. His twelve week study, on 43 post-menopausal women consuming a soy rich diet, containing 60-70 mg of total isoflavines each day also highlighted the anti-oxidant effects of soya.

    Furthermore, on October 20th 1999, the US Food and Drug Administration in the USA approved a health claim for soy protein and its role in the reduced risk of coronary heart disease. This effectively means that food products which contain a minimum of 6.25 grams of soy protein per serving will be allowed to state on the label that in conjunction with a low fat, low cholesterol diet, the product may reduce the risk of heart disease. The health claim was developed by the FDA, which concluded, based on scientific evidence form more than 50 independent studies, that 25 grams of soy protein, included in a daily diet, low in saturated fat and cholesterol, reduces the risk of coronary heart disease.

The Italians are so convinced about the value of soy in lowering cholesterol that it is now provided free of charge by the Italian National Health Service to those with high cholesterol levels.

Cardiovascular disease is a leading cause of death in post-menopausal women, as they are no longer protected by oestrogen. They are particularly at increased risk of high cholesterol levels and heart disease. The benefits of phytoestrogens on lowering cholesterol levels and improving heart health are therefore an extremely important in medecine.

What your doctor can do

- Assess the severity of the condition. Those presenting with angina at a young age, those with severe symptoms uncontrolled by drug therapy, and others with certain risk factors need a detailed assessment often involving x-rays of the coronary arteries – a coronary angiogram.
- Treat the symptoms. Angina may be helped by the use of several types of drugs: nitrates help dilate the coronary arteries and can be given as a spray or tablets under the tongue; beta-blockers slow the heart rate and reduce the demand for oxygen and calcium antagonists also open up the coronary arteries. Many of these drugs will need to be given on a regular daily basis as well as being used for acute attacks.
- Treat a myocardial infarction or a clot. Rapid response by the doctor or emergency services with use of anti-clotting treatments, aspirin, beta-blockers and nitrate drugs has resulted in improved survival. Speed, however, is of the essence in this situation, and all middle-aged and elderly people with prolonged chest pains are suspected of having a heart attack until proven otherwise.
- Assess the main risk factors for atherosclerosis. This will involve measurement of blood pressure, tests for diabetes and measurement of a fasting blood cholesterol level. If the blood cholesterol is elevated then the need for advice about drugs and diet can be assessed. Even if the patient is not enthusiastic she will often do well to use some of the newer drugs as well as diet to lower its level.
- Prevent further myocardial infarction by use of drugs. This often involves giving aspirin which helps prevent blood clotting, beta-

blockers to slow the heart rate, ACE inhibitor drugs for those with a weakened heart, or calcium antagonists. The choice of these depends upon factors such as patient tolerance, blood pressure, diabetes and the use of other drugs.

- Prevent further myocardial infarction by lifestyle changes such as cessation of smoking, reduction in weight, changes to the diet, drugs to lower blood cholesterol, and a carefully supervised exercise regime to improve fitness.
- Consider the need for surgical correction of coronary artery narrowing. In selected patients who have had a myocardial infarction or are at risk of one, either open-heart surgery and by-passing the blockage, or the newer technique of opening up the blockage from within the artery – coronary angioplasty – can be highly successful, and be associated with an improved life expectancy. Coronary artery by-pass graft survival is very much influenced by the control of blood cholesterol and lifestyle factors.

The last 20 years has seen a substantial improvement in the outcome for those affected with ischaemic heart disease. For both the patient who suffers angina on exercising, and the patient who is recovering from their (first) myocardial infarction, there is much they can do to improve their lot and reduce the risk of more angina, another infarction and sudden death. The wise patient should regard the diagnosis of ischaemic heart disease as a signal to make some changes and regard that day as the first day of the rest of life.

What you can do

Plenty!

- Make sure that you get proper medical treatment as above! The provision of good care together with appropriate monitoring are not automatic. Expert assessment is very often needed for those with severe angina, those whose lifestyle is significantly altered as a result of a myocardial infarction, those who have had several infarctions, those with diabetes, those with a high blood cholesterol unresponsive to simple dietary measures and those with a weakened heart.
- Don't smoke. You're crazy.
- Don't be overweight. If you are, lose weight. Never mind the details of the best diet for heart disease, just get the weight off. Follow The Simple Weight-Loss Diet (see page 452).
- If your cholesterol is even slightly elevated then follow The Very Nutritious Diet (see page 437). Make sure that you achieve the following dietary goals:

- ○ three pieces of fresh fruit daily
- ○ two portions of green vegetables daily
- ○ three portions of fish per week with two of these being mackerel or herring
- ○ use mainly soya, rape seed and walnut oil. This latter is good for salad dressings
- ○ use a polyunsaturated margarine rather than butter
- ○ allow yourself some alcohol per day particularly red wine which appears to be particularly good for the heart. Seven units per week (about 4–5 drinks) is the optimum intake for women and twice this for men
- ○ if you can, include garlic, onions and some nuts – walnuts, almonds and pecans – into your diet.

- If this is not effective enough then more specialised dietary advice may be needed. For example a Vegan Diet (see page 455) might appeal to some, but be too difficult for many. You could modify this and add in oily fish to make it a Tunatarian diet (see page 455). Allow yourself one portion of mackerel, herring or salmon daily. A strict vegan diet has been used as part of a highly successful non-drug treatment for severe angina.

- Include a daily serving of phytoestrogens to help reduce cholesterol levels. Phytoestrogens predominate in soya beans and soya bean products like flour, tofu and soya milk, golden linseeds and the herb red clover (tablets, or sprouted seeds).

- Regular exercise is a good idea for all. Probably it is best to get some expert advice about this. Ask your doctor, or there may be a post-myocardial infarction exercise group at the local hospital. Some sports clubs run specialised classes for heart patients.

- Nutritional supplements do have some value too:
  - ○ Vitamin E at high dose, 600 IU per day, had been shown recently to reduce the risk of a heart attack but a more recent and large study of 4001 showed no benefit over 4.5 years. Take it but don't think this means you don't have to do anything else. Those who are taking the blood-thinning drug Warfarin will need to check with their doctor first, as vitamin E influences the effects of this drug.
  - ○ Vitamin C as a supplement of around 1 gm per day may help lower an elevated blood cholesterol but probably only if your diet is devoid of fruit and vegetables.
  - ○ Fish oil supplements can be helpful. High doses providing a total of at least 1 gram of Omega-3 EPA and DHA can lower heart disease risk by about 15 per cent.
  - ○ Magnesium might be helpful. Some but not all studies have shown that very high doses help in the recovery from a heart attack. It is

perhaps most useful for those whose blood level is low as a result of diuretic (water) tablets.

○ Chromium is a curious trace element. It is required in tiny quant-ities and it helps insulin in its action of controlling blood sugar. Supplements have been shown to help correct a diabetic tendency and improve elevated blood cholesterol levels. Low levels of the mineral are associated with coronary artery disease. A supplement of 200 mcg per day is worth considering. It will need to be taken long term.

○ Multi-vitamins are worth a mention. Perhaps the simplest thing to take is a modest strength multi-vitamin with vitamin E, 200 IU, and vitamin C, 250 mg. Older patients, those with a restricted diet or those on many drugs may be the most suited to this.

○ Take vitamins B12, folic acid and B6 if the level of the artery damag-ing amino acid homocysteine is elevated. Folic acid appears to be the most important vitamin to supplement in order to normalise homo-cysteine levels particularly in older people.

• Make sure that there is good control of any possible blood pressure, diabetes and any blood stickiness problem.

• Avoid stressful situations at home and at work. These very often precipitate attacks of angina or even a heart attack. Relaxation tech-niques are appropriate for those for whom this is a particular problem (see page 29).

Complementary Therapies

These have not come to the fore for heart disease in the way that they have in other areas. Perhaps it is because of the life-threatening nature of ischaemic heart disease that no great emphasis has been put on these complementary approaches. Any de-stressing therapies are worth consid-ering. They should complement, not replace, conventional treatment. Aromatherapy, massage and acupuncture would fall into this category. Herbalism may prove to have much to offer. The potential of plant prod-ucts to provide a degree of chemical protection from heart disease is slowly being realised. Seek expert advice form a qualified herbalist on this last point.

Kidney Stones

Urine is a chemically complicated fluid. It is obviously composed mainly of water, but dissolved in this are significant amounts of certain minerals including sodium, calcium, magnesium, potassium and phosphate. The yellow colour is due to breakdown products from blood and plant pigments, and sometimes vitamin B2, riboflavin. There is a limit to the amount of a mineral that can be dissolved in a given volume of fluid. If urine volume is decreased, the mineral concentration increases; as a result, some of these minerals may be precipitated out as crystals which then form stones. The stones normally form in the kidney and once released they try and travel along the thin tube connecting the kidney and the bladder, the ureter. If this becomes blocked or goes into spasm, then pain results. Renal colic, as it is known, is one of the most painful conditions known in medicine, and very often patients attend hospital as an emergency with severe gripping pain in the side of the abdomen which may pass down into the groin. The site of the pain changes as the stone passes along the urethra until it eventually passes out into the bladder and hopefully through the urine to the outside world. The stone can be collected using a tea strainer. This is important as chemical analysis of the stone indicates the type of stone and the best treatment for its prevention.

What causes them?

As there are a variety of kidney stones there are a variety of possible causes. Usually there are several at work together and typically a combination of them in any one individual.

The following are all possible factors:

- Infection in the urine. This leads to a change in the urine's chemistry and under certain circumstances can lead to kidney stone formation.
- Too much calcium in the urine which is only rarely due to too much calcium in the diet. An important possibility is an excessive level of calcium in the blood because of changes in hormone chemistry. More usually there is an excessive leaking of calcium out into the urine and this is probably aggravated by a diet high in sodium, sugar and low in magnesium and essential fatty acids.
- Dehydration which is an important cause of kidney stone formation in the tropics.
- Accumulation of oxalic acid. This comes from certain foods in the diet and some people excrete excessive amounts of this acid into the urine.
- An excess of uric acid in the urine. This compound is also the cause of gout (see page 83). Again some of us pass larger than usual quantities out into the urine and because it is hard to dissolve it can easily lead to kidney stone formation.

What your doctor can do

- Treat the acute episode with strong painkillers.
- Investigate the type of stone. This involves analysis of any stones

captured, blood test and urine tests. These tests centre upon measuring the levels of the minerals and compounds previously mentioned.

- Test the urine for infection which is a significant factor in stone formation.
- Give specific recommendation, depending upon the type of stone. This may require expert assessment but some general guidelines can be given (*see below*).

What you can do

The following recommendations will apply almost no matter what the type of stone is:

- Drink plenty of fluid – at least 3 and up to 5 pints (1.75–2.75 litres) of water daily.
- Eat a diet low in sugar, salt and refined foods, and high in fruit, vegetable and wholegrain cereals. This sort of diet reduces the loss of many minerals in the urine, but more specialised dietary advice may be required.
- Supplements of magnesium, which passes out into the urine and generally has stone-inhibiting properties. This is not very effective but is very safe and may be followed on a long-term basis. The reasonable dosage is 200–300 mg per day of elemental magnesium.
- Sometimes a low calcium diet is recommended if there is continuing loss of calcium in the urine.
- Minimise your consumption of animal protein, or eliminate from your diet altogether. A high animal protein diet causes the body to excrete calcium, producing excessive calcium, phosphorous and uric acid in the kidneys and often resulting in painful kidney stones.
- Supplements of bran may inhibit the absorption of calcium from the diet and reduce the amount lost in the urine. This is not recommended if the person is at risk of developing osteoporosis.
- Supplements of evening primrose oil and fish oil, Efamol Marine, have an interesting and useful effect in recurrent kidney stone formation when these are high in calcium. They reduce the loss of calcium via the kidney, and together with the above simple dietary means, may even reduce the rate of stone formation. It is thought that they may do this by preventing the loss of calcium from bone.
- Follow a diet low in oxalate. This compound is found in a variety of foods notably tea, coffee, peanuts, chocolate, rhubarb and spinach. A reduced dietary intake may be required in some adults and children who have this type of kidney stone. Expert assessment is required before beginning this diet.
- Lose weight if you are over-weight.

- Stay active. People who are sedentary tend to accumulate high levels of calcium in the bloodstream. Exercise helps transfer calcium from the blood into the bones, where it belongs.
- Cut down on alcohol, particularly important if you have gout (see page 83).

See also: References.

Loss of Libido

In our youth, before the responsibilities of life settle on our shoulders, many of us take our libido, or appetite for sex, for granted, never dreaming that anything might influence it. However, the passionate nights of a new relationship live on in the dreams of most, but in the reality of only a few. Childbirth, sleepless nights, the stresses and strains of life and general preoccupation, all contribute to a waning sex drive.

Over the years at the WNAS we have come to realise, from dealing with thousands of women of all ages, that women regard their loss of libido as their lot. They accept that it is all part of their fading youth, even if it happens in their late twenties! They don't discuss it with others through embarrassment as they assume they are suffering alone, and it doesn't occur to them that the situation is reversible.

There are no hard and fast rules about what is a normal level of libido, and there is no such thing as a 'normal' libido. What is normal to one couple may be abnormal to another. You can only judge your libido by your own standards, and if you feel that your sexual desire has diminished, for whatever reason, you will need to seek help to restore it.

What are the causes?

Most of us have a natural interest in sex initially. That's the way we were designed. There are, however, a number of reasons why sex drive can decrease either over a period of time or suddenly following a particular incident.

Loss of libido can be due to physical or hormonal problems or mental stress and sometimes a combination of the two. Amongst the causes are:

- After childbirth many women lose interest in sex because of their rapidly changing hormone levels, their disturbed nights and the fact that Mother Nature makes a woman treat her baby as a priority rather than her husband's needs.
- Excessive weight gain, weight loss, irregular periods, hair loss or

excessive hair growth may all signify hormonal problems which can also result in a low sex libido.

- Other hormone disturbances like thyroid problems, or galactorrhea, a white milky discharge from the nipples, can cause low libido.
- Sometimes people are put off sex as intercourse becomes painful. The pain can be due to infection, vaginismus, when the vaginal muscles go into spasm, an enlarged or displaced womb or other conditions.
- Long-term illness and lack of energy.
- Psychologically distressing past experiences which still haunt you.
- Simply a lack of feeling for your partner.
- Stress, worry and depression often take their toll on sex drive. When you are mentally preoccupied with pressing problems the body naturally diverts its energy to helping you through the troubled times and sexual desire may take a back seat.

What your doctor can do

If you feel that the cause of your loss of sex drive may be due to hormonal problems or pain or discomfort, your doctor should be able to offer you some effective treatment. If there is an underlying psychological problem, or you are feeling overwhelmed with stress you will need to get some professional counselling to help overcome the problems before you can expect your libido to return. The doctor can:

- give you routine blood tests, including serum ferritin to check your iron stores.
- give you a physical examination to eliminate any underlying physical causes.
- refer you for some counselling if your relationship is under strain or if you are suffering the effects of past trauma.

What you can do

If, however, you feel that your libido has decreased for no apparent reason, particularly if the situation is worse before your period, then it is possible that you can gain some benefit by attending to your diet.

At the Women's Nutritional Advisory Service we have found that a programme of diet, exercise and nutritional supplements helps some 90 per cent of women get their sex drive back within four to six months.

The body depends on important vitamins and minerals in order to function properly. When under stress there is a significantly increased demand for essential nutrients. Because we lack education about the foods which contain these important nutrients, these increased demands may not be met.

We know, for instance, that the mineral magnesium is necessary for normal hormone function and that B vitamins and the mineral zinc are particularly important in sex hormone metabolism and maintaining your sex drive. So it stands to reason that if your diet does not provide you with a constant supply of good nutrients, the body will eventually stop functioning normally, and your sex drive may well be affected.

- Follow the instructions for The Very Nutritious Diet on page 437.
- Eat plenty of ordinary foods like bread, milk, eggs, meat, chicken, nuts, beans, dried fruit, green vegetables, and fish. Oysters long regarded for their aphrodisiac qualities, are extremely high in zinc, and are vital for sperm and male hormone production.
- It is important to avoid drinking too much alcohol as it knocks most nutrients sideways. Whilst you are trying to consume lots of good nutrients through your diet it would defeat the object to wash them away with alcohol. Alcohol may initially increase the desire but usually reduces the performance. Try to limit yourself to no more than three drinks per week.
- If you are overweight it is important to get yourself back into shape. Apart from the health benefits of being trim, your self-esteem will improve and you are likely to feel more desirable. Losing weight can help improve hormone function in women in particular.
- You will also help your sex drive on its way by taking regular physical exercise. Ideally you need to do four or five good sessions of exercise per week to the point of breathlessness. Adequate exercise helps to elevate your mood and is likely to have a positive effect on your hormones and your energy levels.
- If you lead a busy life and have children to care for it is important to take time out with your partner from time to time. There is nothing like a few days away without any interruptions to rekindle the old flame.
- Watching a video together like *The Lover's Guide* or referring to a book specially prepared to help you improve your sex life, might bring back that old familiar, tingling feeling.
- Plus, you might well speed things along by taking specific nutritional supplements. We use a specially formulated multi-vitamin and mineral preparation, Optivite, which has been shown to help influence hormone levels positively and help women with PMS, and for older women the sister product, Gynovite. Extra supplements of zinc may be useful for those with a low intake.
- St John's Wort has been shown to be helpful for the treatment of libido problems. A German study of 111 menopausal women with libido problems showed that a twelve-week course of St John's Wort restored

libido levels in 60 per cent of the women and improved 80 per cent of psychological symptoms of depression, irritability, inner tension and anxiety associated with the menopause. The daily dose used in the study was 900 mcg. It would be advisable to start with 300mcg daily and then increase the dose accordingly.

- You might like to obtain a copy of Maryon's *Zest for Life Plan*, which will enable you to find the right kind of diet for your body and to lose those extra pounds.

Flagging libido does not signal 'the beginning of the end', it is simply your body's way of telling you that all is not well. Providing there is no underlying cause, self-help measures and patience will bring back the old sparkle! Patience is essential, as these recommendations are not a magic pill, you must expect to work at it over a period of several months.

Diane's story

Diane Preston was a 32-year-old mother of two. She and her husband had enjoyed their sex life until after the birth of their second child she suddenly went completely off sex and couldn't bear to be touched.

'I felt very guilty about losing interest in sex. I'd become very moody and depressed, and was irritated by any approaches made by my husband. I didn't even want to kiss and cuddle which was so unusual for me. He used to creep up behind me and kiss the back of my neck when I was cooking or washing up, and I'd always enjoyed it. Now if I thought he was approaching I'd quickly move out of the way, and if he put his arm around me I would shrug him off.

In bed I'd curl up and pretend to be asleep before he could make a move. When I first pushed him away he looked so hurt and asked if he had done anything to upset me. I just made excuses about being tired or busy as I couldn't face telling him the truth – that I'd gone off him. It was horrible because I knew I still loved him, but I felt I was betraying him by not wanting to make love to him anymore.

Once or twice I thought I would go through with it for his sake which was disastrous as my lack of response made him feel even more rejected. He eventually asked me if I wanted to separate. I tried to convince him that it was because my body felt switched off and not because of anything he had done. He was very supportive under the circumstances and suggested that when I felt ready for sex I should make the first move as he couldn't bear any further rejection.

By chance a couple of weeks later I read about a range of

symptoms which I knew I'd been suffering from – including loss of libido, depression and sore throats. I contacted the organisation mentioned which was the WNAS. I was advised to give up smoking and caffeine, sugar and salt. I didn't think I would manage without these vital lifelines, but I was so determined to succeed. I was also prescribed supplements of Optivite, zinc, vitamin C and Normoglycaemia to help with my cravings for food premenstrually, which was also a problem. I took regular exercise as well and within a few weeks I could feel my symptoms begin to lift. My moodiness vanished and one afternoon I suddenly realised that I wanted sex again.

My first thought was how to break the news to Jeff after so many months without sex. I felt scared of being rejected too. I resorted to the corny old candlelit supper, and over a bottle of wine hinted that I was 'in the mood'. At the end of the evening I said to Jeff, 'I think I'll go to bed now', and with a twinkle in his eye, he said, 'I think I'll join you'.

That night was a great success, and a terrific boost for Jeff's flagging confidence. I've had the occasional relapse, especially if we've been out to dinner with friends and I've binged on all the baddies I'm supposed to avoid. But mostly, our sex life is great – in actual fact it's even better than before! A while ago a friend commented that Jeff and I rarely go out. Jeff told her that was because we always go to bed early. She didn't get the message, so he spelled it out 'we go to bed early, but we're awake for hours . . .'

Complementary therapies

Herbal medicine would be our first choice once nutritional deficiencies have been corrected.

See also: What's wrong with present-day diet and lifestyle?, Nutrition is the key to health, Standard references and Recommended reading.

Liver Disease

There are a large variety of conditions that affect the liver, and they are the province of the hospital-based liver specialist. Some points are worth mentioning in a book of this sort, though. More will be heard of liver problems, as time passes, especially as some types become more commonplace and there is increasing recognition that some disorders of female sex hormones and related problems are due to liver conditions.

What causes it?

- *Viral hepatitis* There are several types of these viruses, termed hepatitis A, B, C, D, or E virus. The first and last cause an acute hepatitis with a flu-like illness and jaundice in some, though not all. The middle three can produce a chronic inflammation of the liver. They are spread through contact with saliva, by sexual intercourse, or from blood to blood transmission as in intravenous drug users. Worldwide there are several hundred million people infected with these viruses.
- *Excessive amounts of alcohol* The risk appears in those drinking more than four units per day. The duration of alcohol excess is a risk factor, and there also appears to be a genetic component too.
- *Exposure to many toxins* These include oil-derived and industrial chemicals, pesticides and many different drugs including anti-cancer preparations, some antibiotics, drugs used to treat psychiatric disorders, the oral contraceptive pill (rarely) and even regular high doses of paracetamol.
- *A wide variety of infections and inflammatory conditions* These include arthritis, colitis, and Crohn's disease. One particular type develops almost only in middle-aged women, and can accompany heavy periods, skin itching, malaise, and prominent blood vessels on the chest and neck.
- *Fatty liver* A relatively mild disturbance in liver function easily develops in some people who are overweight, diabetic or drink too much. If tackled early, then this is completely reversible.

What your doctor can do

Where liver disease is suspected, specialist treatment is essential.

- *Remove the cause* Most usually this means stopping a drug and avoiding alcohol.
- *Give drugs to control the inflammation* These include steroids and powerful immune-altering drugs.
- *Correct nutritional deficiencies* Just about every nutrient can become deficient, so early recognition and treatment are important. Older women may be especially at risk, so calcium and vitamin D may need to be given to prevent osteoporsis and bone softening. The metabolism of the B vitamins is easily disturbed, plus zinc deficiency and vitamin A deficiency are all possible.
- *Consider a liver transplant* Now becoming more commonplace and with a good degree of success. For many the alternative is death.

What you can do

This is really most relevant to those with mildly disturbed liver function which may have been detected on routine blood tests, those with early liver disease or the increasing number who will be found to be carriers of hepatitis C virus which is currently estimated to be many as one million people!

- Don't drink alcohol.
- Don't be overweight.
- Follow the recommendations for The Very Nutritious Diet (see page 437). Eating little and often may reduce the metabolic load of a meal upon the liver.
- Do not take drugs unnecessarily, and avoid illicit drugs.
- Take supplements of vitamin B complex as there are a few studies that have shown small improvements in liver function within the normal population. It is possible that, as most of the B vitamins are processed by the liver, this harmless approach could help some of those with a mild disturbance in liver function.
- Other supplements, especially vitamins C, E and beta-carotene which have tissue-protecting properties, may be needed depending upon the advice of your specialist. High doses of vitamins A and D are to be avoided.

Complementary therapies

Herbalism probably holds the most promise, but you should seek the advice of a qualified herbalist as some herbs are in fact toxic to the liver.

Angela's story

Angela was a plump, pleasant, retired 60-year-old woman. For many years she had been troubled by fatigue and a general malaise. An underactive thyroid had been diagnosed, but treatment for this had not helped entirely. Further investigation revealed that she had persistently abnormal tests of liver function. Specialist investigations had not revealed the cause and she had refused the liver biopsy test that she had been offered. Blood tests showed that the level of various liver-derived enzymes were two- to five-fold the preferred values. She was a non-drinker, but a little overweight at 73 kilos, and those tests that had been performed suggested that there was a degree of fatty infiltration in the liver.

Nutritional tests had shown that a number of nutrients were moderately low including zinc, magnesium, selenium, vitamin E and some of the essential fatty acids.

She took supplements of these together with vitamin B complex,

Biotin, Choline and Inositol. She began a weight reducing diet though this only resulted in her losing one or two kilos.

After a year her liver function tests had become nearly normal and there was some improvement in her fatigue.

It was not possible to know exactly which nutritional factors contributed to the improvement in her liver function tests. It was probably a combined effect.

Mastitis

Mastitis simply means inflammation, which usually comes about when some of the milk ducts deep in the breast become blocked and in some cases infected. You may suddenly notice a red patch on the breast, which is tender to the touch, and have a headache, and/or feel weak and feverish. This can all have an extremely rapid onset, and be very dramatic, with fevers soaring to 104°F (40°C).

What causes it?

- Often the blockage occurs in the lower portion of the right breast of right-handed women, as it is more difficult to latch a baby on to the nipple with the left hand. Very often, because of the sitting position, the base of the breast fails to empty.
- An ill-fitting bra that is too tight.
- Cracked, sore nipples allow bacteria from the baby's mouth to enter the milk ducts and multiply.

What your doctor can do

- Offer painkillers to help with the pain, which is sometimes very severe, and to bring the fever down.
- Prescribe antibiotics to combat the infection, especially if the fever becomes high.

Danielle's story

Danielle is a 32-year-old who has had four miscarriages between her two successful pregnancies, and worked on a voluntary basis as a breastfeeding counsellor.

'I was very keen on breastfeeding after attending National Childbirth Trust classes and got off to a very good start after the birth of our son. I had plenty of milk which let down well, but Alex didn't seem to empty my breasts properly. Consequently I became *susceptible to breast lumps – which repeatedly turned into mastitis. The first episode was very frightening as my fever went up suddenly to 104°F (40°C). I felt very disorientated and nervous. I wanted to avoid using antibiotics if at all possible and managed by using a combination of two homeopathic remedies Bella Donna and Phytolaca.*

I seemed to be particularly susceptible to mastitis whilst feeding our first child as it recurred on ten or eleven occasions. I did succumb to antibiotics on one occasion as I felt too ill to manage without them. In the main I used hot water pads before feeding and a pack of frozen peas after feeding. I spent lots of time massaging my breasts and having warm baths to keep the flow of milk going. I took some vitamins and minerals, in particular vitamin E which I understood would help to prevent further episodes of mastitis. I am so glad that I managed to continue breastfeeding Alex, despite the pain. It is such a precious time, I was determined not to let anything disrupt it.'

What you can do

- Keep feeding your baby, no matter how painful it may be, as emptying your breast will help to resolve the mastitis.
- Feed your baby with its body nestled under your arm and legs tucked behind you, as it may be easier to get the baby's jaws in the proper position.
- Offer the inflamed breast to your baby first, and make sure you empty it fully.
- Use a breast pump to fully empty the breast if necessary.
- Massage the sore parts of your breast with your fingers, encouraging the milk out of the ducts.
- Have plenty of hot baths, with hot flannels pressed directly on to the breast.
- Alternatively, place packs of frozen peas on the breast to reduce the inflammation.
- Try some gentle arm movements to keep the circulation flowing in the area.
- Take plenty of rest in between feeds, you will need all your strength.
- Use a homeopathic remedy, either Lachesis or Belladonna, every few hours until the inflammation and the fever subside.
- Remember that painkillers and antibiotics are there if you need them. If the breast becomes infected, and you feel really unwell, you owe it to yourself and your baby to speed the recovery. Neither the painkillers nor the antibiotics will harm your baby, and neither will the milk from an infected breast.

Some women never experience mastitis, whilst others seem to get it repeatedly, despite taking precautions. Do persist. Your baby gets a far greater start in life by being breast-fed.

See also: Breast problems, Recommended reading (*Healthy Parents, Healthy Baby*).

The Menopause

For at least three-quarters of all women, the menopause brings with it rapid changes and unwanted symptoms which often disrupt life and result in utter misery. Frequent hot flushes during the day, and sweats at night leave them exhausted, disoriented and despondent. A dry vagina and reduced libido can wreck their sex lives, and repeated insomnia can leave a woman wondering whether life as they knew it is over.

The menopause is a transition which signals the end of a woman's monthly fertility cycle, and in order to have a smooth passage through it, our bodies need to be in really good shape.

What is the menopause?

The menopause itself is merely the day menstruation stops, which one can only usually be certain about with hindsight. Therefore many women will experience the actual menopause without really knowing at the time. Most of the symptoms experienced occur whilst in the perimenopausal stage, which means *around the time* of the menopause.

After the age of 40, the supply of eggs starts to run out, and the level of the female hormone oestrogen starts to fall. The dwindling number of eggs then mature irregularly, so that as the menopause approaches, the length of the menstrual cycles start to vary and periods become irregular.

Periods cease when eggs run out. As oestrogen levels fall, the lining of the womb loses its main source of stimulation, and periods stop altogether. The majority of women will have their last natural period somewhere between the ages of 45 and 55, with the average standing at just over 50. In rarer cases women start an early menopause in their late 20s or early 30s, and sometimes women go on having periods until they are in their late 50s. However, statistics do show that smokers may reach the menopause as much as two years earlier than non-smokers.

What are the symptoms?

From a survey of 500 women who had recently gone through their menopause, we at the WNAS discovered that there were three main groups of symptoms that occur at the time of the menopause, but only one group is directly related to the falling oestrogen levels. The other two groups of symptoms that we discovered, were more to do with dietary and lifestyle inadequacies.

Oestrogen withdrawal symptoms

These are are predominantly:

- hot flushes
- night sweats
- vaginal dryness
- loss of libido
- urinary symptoms
- skin changes
- difficulties with intercourse

Physical symptoms

These consisted primarily of:

- aches and pains
- irritable bowel syndrome
- constipation
- fatigue
- migraines and headaches

Mental symptoms

These included:

- anxiety
- panic attacks
- palpitations
- irritability
- aggressive feelings
- mood swings
- depression and confusion

All of the symptoms listed are commonly experienced. What is not widely appreciated however, is that HRT is aiming only at the oestrogen withdrawal group, and not necessarily the physical and the mental groups of symptoms.

We know from research conducted on several groups of younger women suffering with premenstrual syndrome that minerals like magnesium, iron and the B vitamins are often in short supply, which affects the efficiency of brain chemistry and hormone function. The menopause is a great transition, which places extra demands on brain chemistry. If the body is not 'firing on all cylinders' because of previous dietary inadequacies and lack of education, a bumpy ride can be expected. It is thought that approximately 75 per cent of women in the western world will experience adverse symptoms at the time of the menopause.

What your doctor can do

The favoured treatment for menopausal women is Hormone Replacement Therapy, HRT. Oestrogen therapy was initially pioneered in the USA. Oestrogens alone were used for the first twenty years, but then it was discovered that women with an intact uterus had a greatly increased risk of cancer of the lining of the uterus, and so progesterone was added to make it safer.

Guiding principles on the use of HRT

These are intended to help the patient (and doctor) understand the appropriateness of HRT for her particular situation.

- There are many different forms of HRT. Tablets, of varying type, patches, gels, and implant preparations all come with a choice of dose and can be provided in different combinations of oestrogen and progesterone. All are effective at controlling immediate symptoms and most are proven to have beneficial effects upon bone health. The wide choice means that there is considerable flexibility and gives the doctor many alternatives if one preparation is not well tolerated. Women with a uterus will need to take progesterone for twelve to fourteen days per month to prevent endometrial overgrowth and cancer developing. This applies also to those women receiving vaginal oestrogen preparations for more than three months.
- HRT brings both short- and long-term benefits. In addition to the control of menopausal symptoms HRT reduces the risk of osteoporotic fracture and *may* bring other benefits including a reduction in the risk of heart disease and dementia, but this is by no means certain at present. Large detailed trials to answer these and other questions are underway in Europe and the USA. The results will not be available for nearly ten years.
- HRT use can bring both short- and long-term health problems. Common initial side effects include breast tenderness, aggravation of pre-existing breast disease, mood changes and in those receiving cyclical progesterone, cyclical mood changes akin to premenstrual syndrome, headaches and irregular vaginal bleeding. These problems are of course similar to those experienced with the oral contraceptive pill. They may become tolerable, diminish with time or can be controlled by a change in dose or preparation. The longer term side-effects are more serious and include an increase in the risk of breast cancer and thrombosis.
- To some degree the increased risks of breast cancer and thrombosis are predictable. The increase in breast cancer is between ten and twenty per cent after ten years continuous use with very little increase in the first five years. Furthermore five years after ceasing treatment the risk returns to that of non-users. The increased risk of thrombosis may become apparent after just a few weeks of HRT use and results in the risk of one in 10,000 per year for a non-HRT user rising to three in 10,000. Occasionally this may lead to blood clot on the lung which in

one to two per cent of cases can be fatal. The risk of thrombosis rises significantly with the higher dose preparations, particularly if the woman is overweight, a smoker or has had a thrombosis in the past.

- Some conditions call for additional attention on the part of the doctor. There are a number of situations where HRT is not prohibited but special care needs to be taken either because there is an increased risk of thrombosis developing, or because the condition may worsen as a result of HRT. In the former category are: being very overweight (Body Mass Index greater than 30) or being immobilised, especially if the woman is also a smoker, and following major trauma or surgery. In the latter category are a wide variety of conditions including: uterine fibroids, mild chronic liver disease (blood tests to monitor liver function every eight to twelve weeks), gallstones, otosclerosis (hormone dependent hearing loss), migraine, multiple sclerosis, epilepsy, diabetes, high blood pressure, kidney disease, uterine fibroids, the rare metabolic condition porphyria, and tetany.

- For the control of menopausal symptoms most women will need treatment for between one and five years. The majority of patients will be between 40 and mid-50s with younger patients typically having more severe symptoms often requiring a higher dose of HRT and for longer. Stopping treatment after a maximum of five years will minimise the increase in the risk of breast cancer and thrombosis and by this time many symptoms will have lessened. Younger patients with a premature menopause, before the age of 45 years, may well need or wish to take it for longer. However as a rule it would seem inappropriate to continue HRT past the age of 55 years unless a women is known to have or are at high risk of developing osteoporosis, and even then, there now exists alternative approaches as you will see from page 345.

- For the treatment of established osteoporosis and its prevention the treatment will be needed for between five and ten years. The majority of such patients will be elderly and five years is probably the minimum time period needed to achieve a reasonable effect. Going beyond ten years may either not be necessary or may add to the risk of breast cancer and thrombosis with little additional benefit in terms of bone protection.

- The benefits of HRT are not unique to HRT. There are alternatives to HRT of a pharmaceutical and non-pharmaceutical nature. Hot flushes can be helped by a low dose of the drug Clonidine, by relaxation techniques and dietary change including the consumption of certain foods or preparations containing phytoestrogens which in part perform some of the functions of HRT, see page 480. Osteoporosis can be treated by other drugs, calcium with additional vitamin D for the elderly and helped by regular exercise. Furthermore regular exercise and a healthy diet will almost certainly protect against both osteoporosis and heart disease to at least the same extent as HRT and bring with it many additional benefits, see pages 233 and 345. If a doctor is prescribing HRT for its long-term preventative benefits then he or she should also be advising about other ways to minimise the development of both osteoporosis and heart disease.

- Certain situations call for the immediate cessation of HRT. This is needed if there is:
  - ○ a thrombosis, a blood clot, in any part of the body: leg, lung, brain or heart or if there is an injury which is likely to result in a thrombosis.
  - ○ severe migraine headaches developing for the first time or any other frequent or severe headaches especially if they are associated with visual disturbance or the development of symptoms such as numbness or tingling in a part of the body.
  - ○ the development of jaundice, high blood pressure or pregnancy. These are all other reasons to stop HRT without delay.
  - ○ HRT should also be stopped six weeks before any operation or if there is prolonged immobilisation.
- Abrupt cessation of HRT can cause a marked return in symptoms. Research shows that women who come off HRT suddenly often experience severe hot flushing. The return of hot flushes and night sweats when HRT is stopped abruptly is not 'proof' of oestrogen deficiency but merely testimony to the intolerance of many women's bodies to sudden and substantial hormonal change. Gradually reducing the dose may produce fewer symptoms and may need to be done for many women coming off HRT in their early to mid-50s. Some of these women may return to HRT a decade or two later for the treatment/prevention of their osteoporosis.
- The duration of HRT treatment often cannot be decided until after an initial test phase. Only after several months of trying HRT can the full balance between risks and benefits for the individual be made especially if it has been necessary to adjust the dose or type of HRT to control initial, adverse symptoms. This means that each woman should be advised when initially commencing on treatment that they are not necessarily committing themselves to long-term treatment but actually undertaking a therapeutic trial. At the end of the first few months or year of treatment there can then be a more detailed assessment of the appropriateness of continuing with HRT in the medium to long term.

Assessing the appropriateness of HRT

Having absorbed these guiding principles we can now make some kind of a planned approach to assessing the appropriateness of HRT for an individual woman. A lot of the following factors will need to be considered, albeit briefly, but in the logical sequence that is presented here. Each case should be considered as a therapeutic trial unique to that individual. Assessing these factors carefully and explaining them to the patient will often take more time than a typical short consultation with the family doctor will allow.

The initial assessment will include blood tests to diagnose the menopause. The tests at the GP's disposal, to confirm a diagnosis of 'menopausal' are as follows:

- FSH and LH. These are tests of pituitary function and will be elevated as the pituitary gland works hard to try and stimulate the failing ovary. In perimenopausal women these levels rise before the oestrogen level falls.
- Oestradiol. This is the main type of oestrogen in the body and levels will fall at the time of the menopause. A low normal level, in conjunction with elevations of FSH/LH are found in perimenopausal women.
- Other tests. Most commonly these will include blood tests of thyroid function and anaemia especially if some other health problem is also suspected. Other tests will rarely be needed.

Should the woman be given an initial trial of HRT? This should be considered:

- If there are symptoms of *hot flushes, night sweats* or *vaginal dryness*. These are archetypal symptoms of oestrogen withdrawal. Other symptoms such as depression, low libido and muscular aches and pains have many other causes and by themselves are not a good guide as to the suitability of HRT.
- If there is a high risk of developing osteoporosis especially if combined with an early menopause.
- If there are no major contraindications to HRT or if there is a relative contraindication to HRT, but the client is willing to accept the associated increased risks.
- If the individual is psychologically prepared to take HRT. This means that she has not been scared off by stories that she has heard or read and is willing to accept the use of a physiological replacement initially for a short-term trial. Importantly there should be no pressure for her to agree to take it on a long-term basis until she has seen how she gets on with it in the short term.

Major contraindications to HRT

There are some women who should not even attempt to try HRT. This is because they have a pre-existing condition that is likely to be worsened by HRT or they have a history of marked intolerance of oestrogen preparations.

The contraindications listed below are taken from standard texts including the prescribing handbook *MIMS* (The Monthly Index of Medical Specialities) which sits at the elbow of most consulting doctors, and from the relevant reference texts.

- **Pre-existing breast cancer.** The growth of breast cancer is usually hormone dependent especially in young women, and HRT would conflict with treatment for the cancer, especially with the oestrogen modulating drug Tamoxifen.
- **Pre-existing uterine, ovarian, or cervical cancer.** Again these are hormone-dependant cancers and HRT should not be given.
- **Undiagnosed vaginal bleeding.** This could be due to cancer of the genital tract. Heavy or erratic bleeding or bleeding after intercourse should arouse suspicion.
- **Endometriosis.** When the endometrial lining has extended outside the womb there is usually considerable abdominal pain with menstruation and typically a day before the onset of bleeding. Abdominal pain and swelling are likely to worsen with HRT.
- **Previous thrombosis when taking oestrogen.** Oestrogen causes an increase in blood clotting factors which in a few individuals will lead to a blood clot developing in a vein, a venous thrombosis, which will cause a swollen and usually painful leg. However sometimes this process is silent until a clot breaks off and travels to the lung causing a pulmonary embolus. If large, this may occasionally be fatal. Smaller ones will usually cause, chest pain, shortness of breath and a cough often resulting in blood stained sputum. Multiple small pulmonary emboli, if unrecognised, can damage the lung and heart. The risk of thrombosis rises with increasing age, obesity, smoking, immobility, recent trauma or surgery, and any of several otherwise silent blood conditions that predispose to blood clotting. These may only be suspected because of a previous personal history of thrombosis especially in association with the oral contraceptive pill or HRT, or because a first degree relative has suffered a thrombosis spontaneously or when taking an oestrogen preparation. Rarely such individuals may have experienced a stroke or stroke-like episode when on the oral contraceptive pill. Sophisticated and expensive blood tests exist to detect the different forms of thrombophilia as these blood conditions are known. However they are not widely or always easily available, which is a situation that will have to change in the future.
- **Active thrombosis or embolism.** For the same reasons.
- **Severe migraine or visual disturbance when taking the oral contraceptive pill.** These symptoms could mean an impending stroke linked to increased risk of thrombosis when taking the pill.
- **Severe heart, kidney or liver disease.** HRT can aggravate the fluid retention that occurs with these conditions.

- **Some liver diseases.** These may alter the metabolism of oestrogen.
- **Pregnancy or lactation.** Not all older women have ceased menstruating because of the menopause. It is prudent to enquire whether they might become or be pregnant!
- **Likely to have an operation within the next six weeks.** An operation increases the risk of thrombosis and whenever possible HRT should not be taken during this time.

Relative contraindications to HRT

The majority of these conditions will usually have been previously diagnosed in the individual because of some prior episode of ill-health. They include:

- **Uterine fibroids** which could cause heavier bleeding as a result of HRT use.
- **Mild chronic liver disease.** Further monitoring of liver function tests will be needed every eight to twelve weeks.
- **Gallstones.**
- **Porphyria,** a rare metabolic condition that alters liver metabolism.
- **Otosclerosis** – deafness in pregnancy or in association with the oral contraceptive pill.
- **Hypertension.** Rarely this may be made worse by HRT but is usually unaffected.
- **Migraine** which again may be made worse by HRT.
- **Epilepsy** might be made worse by HRT and some anti-epileptic drugs will increase the required HRT dose.
- **Multiple sclerosis** may very rarely be worsened by HRT.
- **Diabetes.** There may be minor changes in blood sugar control following treatment with HRT.
- **Renal impairment,** as HRT might aggravate fluid retention
- **Premenstrual syndrome** either currently or in the past may mean that the woman will be prone to cyclical mood changes when taking HRT. This is quite variable and not easily predictable, but it is thought that one third of women who try HRT can expect to experience premenstrual symptoms.
- **Breast cysts or pain** may worsen with HRT. All such women should be examined before commencing treatment and if the diagnosis is in doubt be sent for mammography.
- **A strong family history of breast cancer.** The increased risk of breast cancer developing following the use of HRT is small, especially when it is only taken for a short period of time, but not insignificant. In women with a strong family history of this cancer careful and sympathetic discussion is often required, and alternative approaches may well be preferred.

Most of these points can be quickly assessed by your own family doctor. The most tricky one is when there is a personal or family history of thrombosis, as at present there are no clear guidelines as to how to assess the risk in individual cases.

Medical survey on the menopause

A recent survey of a thousand general practitioners was carried out in an attempt to assess the help that is currently available for menopausal women. The questions focused on HRT, the frequency of use, side effects experienced by patients and their knowledge and incorporation of alternative treatments for the menopause. The survey revealed some interesting and surprising statistics, which are detailed below.

Analysis of the survey revealed that 36 per cent of all women who seek help for the menopause are prescribed HRT. However, 54 per cent of those recommended to take it actually do, and 46 per cent don't, which would indicate a degree of dissatisfaction with the treatment! In fact, according to GPs, 21 per cent of women taking HRT actually come off of it within a year of commencing, so overall, less than 50 per cent of the women who were advised to take HRT are still taking it.

We were particularly surprised that doctors were divided over issues like inactive breast cancer and family history of thrombosis. We were also amazed that so few were concerned about prescribing HRT to women with high blood pressure.

Clearly there is a lack of education about the effectiveness of HRT in preventing heart disease and alzheimers. Whilst there is some evidence to support the theory that HRT helps to prevent heart disease, the jury is still out. In fact, at the 3rd International Symposium on the Role of Soy in Preventing and Treating Chronic Disease (1999), it was broadly agreed that the research on phytoestrogens preventing heart disease was much stronger than the research on HRT and heart disease. As for alzheimers, the research is yet young. There was also a great variation in the number of doctors who use HRT to treat fatigue and depression.

When questioned as to the side effects attributable to prescribing HRT:

- 85 per cent of patients suffered with breast tenderness.
- 72 per cent put on unwanted weight.
- 39 per cent experienced mood swings.
- 21 per cent of patients were affected by depression.

On a more serious note, HRT caused a rise in blood pressure in 17 per cent, six per cent lost hair from their head and six per cent had thrombosis.

It was interesting and enlightening to learn that the doctors who participated in the survey were knowledgeable of, and even incorporated natural treatments for the menopause. The more conventional treatments like Dixarit, a drug to alleviate hot flushes appeared to be as little as 27 per cent effective. Advising their patients to reduce caffeine, alcohol and smoking were nigh on as effective for reducing flushes.

It was quite amazing to see that as many as 17 per cent of doctors were recommending a soya rich diet, 18 per cent advised taking a phyto-estrogen rich diet, which compared favourably with prescribing vitamin supplements and referral for psychotherapy, recommended by only eight per cent of doctors.

Since we carried out our first GP survey in 1994, it would be fair to say that knowledge of complementary therapies for treating menopausal symptoms is increasing, perhaps not significantly, but at least the trend is moving in the right direction.

Phytoestrogens and the menopause

Much more exciting research has since been conducted on the effects of phytoestrogens to the point where it has been discovered that they have certain similarities to the 'designer hormones' – the Selective Oestrogen Receptor Modulators (SERMS). This group of hormones are being developed to retain their beneficial effects on the cardiovascular system and the skeleton, without having cancer promoting effects on the breasts or the lining of the womb. However, unlike phytoestrogens which help to relieve hot flushes, the down side with the SERMS is that they seem to *cause* hot flushes.

A study on phytoestrogens and the menopause, conducted by researchers at the University of South Manchester, England, also found positive results. They fed menopausal women a 60 gram soya protein drink daily for two months, and were able to reduce hot flushes by half, and the remaining flushes were 30 per cent less severe. Another soya protein experiment was set up by Professor Burke, of the department of public health science at the Bowman Gray School of Medicine, Winston-Salem, North Carolina. He fed 43 American women, aged between 45 and 55, 20 grams of soya protein, sprinkled over their morning cereal, for six weeks. They found that symptoms significantly reduced, although they did not entirely disappear. As a result they have a larger ongoing study, who are being given much higher doses of soy.

In 1998 Dr Albertuzzi confirmed the value of soya protein in helping to control hot flushes. His study of 104 post-menopausal women, who took either 72 mg of isoflavones or a placebo, each day for twelve weeks, showed that soy was significantly superior in reducing the number of hot flushes experienced. Women taking soy decreased their hot flushes by 26 per cent after three weeks, 33 per cent by week four, and 45 per cent by week twelve, compared with a 30 per cent reduction in the hot flushes of women in the placebo group.

A few years ago, an Australian study of menopausal women consuming bread rich in both soya and linseeds, showed a 40 per cent reduction in hot flushes and a small increase in bone mass. This preliminary research indicates that these phytoestrogens may well be as powerful as HRT, not just in their effect on vaginal tissue, but also in protecting us against both osteoporosis and heart disease.

There is a whole array of phytoestrogenic foods on the market claiming to alleviate menopausal symptoms while reducing the risk of breast cancer and heart disease. However we need to be discerning, as many foods may well contain phytoestrogen rich ingredients in principle, but it is very difficult to standardise food, as became apparent to me after becoming familiar with the results of a survey conducted by Novogen in Australia. They analysed a long list of common phytoestrogen-rich foods including soya products, chickpeas, lentils, and found a terrific variation of phytoestrogen content. Amazingly some of the tested foods contained very little phytoestrogens indeed.

The phytoestrogen content of food may vary considerably depending on the crop, the time of year it was grown, the climate, and a number of environmental factors. Foods that have been put through scientific analysis will state the phytoestrogen content on the label, so once again it is down to label reading.

It seems that Mother Nature has provided us with foods that allow us to top up on our oestrogen levels, at the time of the menopause and beyond, quite naturally, without having to resort to Hormone Replacement Therapy. The only problem I have encountered, it that women are generally unaware of which foods contain phytoestrogens, and as a result our intake in western countries are negligible, compared to Asian women who consume between 50–100 grams of phytoestrogen or phytoestrogen-containing food per day.

So far research does tell us about many of the foods that contain plant oestrogens and other important phytochemicals. Although we are beginning to know about the precise quantities of isoflavones and lignans is some of the foods, we have yet to determine the precise values of other foods. Whilst it seemed to be the general consensus of opinion of researchers presenting new data at the 3rd International Symposium on The Role of Soy in Preventing and Treating Chronic Disease, that soya in our diet is only likely to decrease hot flushes by 30 per cent, our experience is that when combined with other aspects of the WNAS menopause programme, it is a valuable part of a highly effective, natural alternative to taking HRT, which aids the control of hot flushes in a relatively short time period.

What you can do

There is a great deal that you can do to ensure a smooth passage through the menopause, and to prevent heart disease and the bone-thinning disease, osteoporosis, without taking HRT. The recommendations that we use at the WNAS are all based on published scientific papers.

If you are aiming to overcome severe and debilitating symptoms at the time of the menopause it is likely, in our experience, that you will need to consume at least 100 mg of isoflavones per day initially, combined with the other important aspects of the WNAS programme. This will enable you to emulate the Japanese in their consumption of daily phyto-estrogens, but in a western way.

- A group of Australian workers published a paper in the *British Medical Journal*, which showed that a group of women going through the menopause, regularly consuming foods and drinks that contained naturally occurring oestrogens, were able to bring about the same positive changes in the lining of the vagina, as women taking HRT.
- Practising relaxation techniques each day can reduce your hot flushes by as much as 60 per cent.
- Taking supplements of calcium, EFAs and marine fish oils, can reduce the amount of calcium lost through the urine, increase the amount of calcium absorbed through the gut wall, and improve the calcium balance in the bones.
- Taking regular low-impact aerobic exercise, like brisk walking, skipping, racquet sports or working out, is good protection against both heart disease and osteoporosis.

Dietary recommendations

It is well established that Japanese women, who already eat a diet particularly rich in plant oestrogen, have far fewer problems at the time of the menopause, demonstrating once again that there is a lot we can do for ourselves.

1. Include the plant oestrogens in your diet, particularly soya products including soya milk with cereals or mixed with fruit as a fruit shake, tofu & silken tofu blended with fruit, Linusit Gold, golden linseeds, chick peas, lentils, mung beans, alfalfa, sunflower, pumpkin and sesame seeds and green and yellow vegetables. Refer to *The Phyto Factor* by Maryon Stewart for further food lists, recipes and details of how to use these products (see Recommended reading, page 490).
2. Apart from a phytoestrogen-rich breakfast, have a 'fix' later in the day, either as a snack or as a dessert. Try a phyto fruit shake, or a fruit whip made with silken tofu and soft fruit in the blender.
3. Reduce your intake of sugar and junk foods. This includes sugar added to tea and coffee, and that in sweets, cakes, biscuits, chocolate,

jam, puddings, marmalades, soft drinks containing phosphates, ice cream and honey. Consumption of these may impede the uptake of essential nutrients and may cause water retention.

4. Reduce your intake of salt, both added to cooking and at the table. Also avoid salted foods like kippers and bacon. Salt causes fluid retention and induces calcium loss from the body in the urine. Use potassium-rich salt substitutes such as garlic, onion, kelp powder, fresh herbs, sesame powder or other mild spices.

5. Over-spicy food, hot drinks and alcohol can aggravate flushes. Let your hot drinks cool down and keep alcohol to a minimum whilst going through the menopause. Alcohol tends to knock most nutrients sideways anyway, and this is definitely a time to conserve essential nutrients.

6. Eat vegetables and salads daily. Three portions of vegetables and a salad should be eaten every day, as they contain plenty of essential nutrients. Where possible use organic, or grow your own.

7. Eat plenty of fresh fruit, at least two servings each day, as these are good sources of nutrients.

8. Concentrate on consuming foods that are rich in important nutrients, especially magnesium, calcium, B vitamins, essential fatty acids and zinc. You will need to refer to the section called The Nutritional Content of Foods that begins on page 483.

9. Limit your consumption of red meat to one or two portions each week. Substitute meat with fish, poultry, peas, beans and nuts. You may like to refer to the Vegetarian, or Tunatarian diets on pages 455, when you learn that meat eaters have a lower bone density than their vegetarian counterparts.

10. Dairy products, such as milk and cheese, are excellent sources of calcium. Use low-fat versions if you need to watch your weight. Aim to drink 600ml (1 pint) of milk per day, or other foods rich in calcium, see page 487.

11. Keep your consumption of animal fat down to 30 per cent of your total calorie intake. For most, this means reducing fat intake by at least one-quarter. Instead use cold-pressed oils such as safflower, sunflower, olive, sesame, rapeseed etc, and use soft polyunsaturated spreads instead of hard margarines or lard.

12. Drink plenty of liquids, preferably the equivalent of six glasses of water daily. Use decaffeinated drinks, or better still alternatives, see page 6, and keep carbonated drinks down to a minimum.

13. If you smoke, try to cut down gradually, or stop completely, as smoking can aggravate some symptoms, especially hot flushes and night sweats. Stopping smoking at the time of the menopause can reduce your risk of hip fracture by as much as 40 per cent.

14. Keep a supply of nutritious snacks to eat in-between meals if you get peckish. Nuts, raisins and fresh or dried fruit are fine.

Other useful self-help tips

- Aim to exercise for at least half an hour five times per week – you need to do weight-bearing exercise that is also aerobic. The benefits are a healthy heart, strong bones and a feeling of well-being (see page 32).
- Try to spend 15–20 minutes relaxing each day to keep the stress levels down and the flushes at bay. Research shows that these simple measures will reduce hot flushes by as much as 60 per cent. See also page 29.
- Wear several layers of thin comfortable clothing during the day so that you can peel them off should the need arise.
- Use lightweight layers of bedclothes so that you can adjust them according to temperature. Wear cotton nightclothes instead of man-made fibres.
- Carry some cool wipes in your handbag until the flushes have abated.
- Take extra care of your hair, skin and nails. Use rich hair conditioner, good moisturising lotions for your skin and nail strengtheners.
- Do toning pelvic-floor exercises once or twice a day by repeatedly holding in the vaginal muscles to the count of ten and releasing slowly.

The value of supplements

At the time of the menopause we often have to put back nutrients that time and nature have taken out. In addition we aim to restore oestrogen levels, through diet and standardised supplements initially, in order to alleviate the hot flushes and night sweats as soon as possible. At the WNAS we successfully use a selection of scientifically based supplements which individually address the variety of common symptoms. The following chart will allow you to assess which supplements you should be trying according to your current symptoms. We usually aim at sorting out the short-term oestrogen withdrawal symptoms initially, and once these are under control move on to address the long-term business of maintaining a healthy heart and strong bones.

Phytoestrogen-rich supplement

A recent US study has validated the effectiveness and safety of Novogen red clover. The study, conducted by Tufts University School of Medicine and New York University School of Medicine, showed that menopausal women who took a single tablet of redclover daily experienced a reduction in the intensity and number of hot flushes. Hot flushes were reduced by 56 per cent (from 8.1 per day to 3.6 per day) after eight weeks. Intensity of hot flushes also decreased by 56 per cent, and night sweats decreased in intensity by 52 per cent. Hot flushes and night sweats are the two most common symptoms in menopausal women. The other good news was that red clover did not cause thickening of the endometrial lining, which is a complication commonly associated with HRT. The women in the study also reported no side effects or weight gain from taking the red clover.

We have now been using Novogen red clover as part of the WNAS menopause programme for the last two years. Within the first few months of experimenting with the product, as we did by giving samples to our patients to try, we discovered that the hot flushes and the night sweats were being controlled much more quickly. It used to take us at least three or four months to control hot flushes prior to using the red clover supplement. Patients began returning for their follow-up appointment, just one month after their initial consultation, delighted that both their flushes and night sweats were far milder. This was excellent news to the WNAS team, as well as the patients themselves who are more than just slightly keen to be restored to normality as soon as possible.

Matching Nutritional Supplements to Symptom

Problem	Type of supplement	Daily dosage	Available from
Hot flushes and nightsweats	*Novogen red clover	1 x 45 mg tablet	WNAS Mail Order Service
	*Natural vitamin E	200–400 IU	Chemists, health-food shops and WNAS Mail Order Service
	*Panax ginseng	1–2 x 600 mg capsules	Chemists, health-food shops and WNAS Mail Order Service
Anxiety, irritability, mood swings, depression	*Gynovite	2–4 tablets	Health-food shops and WNAS Mail Order Service
Eczema, dry skin	*Efamol	1 x 10000 mg capsules	Chemists and WNAS Mail Order Service
Heavy periods	*Gynovite	Dose as above	WNAS Mail Order Service
	Iron-ferrous sulphate	1 x 200 mg tablet with fruit juice	Chemists
Painful periods	*Magnesium amino acid chelate	2–4 x 150 mg tablets	Health-food shops and WNAS Mail Order Service
Breast tenderness	*Efamol/Efamast	As above	Chemists, health-food shops and WNAS Mail Order Service
	Linusit Gold	2 tablespoons	Health-food shops
Osteoporosis	*Efacal	4 capsules	Chemists, health-food shops and WNAS Mail Order Service
	Calcium carbonate, gluconate or citrate	1000 mg elemental calcium	Chemists and health-food shops
	*Magnesium amino acid chelate 1	50–600 mg elemental magnesium	Health-food shops and WNAS Mail Order Service

*Available by mail order through WNAS Mail Order Service, PO Box 268, Lewes, East Sussex, BN7 1QN or visit our website on http://www.wnas.org.uk

Complementary therapies

As well as dealing with symptoms on a nutritional level it is important to address the underlying problems that may well have accumulated over the years. Not meeting your nutritional needs at various stages in life, being pregnant and breast-feeding, coping with stressful situations and perhaps suffering premenstrual symptoms before your menopause, may well have left their mark. Your body may need some extra help in order to recover at the time of the menopause, which can be provided by some of the complementary therapies.

Acupuncture and acupressure

Many problems that occur at the time of the menopause, like hot flushes, night sweats, insomnia, depression, aches and pains, mood swings and headaches, may well respond to acupuncture or acupressure. Acupuncture will need to be administered by a qualified practitioner, and acupressure can be a useful self-help tool. The Council for Acupuncture lists all qualified members (see page 513).

Herbal medicine

The indication for herbal medicine at the time of the menopause is quite strong. Trials have demonstrated that herbs can help to reduce hot flushes, reverse the ageing process of the cells in the lining of the vagina, and speed up the healing process of broken bones. There are herbal preparations that can be purchased in the health-food shop like ginseng, dong quai and agnus castus, with which you can help yourself. However, a qualified herbal practitioner may prescribe a combination of many different herbs. You may even be given herbs that are to be taken at different times of the day, or even different times of the month depending on whether you are perimenopausal or postmenopausal.

Homeopathy

Sepia and sulphur are just two of the many remedies that may be indicated for hot flushes and nightsweats. There is also a wide choice of remedies for poor memory, depression, insomnia, anxiety attacks, irritability, headaches and confusion. To find a qualified practitioner in your area contact The British Homeopathic Association, whose address is listed on page 513. *The Women's Guide to Homeopathy* is an excellent reference book, and details can be found on page 491.

Cranial osteopathy

It is certainly worth paying a visit to a qualified cranial osteopath at the time of the menopause. Not only do they provide help for long-standing back, head and neck problems, but they have been shown to reduce hot flushes. The treatment for women suffering with menopausal symptoms is often aimed at improving pituitary function, the gland found at the base of the brain, and balancing the function of the adrenal glands and the pelvis.

The European School of Osteopathy have a directory of qualified practitioners. You will find their address on page 515.

Creative visualisation

This is a wonderfully simple and most enjoyable method of relaxation, that requires little or no training. It is perfect for those who haven't had the time to learn how to practice yoga or meditation. See page 31 for details.

Shiatsu

Shiatsu is a form of ancient Japanese massage developed in the late nineteenth century, which translates as 'finger pressure'. Although influenced by western medicine, it has its basis in Traditional Chinese Medicine and follows the same principles of energy and meridians as acupressure. The practitioner uses fingers, thumbs, elbows, knees and even feet in a combination of massage techniques, applying pressure to key points to influence and stimulate energy flow in the body. Shiatsu has become very popular in the west, where it is practised both by trained practitioners and as a self-treatment for minor ailments. It is particularly useful for treating musculo-skeletal problems such as arthritis, stress, fatigue and circulatory problems which are often exacerbated during the menopause.

T'ai chi

T'ai chi is a Chinese movement therapy practised by Taoist monks in the thirteenth century, but its exact origins are difficult to trace. Derived from the words for 'great', 'ultimate' and 'fist', t'ai chi can be translated as 'supreme ultimate power'. This therapy was suppressed during the Cultural Revolution (1966–69), but it has since been promoted by the Chinese government as a form of preventive health care. In the West it is now one of the most popular movement therapies of all ages. The key principles of t'ai chi aim to ensure the smooth flow of 'life energy' through the body's meridians. It is recommended therapy for conditions of old age, improving vitality, enhancing mental and physical control and generally promoting optimum health.

Nicola's story

Nicola was a 46-year-old mother of two and part-time conference organiser. She read about the WNAS in a national newspaper and contacted us as she was looking for an alternative to HRT because of the horrendous side effects she had had from it.

'At the age of 44, a blood test showed early menopause. I tried HRT but within days was experiencing panic attacks, depression, feeling totally out of control and suicidal. Within one week I had stopped the HRT and it took me several months to regain my composure. Apart from this, I was suffering from hot and cold flushes, night sweats, headaches, abdominal bloating, constipation, general aches and pains, and continued depression.

At my initial clinic consultation with Maryon Stewart I was given recommendations with regard to my diet and supplements to take. I began the nutritional diet by avoiding wheat and bran, changing ordinary tea to the Rooibosch tea and adding things like oily fish and phytoestrogen-rich foods and herbs. I was advised to take various supplements to boost my vitamin and mineral levels and help reduce my symptoms.

One month later I saw Maryon again at her clinic and was able to say that I generally had more energy and was more positive. My symptoms were reducing and I was satisfied with the nutritional diet.

I travel frequently with my job, staying in hotels but manage quite well to stick to the recommendations. Four months down the line and I am getting on very very well. I feel better mentally, more in control and much more positive. I am relaxing more now and will look into having some massage. My fatigue and irritability have gone, I am sleeping much better, my flushes are very infrequent and constipation is a thing of the past. A bonus throughout the programme at the WNAS is that my weight has dropped to a comfortable level for me at 55 kilos. I am very pleased with myself and people have noticed a more rational person in their midst.'

See also: Osteoporosis, Sample WNAS programmes for normal menopause, early menopause, Prevent osteoporosis, sample high calcium diet, References and Recommended reading (Cruising Through the Menopause, Your Health in Your Hands – The WNAS Guide to Better Bones, The Phyto Factor).

Migraine Headaches

Migraine headaches are a common problem in both adults and children, and are often related to hormonal events like puberty, the onset of a period or the menopause. Migraines can be distinguished from other headaches because they are characterised by a severe, intermittent ache which is often accompanied by a variety of symptoms including nausea, vomiting, disturbance of vision, flashing lights, and other strange feelings, all of which may occur either before or at the start of a headache. Intolerance to light and noise are also common features of a migraine. The attacks can last anything from several hours to two to three days.

As many sufferers know, once an attack has begun, it is virtually impossible to stop it running its course. This is now thought to be due to a series of chemical or electrical changes that occur in the blood vessels of the head and the brain. It seems that there is a strong physical or chemical basis to many sufferers' migraine headaches, which may be triggered by a variety of factors.

What causes them?

Potential triggers for migraine headaches include:

- Stress, such as family or work tensions, or lack of sleep.
- Low serotonin levels – it is though that migraine attacks are caused by chemical imbalances in the brain. Levels of the brain chemical serotonin drop during a headache which triggers an impulse along one of the nerves which triggers inflammation and swelling of the blood vessels.
- Poor posture.
- Muscle tension.
- Glare or eye strain.
- Weather changes, e.g pressure changes, exposure to sunlight.
- Often migraine headaches occur in relation to the menstrual cycle during the build-up to a period, or on the day it arrives.
- The oral contraceptive pill can also trigger migraine headaches in some people, as can hormone replacement therapy.
- Missing meals also seems to be a trigger for migraine, and children may be particularly susceptible to this.
- Doing without your regular cups of tea and coffee can certainly cause withdrawal migraine headaches and these seem to occur particularly at the weekends, when you are out of the office, when going on holiday perhaps, or if there is a change in your daily routine.
- Additionally, there is a wide variety of foods that are known to trigger migraine headaches in susceptible individuals. The commonest foods include cheese, chocolate, most alcohol beverages and particularly red wine, yeast extracts (for example Marmite), pickled herrings and soy sauce, which are all rich in certain types of chemicals called amines. Some migraine sufferers seem to be particularly sensitive to amines. Other less common triggers include certain fruits, in particular citrus fruits, bananas, plums and pineapples, broad beans, artificial colourings and monosodium glutamate, that favourite flavour-enhancer of many a Chinese meal and savoury snack.

Some migraine headaches can also be due to a sensitivity to milk and wheat, even though they do not contain these chemicals.

What your doctor can do

- Measure your blood pressure, as occasionally migraine headaches are due to the presence of high blood pressure or other conditions affecting the nervous system.
- Examine you, and if your symptoms are severe or persistent, refer you to a neurologist to determine whether there is an underlying medical cause.
- If severe migraines occur as a result of taking hormones or the oral contraceptive pill, then a change in treatment may well be needed. We often find that hormone replacement therapy, prescribed at the time of the menopause, produces more frequent and more severe migraine attacks.
- Suggest you take aspirin on a regular daily basis, as this may ease the mechanics of a migraine. Research shows that blood platelets of migraine sufferers clump together more than they do in non-sufferers, particularly between attacks. Aspirin has been shown to reduce the degree to which platelets stick together.
- Prescribe medication specially designed for migraine headaches like Migril or Migraleve which often ease the symptoms, but do not address the root cause.
- Give you some dietary advice, as there is plenty of evidence to show that certain foods can trigger platelet stickiness, and thus precipitate an attack.
- Offer some other drugs which may be useful in preventing migraines. They include low doses of antidepressants, anti-arthritis drugs and beta-blockers used for high blood pressure.

Deborah's story

Deborah Crean was 52 when she approached the WNAS. She had two grown-up daughters and was just beginning her menopause. She had suffered migraine headaches, for at least two weeks per month, for over 20 years.

'I was in a real state when I went along to the WNAS for the first time. My migraines were ruining my life, and no amount of Imigran or Migril seemed to control them. Things went from bad to worse when I was put on HRT eighteen months ago for the start of my menopause, as the frequency of the migraines accelerated until I was experiencing daily migraines. My doctor had no other suggestions

which made me feel very depressed, especially as both my mother and one of my daughters suffered with migraine as well.

I read about the work of the WNAS in a national newspaper and in desperation made contact. I was given lots of information about my body's requirements during my first consultation, and was then sent off for a month to follow an exclusion diet, take gentle exercise and some supplements. I didn't get on very well with some of the supplements, as they seemed to make the headaches worse, but I continued with the others.

I had awful withdrawal symptoms for the first week , but after a month I realised that my hot flushes had gone, and so too had the giddy feelings and lack of energy. Within three months of starting the programme, I had two normal periods, which had been missing for several months, and no migraines for the first time in 20 years. It felt like nothing short of a miracle to me. I felt marvellous. It turned out that caffeine and chocolate brought the headaches on and I obviously avoid them like the plague now that I know.

My husband was so delighted that he had got his partner back, he booked a Caribbean Cruise as a second honeymoon! It has been nearly four years now, and I haven't looked back.'

What your dentist can do

Primarily, he can check to see whether you are grinding your teeth or clenching them at night, as this can send the jaw muscles into spasm. Also the jaw can sometimes be out of alignment (this can be corrected by wearing a plate designed by a dental specialist).

Just how spasms trigger headaches is not clear. One theory is that the exhausted muscles build up waste products, and instead of draining into the circulation they flow up the venous system into the head, irritating the brain. Another theory is that the muscles and jaw joints are sending a continuous stream of unconscious messages to the brain that they are not 'comfortable', and in an attempt to block out the flood of information, a migraine is started. Ear aches, neck aches and even sore throats can also be triggered by temporo-mandibular (jaw bone) joint dysfunction.

What you can do in the short-term

If you feel a migraine headache coming on:

- The first thing to do is to rest and avoid stress, if at all possible.
- Take a simple painkiller, such as paracetamol or aspirin; certain special forms of these are available for migraine sufferers. There is also a variety of other stronger drugs which can be taken and these can switch

off a migraine attack. You will need to ask your doctor about these as they are available on prescription only.

- Sometimes taking one or two teaspoons of sodium bicarbonate in a glass of water can help to relieve a migraine. This loads the system with carbon dioxide.
- Another way of loading your system with carbon dioxide is to place a large paper bag over your mouth and breath in and out of it slowly for five or ten minutes.
- Massage your temples, forehead, ears and skull gently whilst breathing regularly and deeply.
- The herb, feverfew, has been shown to be helpful with migraine headaches. You can buy feverfew pills in health-food shops.
- Another very simple but useful remedy is to chew on some crystallised ginger and use root ginger in your cooking. Ginger helps to dilate the blood vessels that have constricted during a migraine attack.
- Always seek and treat the cause of the headache, rather than the symptom, as long-term reliance on pain-killers can switch off the brain's natural ability to fight the pain.

What you can do in the longer-term

- If you suffer with migraines it would be a good idea to eliminate the foods associated with migraine from your diet, and also to limit intake of tea and coffee. Reduce your intake gradually, eat regularly, and avoid stress where possible. Follow the recommendations and suggested menu on page 473. The success of diets excluding these and other foods can be very high. Reduction rates of 90 per cent of migraines have been recorded, but this does vary a lot from individual to individual.
- If after a few weeks that doesn't seem to do the trick, then follow the recommendations in The Simple Exclusion Diet on page 460, for four weeks.
- If you smoke, cut out the cigarettes.
- If you take the pill, try another method of contraception for a few months to see whether there is any relationship between this and your migraine headaches.
- Low magnesium levels may also play a significant role in many cases of headache. It is particularly important in the relief of tension headaches as the mineral has muscle relaxant properties.
- Taking an essential fatty acid supplement can significantly improve migraine headaches by reducing platelet aggregation (red blood cell clumping) associated with the prevalence of headaches.
- Never miss a meal – make sure you eat wholesome food little and often to maintain your blood sugar levels.

- Take plenty of aerobic exercise, at least three times per week, as studies have shown that this will reduce the number of migraine attacks.
- Get out into the fresh air when possible, and make an effort to look at distant scenery, to give your eyes a different perspective to your everyday chores, particularly if you are doing lots of close-up intricate work.
- Learn to manage your stress with regular relaxation (see page 29).
- The herb ginkgo biloba is useful for treating migraines because it enhances cerebral circulation. Other effective remedies include chamomile, ginger, peppermint and valerian. Consult a qualified practitioner before taking ginkgo biloba.

Do not take any herbs if pregnant.

Complementary therapies

Herbs like feverfew and ginger are particularly helpful, and can be tried without advice. Your herbal practitioner will prepare a prescription for you which may well relieve your symptoms. There are many homeopathic remedies to try, which may also be of help, both in the long term, and in the shorter term, when you feel an attack coming on.

Acupuncture, acupressure, Alexander technique, massage and cranial osteopathy are all likely to be of help in relieving and managing the symptoms of migraine. It is very much a personal choice, and a question of assessing what suits you.

See also: Stress, Allergy, What's wrong with present-day diet and lifestyle?, The simple exclusion diet, Menu for migraine, The caffeine-free diet, References and Recommended reading.

Miscarriage

The definition of a miscarriage is the loss of any pregnancy before twenty weeks' gestation. Approximately 15 per cent of all recognised pregnancies miscarry. However, a pregnancy which miscarries within the first two weeks of conception is unlikely to be recognised as a miscarriage. As many as 60 per cent of conceptions may miscarry within days of fertilisation and the rate of spontaneous miscarriage in the general public is 25 per cent.

The majority of women who miscarry once, go on to have a successful pregnancy next time around. However, there are others, approximately one per cent, who suffer recurrent miscarriages, three or more failed pregnancies before twenty weeks' gestation. Even so, over half of these women do go on to have a successful pregnancy, despite their frustration and disappointment along the way.

What causes it?

There are many factors that can be the underlying reasons for miscarriage:

- *Genetic problems* Defects in chromosome or material from either partner is probably the main cause of sporadic or one-off miscarriages, accounting for 55 per cent of miscarriages. It is nature's way of deciding not to continue with a pregnancy that might have resulted in a handicapped or significantly deformed child. The risk of miscarriage increases if there is a history of genetic illness in either partner's family.
- *Increasing age* of the mother is associated with an increase in miscarriage rate, possibly because of the greater likelihood of chromosomal damage to the eggs, which occurs in Down's syndrome, for example.
- *Environmental factors*, including smoking and drugs. Smokers are 25 per cent more likely to have a pregnancy end in miscarriage than non-smokers. It is the most common environmental hazard associated with miscarriage. Passive smoking might also increase the risk of miscarriage. If you want a successful pregnancy, live in a smoke-free environment.

  Alcohol and illicit drugs carry a similar risk. Those who smoke heavily and/or consume excessive amounts of alcohol or street drugs are far more likely to have a lower intake of good nutrients, which can be a contributory factor to a miscarriage. The importance of adequate levels of nutrients should not be underestimated. Some women with recurrent miscarriage have recorded a relative lack of a chemical called prostacyclin, necessary for the growth and development of the growing baby. Adequate supplies of zinc, B vitamins, magnesium and other nutrients may also be necessary for the right biochemical environment for the developing embryo.
- *Toxic metals* Abnormally high levels of cadmium, present in cigarette smoke, and lead from petrol have been found in the tissues of still-born babies. These metals are more toxic if the diet lacks essential nutrients like calcium, iron and zinc, and a poor intake of these nutrients is associated with an increased risk of miscarriage.
- *Hormonal abnormalities* Severe hormonal imbalances, often associated with infertility, can also result in miscarriage. Additionally obesity, poor diet and lack of essential nutrients that contribute to normal hormone function, might also disturb the delicate hormone chemistry required for the survival of a pregnancy. Disturbances in thyroid function can also increase the risk of miscarriage, but the risk is minimised when the thyroid is treated.
- *Pre-existing disease* Diabetes, high blood pressure and rare diseases that affect metabolism, may be associated with increased risk of miscarriage, which makes careful control of these conditions essential.

Blood abnormalities associated with arthritis contribute to the rate of miscarriage, as does a condition known as SLE – systemic lupus erythematosus – that causes arthritis, skin disorders and other problems in young women. The blood of female sufferers, who may be identified only because they have recurrent miscarriages, may contain what are known as antiphospholipid antibodies. Anyone who has endured three consecutive miscarriages should be tested for SLE, or related blood abnormalities, as these may lead to disturbance in the blood formation in the blood vessels in the placenta, and result in miscarriage or still-birth later in pregnancy. If the tests are positive, specialist treatment prior to conception would be necessary.

- *Anatomical problems* Abnormalities of the genital tract like a soft weakened cervix (neck of the womb) will allow a miscarriage to occur. Surgical treatments before attempted conception, or a stitch in the cervix once pregnant, may be needed.
- *Infection* It is acknowledged that a variety of infections, including rubella (German measles) and listeria, an infection from 'live' soft cheeses, if contracted during early pregnancy can lead to miscarriage or congenital deformity. Low grade mild bacterial infection of the vagina has also be linked to recurrent miscarriage more recently.

What your doctor can do

- Examine you to determine whether you have any anatomical abnormality that needs attention.
- Check your hormone levels, as recent research has shown that increased levels of the pituitary hormone LH (lutenising hormone), close to conception, and a low level of the ovarian hormone progesterone shortly after conception, may reduce your chances of a successful pregnancy.
- Take a vagina swab to assess the possibility of infection.
- Investigate the possibility of an hereditary genetic defect.
- Following three consecutive miscarriages, measure your anti-cardiolipin antibodies, and lupus anti-coagulant.
- Give you some reassurance.

What you can do

- Try not to worry unduly.
- Follow the instructions for A preconceptual programme on page 386. This will mean ensuring you are eating a good diet, taking regular exercise, living and working in a wholesome environment, and keeping away from the 'social poisons'.
- Give your body a rest and recover after miscarriage, before trying to

conceive again. It is preferable to give yourself at least four to six months between pregnancies.

- Take the opportunity to have any medical problems checked by your doctor or a specialist.

Complementary therapies

It is worth investigating what herbal medicine has to offer, especially if you have had more than one miscarriage. Acupuncture may be able to help your body back to normal function, and to speed the recovery process from the last miscarriage. Certainly an appointment with the cranial osteopath will be useful, and aromatherapy massage will help to soothe away your anxiety.

Whilst investigating what these complementary therapies have to offer, it is important to have any medical investigation that is indicated, especially if you have suffered recurrent miscarriage. Don't despair, the chances of you having a live baby after a single miscarriage are 80 per cent, only falling to 74 per cent after three miscarriages.

Denise's story

Denise is a 32-year-old who has had four miscarriages between her two successful pregnancies.

'I had the first miscarriage ten years ago. I was three months pregnant at the time and we had not really planned a baby. It wasn't until after I had miscarried that I realised how much I would have liked a baby. My husband felt ready for children three years later and we then spent three years trying to conceive without any luck. We both had investigations and everything seemed to be normal. As luck would have it, as the investigations finished I fell pregnant naturally, and although I bled through the first part of the pregnancy, I managed to produce a healthy baby boy.

I had subsequent miscarriages when Alex was eighteen months old and again at two and a half and again when he was three and a half. Usually I was between nine and twelve weeks pregnant when I lost the baby. I would always start with spotting and gradually I would miscarry. Twice I ended up having a D&C, and on another occasion I managed with scans to ensure that I had fully miscarried. I was then given a laparoscopy to check to see why I kept miscarrying and the only thing the doctor found was a slightly mis-shapen uterus which was apparently somewhat flat on one side. Whilst investigating he also found adhesions on the ovaries and on my tubes which he removed after the fourth miscarriage.

I was advised to ask my doctor to test my anti-cardiolipin antibodies and lupus anti-coagulant as this might throw some light on *the underlying reason for the miscarriages. The doctor would not conduct the tests as he said I had already been investigated for inflammation. I felt pretty desperate about having another baby which obviously was affecting my relationship with my husband.*

I heard about the work of the WNAS on the radio and wondered whether I might be nutritionally deficient after so many miscarriages. I went along to the clinic and was given a dietary programme to follow with nutritional supplements and a recommendation to do lots of exercise, which I used to do regularly. I enjoyed the programme immensely and managed to get myself back into really good shape, within four months. I felt like a different person.

The following month I managed to fall pregnant again – although I did experience some spotting I rested a great deal and managed to carry the baby until full term. She was a beautiful wide eyed little girl and was well worth waiting for.'

See also: Standard references and Recommended reading (*Healthy Parents, Healthy Baby*).

Mouth Disorders

The most common diseases in the world are those of the mouth, such as dental caries or tooth decay, and periodontal or gum-disease.

- Every year in the UK, about two million days are lost from work because of dental disease.
- Twenty-nine per cent of people over the age of sixteen years (rising to 39 per cent in Scotland) have no natural teeth remaining.
- Amongst those over 35 years old who still have some teeth, over 90 per cent show signs of gum disease.
- Seventy per cent of five year olds and 97 per cent of fifteen year olds have had some tooth decay.

According to the figures (1982/83), about £612 million, which is just under 5 per cent of the health budget, is spent each year on dental treatment in the UK, representing 34.1 million courses of treatment. Except for mental health, this is the largest amount spent on any single group of diseases.

The mouth

Each tooth in the mouth contains a crown, which is the part visible in the mouth, and the root, which is anchored in a socket in the jaw bone and covered by the gums. Teeth are composed of a number of different layers, and each serve a function.

Enamel covers the crown of the tooth and is the hardest structure in the body. It reaches to just below the edge of the gum, and joins the cementum, which is the thin layer of bone-like tissue covering the root of the tooth and which helps to secure the tooth in its socket. *Dentine* is the hard, bright yellow, primarily non-living tissue that forms the bulk of the tooth. It reaches from the crown down through the roots. Finally, the *pulp* is the living centre of the tooth, which contains the nerves and blood vessels, and is therefore the part of the tooth that registers pain or thermal changes.

The supporting structures of the teeth are known as the periodontium, and comprise:

- part of the jawbone which surrounds and supports the roots.
- the membrane which acts as the attachment between the cementum and the socket in the jawbone.
- the gum, known as the gingiva.
- the pink membrane and underlying tissue that covers the bone.
- the cuff of gum around the tooth, which is an important feature in gum disease.

Saliva

This is the watery fluid that is produced by salivary glands within the mouth. It is Mother Nature's own mouthwash. There are three pairs of glands in the mouth from which saliva is secreted. Amongst its other functions, saliva dilutes the amount of sugar-produced acid present in the mouth because of the calcium and phosphates it contains. Both these minerals in the saliva act to repair some of the damage done by dental decay.

Plaque

We all have a thin, sticky film, composed mainly of bacteria, called plaque, covering our teeth. It continually forms in the mouth and sticks on rough surfaces on the teeth. It is most commonly found in the little crevices between our teeth, on the backs of our teeth, and at the gum margin, where gums and teeth meet. Plaque feeds on sugary deposits from our diet, and the by-products of this cause both tooth decay and gum disease.

TOOTH DECAY

When plaque is exposed to sugar from the diet, the bacteria contained in it convert the sugar into acids, which attack enamel on the teeth. After repeated acid attacks a cavity forms which becomes deeper as more acid is released from the plaque. The cavity eventually works its way through the enamel and the dentine and into the pulp chamber, which then becomes infected with bacteria. The pain of toothache is generated from the pulp, and if nothing is done the pulp dies, and the infection then infiltrates the root of the tooth forming an abscess in the bone surrounding it.

GUM DISEASE

There are a number of stages to gum disease, the most minor of which is gingivitis.

Gingivitis

Plaque accumulates around the margins of the gum and the teeth, and between the teeth in the crevices, and if left to stagnate, produces poisons which in turn cause inflammation of the gums known as gingivitis. The gums become red, swollen and shiny and have a tendency to bleed easily. If you notice blood after you brush your teeth, you should consult your dentist.

Periodontitis

When plaque is left to stagnate it gradually absorbs calcium salts from the saliva and hardens to become calculus, or tartar. This sits around the gum margin and is a constant source of inflammation to the tissues. As the disease progresses the calculus works its way down between the gum and the tooth into a pocket, and this stage is known as periodontitis.

Younger people experience gingivitis when they are being careless with their oral hygiene, and this is how the disease process begins. An improved oral hygiene regime can reverse the disease process, until, with age, the gums recede and bone is lost. Neither of these tissues, gums or bone, can be replaced once lost, and so it is vital to remove the plaque thoroughly each day in order to prevent diseases of the mouth.

Acute ulcerative gingivitis

This is an infection of the gums which is possibly bacterial in origin, but it seems it can also be attributed to some underlying nutritional cause. It was given the name 'trench mouth' following widespread outbreaks amongst soldiers who were sharing utensils in the trenches during both the First and Second World Wars. However, it is acknowledged that many of these soldiers were also suffering from scurvy, the result of severe vitamin C deficiency. The gums become infected, turn a greyish colour, the top surface often rubs away leaving sore, painful patches, and it feels like something is wedged between your teeth, particularly the back teeth. As the surface of the gums is attacked and the cells die, a tremendous odour is created. This condition needs to be treated urgently with Flagyll, a special form of antibiotic. You would be feeling unwell enough to seek dental or medical advice if you were suffering, and not able to enjoy a meal because of the pain and soreness.

Ninety percent of adults in the UK have gum disease and many suffer with halitosis or bad breath! Unlike toothbrushes and mouthwashes, dental floss can reach the plaque bacteria, decaying food and toxins, hidden beneath the gum line, which cause bad breath, gum, disease and can lead to tooth loss. Dental floss should be used daily in conjunction with tooth brushing by anyone who is keen to reverse gum disease, maintain oral health and prevent the stage of inevitable tooth loss. Not enough incentive? What about recent research linking gum disease to heart disease, osteoporosis and premature birth?

Few people in the UK use dental floss. Perhaps this is because traditional nylon floss is difficult to use – it's messy, it hurts, it takes too long, and the floss breaks and can catch between teeth.

One brand only is accredited by the British Dental Association. Made from polytetrafluorethylene (PTFE), Glide dental floss has an advantage over nylon in that it slides comfortably between teeth without shredding and leaving fibres behind. Regular flossing as part of a professional oral hygeine routine will prevent gum disease, may reduce the risk of heart disease and even save your life.

Brush your teeth with natural toothpaste containing either fennel or coenzyme Q-10 which both promote oxygen transport throughout the gums.

HERPES SIMPLEX

This is the most common virus of the mouth. The initial infection, which often affects young children, appears as blisters and ulcers on the gums, lips and soft tissue inside the mouth, and often remains undetected. It can cause a fever and make the child feel lethargic for up to fourteen days. This initial phase of herpes is called 'herpetic stomatitis', which simply means herpes in the mouth. This same virus can also cause genital herpes in children, but more commonly in adults, (see page 216).

What you can do

- Give a soft liquid diet as it may be too uncomfortable to eat normally.
- Analgesics, such as Junior Disprol, will help to reduce the discomfort.
- Chlorhexidine-based mouthwashes or dental gel will help to reduce the accumulation of plaque at a time when toothbrushing is too uncomfortable.
- Vitamin and mineral supplements should be given, with extra vitamin C and zinc to help promote healing.

- If you smoke, stop, as tar irritates the gums and reduces the peripheral blood supply to the gums.
- Brush your teeth with fennel toothpaste or aloe vera with added co-enzyme Q-10 which enhances oxygen supply to the gums. Echinacea toothpaste has anti-bacterial properties.
- Chew some sugar-free gum which increases the production of saliva, helps relieve jaw tension and ensures correct loading on the teeth.
- Mouth washes containing aloe vera and tea-tree oil have beneficial anti-viral and anti-bacterial properties.

COLD SORES

Following an initial attack of herpes in the mouth, the individual is likely to develop cold sores on the lips or face, which are secondary outbreaks of herpes simplex. They can be precipitated by numerous external factors:

- excessive sunshine
- emotional stress
- fatigue
- inadequate diet
- periods of ill health

HERPES ZOSTER

This form of herpes may affect the tissues in the mouth during a primary episode of chickenpox. Subsequent attacks can appear in the form of shingles, and may affect the nerves in the head, face and any part of the trunk, chest or abdomen, causing an outbreak of a typical rash with small blisters, which may ulcerate and crust with blood. Ulcers may also form on one side of the mouth, (see page 329).

What you can do

- Make sure you are well nourished – follow the recommendations for The Very Nutritious Diet on page 437.
- Get adequate sleep.
- Don't spend long periods of time sunbathing.
- Protect your lips with petroleum jelly in the sunlight, or other herbal creams like VyrBrit, a German product which has shown to restrict the growth of a cold sore if caught in time, and seems to be as effective as the pharmaceutical preparations like Zovirax.
- Avoid oral sex completely whilst you are infected.
- Try supplements of Lysine, which is an amino acid found in foods and can replace the chemically related amino acid Arginine, needed by the virus to replicate itself.
- Follow a diet rich in lysine and low in arginine. This means avoiding

nuts, chocolate, carob, oats, wholewheat, and soya beans. Instead eat more fish, chicken, meats, milk, cheese, mung and other beans (but not soya).

ACUTE THRUSH

The digestive tract is like a hose-pipe that leads from your mouth to your tail end. If thrush is present in one part of the tube, it can travel to other areas. Thrush can be found in the mouth, appearing as soft white masses on the surface of the tissue, which when scraped off, leave a red or bleeding patch. Occasionally it is a feature of diabetes, or can occur in a patient whose salivary glands are malfunctioning. It can be treated with antibiotics and you would be advised to follow the instructions given in Thrush (see page 124).

MOUTH ULCERS

Approximately 10 per cent of the population experience apthous ulcers (mouth ulcers) at some time. They are little sores that have a yellowish white appearance, and can appear singly or in crops. They also vary in size, but as a general rule the larger they are, the more pain they seem to cause. There is no recorded pattern to their occurrence, except that many women seem to get them in their premenstrual phase.

What causes them?

Although there is no specific agreed cause, there are a number of precipitating factors:

- Undue stress.
- Fluctuating hormone levels. The vast majority of the women we see with ulcers have an outbreak in the two weeks before their periods. The conclusion is that a relationship exists between hormone levels and apthous ulcers. However, in our experience hormone levels may fluctuate abnormally when brain chemical metabolism is disturbed.
- Nutritional deficiencies. In the absence of adequate nutrients, brain chemistry is often disturbed and the immune system may become impaired, rendering the body more susceptible to conditions like mouth ulcers. In our experience when the deficiencies are corrected the outbreaks of ulcers diminish.
- Food allergies. We have observed a relationship between food sensitivities and mouth ulcerations. We very often find that women sensitive to wheat get a recurrence of ulcers when they try to reintroduce it into their diet.
- Accidental trauma to the tissue. Sometimes hitting yourself with a toothbrush or knocking into something can result in ulceration.

What your doctor can do

Prescribe a chlorhexidine- or zinc-based mouthwash, or hydrocortisone pellets or cream, which can be placed over the ulcerated areas to reduce the inflammation.

What you can do

- Get your diet in order. If you have PMS as well, follow the recommendations on page 394. If you suspect you may have some food allergies, follow the recommendations for The Simple Exclusion Diet on page 460. If neither of these apply, then follow the recommendations for The Very Nutritious Diet on page 437.
- Take multi-vitamin and mineral supplements, and perhaps extra zinc and vitamin C.
- If the ulcers continue for more than four weeks, get your doctor to examine them as it is possible to get cancer in the mouth, and it is obviously better to be safe than sorry.

Susan's story

Susan Duncan was a 51-year-old women with two grown up children. She had been experiencing problems with her periods, constipation, general lack of vitality and lichen planus which is a chronic inflammatory disease of the mucous membranes and usually affects the mouth.

'I had not been feeling well in myself for some time and had put on 9.5 kg (a stone and a half) in weight and was experiencing hot flushes. My cravings for food, particularly sweet food, had begun to get out of control and I found myself bingeing on biscuits, cakes, chocolates and sweets, which was particularly worrying as my parents were diabetic and obese. I had an outbreak of very sore ulcers in my mouth but instead of clearing up in the usual way they seemed to spread and become more extreme, to the point where my eyes were affected too. They felt painful and swollen, irritated and sore.

I went to my doctor for some advice. He was somewhat mystified and wondered at first whether it was thrush. He tried me on various different types of medication but the symptoms did not respond at all. My daughter suggested that I visit my dentist, which I did and he diagnosed lichen planus. He referred me to the local district hospital. The diagnosis was confirmed and it was suggested that I either take steroids or learn to live with the problem. When I went back to my dentist and told him I didn't really want to take the steroids he told me that he had heard that diet might help. By this time I felt that my nerve endings had become hypersensitive too so I stopped drinking coffee and approached the WNAS for some help.

After a thorough examination I was given a programme consisting of modifications to my diet, daily relaxation, regular exercise and supplements. I followed the advice I was given by the WNAS and within a matter of a few weeks the lichen planus had calmed down and my eyes were not affected at all. I am not in any pain now. I still have the lichen planus mildly but it does not hurt at all or bother me. In addition to overcoming the chronic mouth problem, I also managed to sort out my constipation, food cravings and flushes and lost the excess weight. I feel very well and have sufficient energy to cope with life.'

BURNING MOUTH SYNDROME

A burning sensation from the oral tissues is a fairly common complaint. It is not usually present in the morning, but seems to get worse as the day goes by, and may be relieved by eating or drinking or removing dentures.

What causes it?

There are, once again, numerous factors associated with burning mouth syndrome:

- problems with dentures
- deficiencies of the blood
- diabetes
- dry mouth
- the menopause
- candida or thrush
- anxiety
- fear of cancer
- depressive conditions
- sensitivity to a mouth wash or over-use of mouthwashes
- esophageal reflux – where partially digested food is brought back.

One factor not given much attention is that a significant proportion of people who suffer burning mouth syndrome are likely to be suffering from a vitamin B1, B2, or B6 deficiency. In a Scottish study of those who were deficient, replacement therapy produced a resolution of symptoms in the majority of cases.

What your doctor can do

- Offer a routine check-up to eliminate the possibility of diabetes, thrush, blood insufficiency or depression being the underlying cause.
- An enlightened doctor would hopefully check your B vitamin levels, and prescribe the appropriate B vitamins if the results indicated a need.
- If you wear dentures your dentist should check to make sure they are not causing an adverse reaction in your mouth.

What you can do

- Follow the recommendations for The Very Nutritious Diet on page 437, unless you feel your symptoms are associated with the menopause, thrush, or anxiety, in which case refer to appropriate dietary recommendations.
- Take strong multi-vitamin and mineral supplements daily, and possibly extra vitamin B complex.
- Get regular exercise and relaxation.
- If you have your own teeth, follow The Good Oral Hygiene Plan outlined here.

The good oral hygiene plan

Keep your breath fresh by brushing your teeth and gums carefully, twice a day, for at least three minutes each time. If your gums are really inflamed and sore, you can start by using a soft-headed brush, aiming to change over to a medium-headed brush to maintain the health of the gums. Gums need to be massaged to create a hard skin layer on the surface, a bit like that on the palms of your hands. Massage in little circles on the spot at the place where the gum and teeth meet, the gingival margin. If you are not sure about brushing techniques, check with your dentist or hygienist.

- You also need to floss between your teeth each day, in front of the mirror to ensure you don't damage the gums. This disturbs the plaque and food debris which build up between the teeth, and are out of the reach of your toothbrush.
- Dental floss should be used daily in conjunction with tooth brushing by anyone who is keen to adopt a thorough, comfortable and effective oral hygiene routine.
- Use a mouthwash to loosen the plaque before cleaning your teeth.
- Rinse your mouth with water after meals, taking care to swish the water around your mouth to loosen any remaining particles of food.
- Eat raw vegetables and fruit regularly as snacks as these exercise your

gums, and unlike sweet processed carbohydrates, don't feed the plaque in your mouth.

- Drink lots of fluid to keep the saliva in your mouth flowing freely.
- Have checks with your dentist and hygienist at least every six months.
- Stop smoking.
- Brush daily with fennel or aloe vera with added coenzyme Q-10 toothpaste.
- Use a mouth wash containing aloe vera and tea-tree oil daily.
- Follow the recommendation for The Very Nutritious Diet on page 437, or if you suspect you may be suffering food intolerances, follow the recommendations for The Simple Exclusion Diet on page 460.
- Take supplements of multi-vitamins and minerals and additional vitamin C, at least 1g per day.

Multiple Sclerosis

This is a common and well-known disease which affects the nervous system. It is primarily a disease of northern Europeans, and occurs infrequently in other races. It is rare in Afro-Caribbeans unless they are born and raised in the UK, and is rarely diagnosed in Aborigines or Maoris. There can be strong family tendencies, with the risk rising as high as one in three for the partner of an affected identical twin. The prevalence is also less in areas remote from Europe. White South Africans and Australians of European origin have only half the rates of those found in many parts of northern Europe. It is sometimes linked with virus infections including measles, mumps, rubella and the Epstein-Barr virus (causing glandular fever), but the link is not proved.

What causes it?

Multiple sclerosis (MS) is due to a loss of the insulating fatty sheath around nerves. This fatty material, known as myelin, facilitates the rapid conduction of impulses along the nerves. Its loss in either the brain or spinal cord means that messages do not get through, with consequent disturbances in sensation, movement and vision. Typical features include:

- loss of vision affecting one or both eyes
- weakness in an arm or leg
- spasm in the major muscles of the arm or leg
- loss of sensation almost anywhere in the body
- disturbance in bowel or bladder function

- double vision
- a variety of other unusual neurological symptoms
- depression and mood changes.

In four out of five patients the disease waxes and wanes. In each attack a different part of the nervous system may be affected producing new problems. These may last for several weeks or months, with slow and sometimes complete, sometimes incomplete, recovery. After many years, ten or twenty, there may be slow but progressive deterioration. In young women the disease is often very mild, and disabling events occur only very rarely. However, up to 15 per cent become severely disabled within a short time due to aggressive disease.

What your doctor can do

- Refer you to a specialist for a variety of investigations in order for the diagnosis to be made. There are a variety of other possibilities in patients who appear at first glance to have multiple sclerosis.
- Exclude vitamin B12 deficiency by measuring its level in the blood or performing specialised tests of vitamin B12 usage.
- Treat the symptoms, which may involve a variety of medical basics to aid with constipation, incontinence, and reduction of muscle spasm, and drugs to control tremor and to minimise feelings of giddiness.
- There have been a number of attempts to influence the course of the disease using drugs that alter or influence the immune system, as this is involved in the initial episode of tissue injury. Preliminary evidence suggests that these powerful drugs may be useful but at present they tend to be used in those who have rapidly progressive MS. Just recently, beta-interferon, a naturally occurring immune altering chemical, showed a one-third reduction in new episodes, but without any measurable reduction in disability or overall course of the disease. This is now available for some patients within the UK and the USA.

What you can do

- *Change your diet* There is some preliminary evidence that diet changes may help. This is taken from pulling the results of three trials where increased doses of linoleic acid, the parent Omega-6 series essential fatty acid, was given in substantial amounts to MS sufferers. This essential fatty acid and its biochemical by-products are found in high concentrations in the nervous system and influence its structure and function. Not all patients benefited but there is a suggestion that those with early disease and relatively mild disability could benefit from a diet rich in these fats (see High Essential Fatty Acid Diet, page 446).

- *Take supplements of evening primrose oil* This, with or without fish oil, may assist the above diet. Unfortunately, there are no large published trials and the effects are likely to be slow. A reasonable dosage of 4–6 x 500 mg capsules daily will probably need to be taken for many years.
- *Take supplements of vitamin B and multi-vitamins* These nutrients are involved in maintaining the chemistry of the essential fatty acids. It is conceivable that some patients with MS lack nutrients involved in fatty acid metabolism. A supplement of 400–600 IU of vitamin E together with a moderately strong multi-vitamin supplement should ensure adequacy of these factors needed for normal essential fatty acid metabolism. Vitamin B12 is particularly important for the health of the protective outer layer of the nerves – the myelin sheath. Demyelination or progressive deterioration of the myelin sheaths means that messages are less efficiently transmitted along the neurones (nerves).
- *Take a supplement of co-enzyme Q10* necessary for improved circulation and tissue oxygenation.
- *Limit exposure to environmental toxins* This means not smoking, and drinking moderately. Rarely, assessment for environmental poisons, such as lead, cadmium and mercury, is needed. Some researchers have linked the presence of mercury amalgam fillings in teeth with increased risk of multiple sclerosis in some communities, but this is not certain. Similarly no firm link has been made between food allergy and multiple sclerosis.
- *Eat organically* where possible to ensure that your diet is as wholesome and pure as possible.

Complementary therapies

A number may produce symptomatic relief, but it is difficult to give firm guidance. Aromatherapy, massage, physiotherapy, acupuncture, and reflexology will all have their advocates. Try them and see.

Nail Problems

A number of minor nail problems are worth mentioning. Sometimes they indicate a nutritional problem.

- Brittle nails can be due to iron deficiency.
- Spoon-shaped or upturned nails can be due to iron deficiency or to repeated trauma.
- White spots on the nails were thought to be due to zinc deficiency but this is probably only occasionally the case. Repetitive minor trauma such as housework or use of a keyboard are more likely.

- Ridging of the nails can be due to eczema, psoriasis or other skin problems. Mild forms are quite common in normal individuals and have no nutritional significance.
- Fungal infections of the nails are common and respond well to the use of modern anti-fungal agents given either as local applications in the form of paint or as tablets. Additionally a supplement of zinc taken for three to six months might be helpful too.

Skin, Hair and Nail Signs of Vitamin and Mineral Deficiency

Sign or symptom	Can be caused by deficiencies of
cracking at the corners of the mouth	iron, vitamins B12, B6, folic acid
recurrent mouth ulcers	iron, vitamins B12, B6, folic acid
dry, cracked lips	vitamin B2
smooth (sore) tongue	iron, vitamins B2, B12, folic acid
enlargement, prominence of taste buds at the tips of the tongue (red, sore)	vitamins B2, or B6
red, greasy skin on face, especially sides of nose	vitamins B2, B6, zinc or essential fatty acids
rough, sometimes red, pimply skin on upper arms and thighs	vitamin B complex, vitamin E or essential fatty acids
skin conditions such as eczema, dry, rough, cracked, peeling skin	zinc, essential fatty acids
poor hair growth	iron or zinc
dandruff	vitamins C, B6, zinc, essential fatty acids
acne	zinc
bloodshot, gritty, sensitive eyes	vitamins A, B2
night blindness	vitamin A, zinc
dry eyes	vitamin A, essential fatty acids
brittle or split nails	iron, zinc, essential fatty acids
pale appearance due to anaemia	iron, vitamin B12, folic acid, essential to consult your doctor

Martine's Story

A forty-five-year-old mother of three, who worked part-time as a secretary, Martine had been neglecting herself since her mother's death nine months earlier, eating largely junk food, and had put on two stones in weight. She was unhappy, had dry spotty skin and her hair was in poor condition. She also had dry rough red pimples on her upper arms and thighs, split brittle nails and cracking at the corners of her mouth.

'I hadn't been feeling brilliant for some time, so having to cope with my mother's death on top of that was probably the final straw. My eating got out of control and over a period of nine months my weight gradually went up to nearly 75 kg (12 stone). My normal weight was around 60 kg (9¹/2 stone), so I felt uncomfortable, and obviously couldn't fit into any of my clothes, which was very depressing. I also noticed that my breasts became incredibly sore each month before my period.

As well as being overweight, I experienced mood swings and noticed that my skin, hair and nails had deteriorated. My nails were split and brittle, my skin became very dry and spotty, and my hair became dull and split. I felt like a walking wreck. I tried dieting, but found I couldn't stick to a diet for more that a few days which was very demoralising.

I read that cravings for food may be a physiological problem in a report on some research conducted by the WNAS, in Here's Health magazine. I contacted them for advice and was given a programme to follow that involved eating good food little and often, exercise and nutritional supplements. I started in December, which was difficult because of Christmas. But once the new year came, I found I was able to stick to my programme, in fact I was surprised how much I enjoyed it.

I lost weight gradually, without counting calories, and my vitality returned. Within four months I had lost 6 kg (1 stone) in weight, my skin was clear, my nails had grown beautifully and even my hair had got its old shine back. The breast symptoms had cleared up too. I felt like a new woman and totally in control. I've had some ups and downs since, but I feel that I now know what my body needs, so it's much easier for me to get back on the right road again.'

See also: Standard References.

Obesity

Despite the fact that in January each year the media attempt to seduce women with even more 'new' methods of restricting their intake of food in order to look more like supermodels, an international effort to halt the worldwide obesity epidemic has recently been launched. According to the World Health Organisation, 'obesity is rising sharply and the current management or prevention strategies are not capable of arresting this epidemic'.

- In the UK alone it is estimated that over one in four people are overweight to some degree. The rate of obesity – those seriously overweight – doubled in men and women from 1980 to 1996 in the UK. In 1996 16 per cent of men and 17.3 per cent of women were classified as obese and many more were moderately overweight. By 1998, 58.2 per cent of people were classed as overweight or obese.
- In the USA and Canada one-third of the adult white population is judged to be obese, and one estimate is that on present trends the entire population of America will be obese by the year 2234!
- Australia and New Zealand follow in the polls; European countries also scored highly, and obesity is even becoming a problem in developing countries.
- According to the Risk Factor Prevalence Study Management Committee Report prepared in Canberra in 1989 obesity in Australia increased between 1983 and 1989 by 15 per cent for women and slightly more for men, bringing the totals to 11.1 per cent for women and 9.3 per cent for men. Additionally, the overweight population increased by between five to seven per cent to 22.4 per cent for women and 36.8 per cent for men.
- The Australian Institute of Health & Welfare's unpublished report of 1993 estimated the direct costs of obesity in 1988-89 at $672 million, with obesity-related coronary heart disease and hypertension accounting for 62 per cent of that amount. The cost of treatment of obesity within the health-care system was $393 million.

One could be forgiven for wondering how these trends have come about when millions of people begin weight-loss diets each year all over the world. Booksellers fill their shelves with new diet books which they hope will catch the wave of New Year resolutions, and millions of hopeful, unsuspecting people will fall for the hype.

The majority of people who start a diet this month will be starting new diets again this time next year, hoping that their new shape will make them feel good. Fitting into a new outfit may be the goal of many, but the 'feel good' factor does not necessarily follow, and the lost pounds return all too soon. It is acknowledged that weight-loss diets slow down our metabolic rate, which then makes it difficult for us to return to our normal way of eating without putting on more weight than we started with. It follows that after several episodes of 'yo-yo' dieting we will be restricted to consuming very few calories and insufficient nutrients in order to maintain either our weight loss or our sense of well-being.

What is obesity?

In developed countries, obesity is now probably the most common diet-related disorder, while in developing countries obesity is usually a mark of prosperity. Being overweight may be a distinct advantage in a country or community that is used to food shortages; those who are thin and lean may fare less well than their plump counterparts at times of shortage. Unfortunately, we cannot use such excuses for ourselves, and so let's get down to some hard facts; facts which we think will give you an understanding of why you are overweight, and how this can best be tackled, in the short and long term.

First of all, how is obesity defined? The graph below gives measurements for height and weight. It is divided up into five sections, -1, 0, 1, 2, and 3. These are grades of obesity based on weight and height taken from the formula originally devised by a Belgian scientist, Quetelet. Quetelet's Index, which is more usually known as Body Mass Index (BMI), is widely

Height/Weight Chart Showing the Quetelet Grades of Obesity

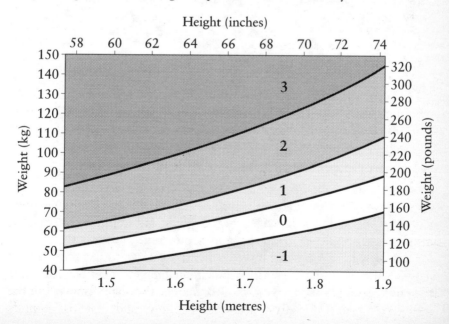

used in the assessment of obesity. The formula is derived by multiplying the weight in kilos by itself and dividing by the height expressed in metres. The categories are as follows:

-1: less than 20
 0: 20–25
 1: 25–30
 2: 30–40
 3: greater than 40

Normal or ideal weight is grade 0. Grade 1 is overweight, usually between 10 and 20 per cent above the ideal weight; grades 2 and 3 are regarded as obese – more than 20 per cent above the ideal weight.

As measured by Body Mass Index, the range associated with the greatest life expectancy and lowest death-rate is 20–25. There is a very slight rise in death rate in those who are mildly overweight, grade 1, but this low rise is so small as to be insignificant. It is grade 2 and especially grade 3 obesity which carry the greatest risk to health. An adult with a BMI of 40 has three times the risk of dying in a year than someone whose weight is ideal. An individual with a BMI of 35 has approximately twice the death-rate of his or her ideal counterpart.

For the majority who are just slightly overweight, grade 1 obesity, the major reasons for dieting are cosmetic and a sense of well-being. Not being overweight, and having a slim, attractive shape, is highly desirable in current fashion. Many of us feel better psychologically when that spare tyre has been whittled away, and if the diet is combined with an exercise programme, there can be a very real improvement in feelings of overall fitness. Medically, there is little change in factors such as blood pressure, and risk of heart disease, though there could be a moderate fall in blood cholesterol level if this is elevated at the start of the diet.

For those with grade 2 or 3 obesity, the potential benefits of losing weight are very real, and the effects on the psychological state of a successful weight loss programme can be dramatic. For example, normal employment may be very different for those who are grossly overweight (grade 3 obesity).

The health risks of obesity

Those who are obese, grades 2 and 3, have a shorter life expectancy, and an increased risk of many illnesses, including diabetes, high blood pressure, heart disease, osteoarthritis, gout, gallstones, reduction in exercise tolerance/level of fitness, and depression. Furthermore, general medical problems may be more difficult to treat in those who are obese. Gastrointestinal disorders, including indigestion, heartburn and constipation, may be more difficult to assess in an obese individual, as the information obtained from a medical examination may be limited.

Additionally, the survival rate of the obese woman with breast cancer is lower than her slim counterpart.

The young obese individual who loses weight to normal or near-normal value may have a substantial improvement in life quality and expectancy, and reduction in risk in practically all of the above. The improvement in arthritis, gout, blood pressure, diabetes, or blood cholesterol level may be dramatic, and evident within a few weeks or months of a dietary programme.

What causes it?

Genetic factors are involved. Analysis of families shows that if both parents are obese, 70 per cent of the children will be obese. If one parent is obese, 40 per cent of the children will be obese, and if both parents are lean, then only 10 per cent of the children will be obese. The predisposition of the parents is thus carried down partially to the children, but of course, we could argue that obese parents eat too much, and thus are likely to over-feed their children, making them obese in turn, and that this has nothing to do with genetics or inheritance. However, in studies of children who have been adopted, the adopted children take after the weight characteristics of their biological parents, rather than those of their adopted parents. This and other work lends substantial support to the idea that the tendency to obesity is to a large degree genetic.

Environmental factors are significant as well. By environment is meant all the factors around us that potentially influence our internal metabolism which we have already seen is initially determined by genetic make-up. With regard to obesity, the most important environmental factors are the food supply, level of exercise, lifestyle and social pressures.

If the food supply, for example, is so meagre that there is barely enough to go round, or starvation conditions exist, then obesity will obviously disappear from the community at large. In such a situation, with a limited food supply, environment is more important than any genetic factor. However, when there is an abundance of food, this allows the obesity tendency to express itself fully. When food is plentiful, some 25 per cent (or more as we have seen in countries like Australia and the USA) of the population may become obese.

The majority of obese individuals will have one parent who is overweight, and only a minority would be the offspring of two obese or two thin parents. At this point you might feel like blaming your mother and father, but this isn't very practical! The only practical solution is in some way to limit the calorie intake of those who are overweight, while taking other steps to improve their rate of weight loss.

In conclusion, it does seem that some people were born to be fat, but are only able to be fat because of the relatively affluent society in which they live.

What your doctor can do

- Check your thyroid to see whether it is underactive.
- Check to ensure that you are not suffering with diabetes.
- Take your blood pressure to determine whether it is high.
- Offer you a simple diet, or refer you to the local dietician.
- Consider drug treatment given with dietary advice over twelve weeks. Many of the older-style appetite suppressants are now banned in the UK. A new drug *Orlistat* acts by inhibiting fat absorption and will cause diarrhoea. It helps approximately one third of patients but prolonged used may lead to vitamin deficiencies and loss of minerals and essential fatty acids.

At the WNAS we have been treating and giving advice to women, many of whom were failed dieters, for some twelve years. We have come to understand that finding the right programme for each individual is the key to both long-term weight loss and, more importantly, good health. Without calorie-counting, we have managed to help thousands of people to understand their body's needs, and as a result to lose weight and reclaim their health. Using our methods people have not only lost weight, but have also overcome common symptoms like migraine headaches, irritable bowel syndrome, fatigue, acne, premenstrual syndrome, eczema and a whole host of other ailments, as well as feeling fitter. The WNAS programme is not just about diet, it encompasses lifestyle, exercise, nutritional supplements when appropriate, and relaxation.

Josephine's story

Josephine was a 46-year-old mother of three who moved with her husband to Geneva thirteen years ago. Her two main problems were gaining an extra 16 kilos and problems with heavy sneezing, especially in the mornings.

'I found it difficult to cope in Switzerland in some respects as our children were still in school in the UK and I think the depression concerning that led me to comfort eat. My usual weight was around 60 kilos until the year we moved house. In that year I suddenly gained 16 kilos. Ever since then I have been struggling with my weight. I managed to lose the weight again a year after I had put it on. Then unfortunately it crept back on again and I have been saddled with it ever since. Another problem I have had for many years is constant sneezing. It feels as if I sneeze a million times a day from the minute I get up in the morning. I have been treated with all sorts of anti-histamine preparations and have had tests for asthma in the past.

I contacted the WNAS for help after seeing a piece on television. One of the WNAS patients spoke of similar problems that had been sorted out. I sent for information and made an appointment for my first telephone consultation. I was given a programme aimed at keeping my blood sugar level constant so that I did not get cravings for sweet food and cheese, as I had done previously. I followed the Vitality Diet which is a plan written by the WNAS which involved cutting out all sorts of things initially and then adding them back gradually.

During the first week of the programme I felt half-drugged and had an awful headache. This gradually wore off until I suddenly felt as if I had come out the end of a tunnel. I lost 5 kilos in the first month – the weight seemed to fall off me and then the weight loss slowed down to a more gradual pace. As a result of the diet I found that I could not tolerate chocolate or vinegar, and alcohol made me feel as if I had a hangover. I had also been suffering with irritable bowel syndrome for four years and cutting out wheat, oats and coffee seemed to sort all those symptoms out as well. I reached my target weight and everyone commented on how well I looked and I certainly felt brilliant. I have had no stomach ache or headache since then, as long as I stick to the diet. It has been three years since I followed the diet and I really do feel like a new woman.'

What you can do

- Follow the instructions for The Simple Weight-Loss Diet on page 452.
- Start the diet when you are ready to do so. You will need time; this is not a diet to do in a hurry. You need to plan and set aside time for shopping, preparation and consumption of meals. Go shopping before beginning your diet, preferably after you have eaten so that you are not starving hungry and tempted to cheat. Take a list with you and make sure you stick to it.
- Eat regular meals, at least three meals a day, preferably with two small snacks in between.
- Never miss meals: irregular eating leads to less healthy weight loss and increased feelings of hunger.
- It is useful to eat from a small plate not a large one. A well-stocked medium-sized lunch or breakfast plate looks more satisfying than a large dinner plate only half filled.
- Chew your food well and savour each mouthful. Try not to hurry your meals.
- Eat fresh foods whenever possible. If at all possible, prepare one meal at a time. If this is not practical, try cooking a chicken, for example, to eat cold over a period of several days.

- Grill food rather than fry to keep your fat consumption low and to preserve the nutrients.
- Do at least four session of exercise per week to the point of breathlessness, which will help to speed up your metabolic rate, and thus burn the fat off! If you haven't been exercising regularly for some time, take it easy to begin with (see page 32).
- Fibre promotes weight loss by binding with water in the stomach, forming a gelatinous mass which induces a feeling of satiety. The theory is that appetite is switched off and less food is consumed. However, this does not work with individuals who do not have this appetite mechanism, and can eat regardless of whether they are hungry or not. Good fibre supplements are golden linseeds, psyllium and glucomannan.
- Supporting blood sugar levels is important for weight loss. If blood sugar levels are up and down all day, snacking on high fat and sugar foods can be a temptation to provide a quick 'fix' of energy until the next dip. Foods with a low to medium glycaemic index factor (see page 172 for more information) should be eaten primarily. Foods in this category are broken down into sugar slowly, therefore keeping blood sugar levels stable for longer.
- The mineral chromium plays an important role in healthy blood sugar control as it improves the sensitivity of the cells to the hormone insulin. Insulin's action is to drive the glucose out of the bloodstream into the cells for energy. GTF chromium is thought to be the most efficient as it is bound with vitamin B3 and amino acids to facilitate its action.
- 5-HTP, precursor of the amino acid tryptophan plays an important role in the appetite control mechanism. Research shows that those with a lower level of tryptophan never get the message to stop eating, even when they are full. This amino acid appears to function by promoting satiety.
- Consider spending a week at a health retreat to get yourself started – perhaps as part of your annual holiday. Having the appropriate food handed to you literally on a plate, and spending your time being pampered will undoubtedly help you to focus on a new sense of well-being.
- If you have tried endless diets without success, and feel you have a psychological block about losing your weight, ask your doctor about the possibility of having some counselling.

Complementary therapies

If your problem is related to an underactive thyroid or sluggish metabolism, it may be worth investigating what our recommended therapies have to offer. The acupuncturist would be my first port of call, as unblocking the energy channels will help you back to optimum metabolism. The nitty gritty on overcoming obesity though is to eat less and exercise more.

See also: What's wrong with present-day diet and lifestyle?, The simple weight loss diet, References and Recommended reading.

Osteoporosis

As a result of osteoporosis one in three women and one in twelve men will suffer fractures of the hip, spine or wrist. Apart from the obvious pain and disability, osteoporosis often brings with it a loss of height and curvature of the spine, known in the UK as 'dowager's hump'. Within six months of sustaining a hip fracture it is estimated that some 20 per cent of patients will die from complications associated with the injury itself, or the enforced immobility. This applies mainly to the elderly. However, osteoporosis is both preventable and treatable.

What is osteoporosis?

Osteoporosis is literally a thinning of the bones. The bones are composed of a 'skeleton' or scaffold of connective tissue around which minerals in crystalline form are laid down, rather like bricks being built up on a steel framework. The framework has certain flexibility as well as great strength, and the minerals give the structure resistance to pressure or crushing. So the structure of bone is rather similar to that of reinforced concrete.

We have two types of bone: trabecular, accounting for about 20 per cent of our bone mass, and cortical, which accounts for the other 80 per cent. Trabecular bone is found mainly in the spine, pelvis and ends of the long bones, such as the head of the femur. It is the type of bone most quickly lost after the menopause. Cortical bone is found in the shaft of long bones and the skull, and is lost more gradually. We are continually losing small amounts of bone throughout our adult life, but about 10 per cent of our skeleton is remodelled during the space of a year.

In osteoporosis an imbalance develops between bone loss and the rate at which new bone is deposited. There is a reduction in both the amount of connective tissue and the mineral content of the bone. The loss of bone mass reduces its strength and increases the likelihood that the bone will break when pressure is brought to bear on it.

You are at risk of osteoporosis if you have ever had or suffered from:

- poor diet, low in calcium, especially dairy products
- an early menopause, spontaneously, or following surgery

- thyroid or other hormonal problems
- low body weight, or suffered with anorexia
- petite build
- cigarette smoking
- regular and excessive alcohol consumption
- lack of exercise and sedentary lifestyle
- excessive physical activity, as in athletes or ballet dancers
- steroid drugs
- suffered more than one fracture since the menopause
- a close relative with osteoporosis
- chronic illness affecting digestion, kidney and liver function.

Bone density

There are a number of dietary, lifestyle and environmental factors that influence the strength and density of bones. The mineral content of a woman's bones at the time of the menopause is not so much influenced by her current dietary intake, but by her past intake of calcium over the previous 40 or 50 years.

The strength of bones is determined by:

- diet, especially the intake of calcium during the growing years
- physical activity, particularly weight-bearing exercise
- hormonal factors, particularly the balance of oestrogen
- genetic factors, which determine the size of bones and muscles.

Modern diet has much to do with the risks of developing osteoporosis in the same way as it influences heart disease and cancer. Many of us consume a diet which, though adequate in the short term, does not provide a good or optimum intake of nutrients in the longer term, thus predisposing us to diseases such as osteoporosis.

Calcium

Calcium is particularly important. Average intakes in the UK, for women, are around 700 mg per day, the amount provided by just over a pint of milk. However, many consume less than this and doing so during childhood and early adult life will mean that they reach middle and old age with a low bone mass and a high risk of osteoporosis. A study published in the *British Medical Journal*, by Professor John Kanis, from the Medical Research Council in Leeds, showed that long-term dose in excess of 1,000 mg of calcium per day decreased hip fracture rate by 25 per cent. This amount of calcium is only achieved by a modest percentage of the UK population.

Up to two-thirds of our calcium intake may never reach the bone because of certain dietary factors. Common foods such as bran and fizzy drinks contain high amounts of phosphates and can interfere with the absorption of calcium from the diet. A diet rich in salt and animal protein can increase the loss of calcium from the urine.

It is vitally important to concentrate on a diet rich in calcium. You will note from the Calcium List of Foods on page 487 that Cheddar cheese contains ten times more calcium than cottage cheese, for example. You will need to take a close look at the list and chose the foods that you enjoy, knowing that they are rich in calcium and other important nutrients.

- *Calcium* in bone also needs phosporous, another mineral, which is abundantly supplied by both healthy and convenience foods.
- *Vitamin D* This is mainly derived from the action of sunlight on our skin, and only small amounts come from the diet. It is needed to enhance the absorption of calcium from the diet.
- *Essential Fatty Acids* Recent research suggests that the essential fatty acids, EFAs, which are part of a healthy diet, also influence the balance of calcium in our bodies, especially in our bones. There are two types of essential fatty acids, the Omega-3 series and the Omega-6 series. The Omega-3 series are derived from fish oils, oily fish including mackerel, herring, salmon, pilchards and sardines, as well as from some cooking oils such as rapeseed, from linseed, soya beans and walnuts. These oils may help to reduce the risk of heart disease and benefit arthritis, but also may slow the natural loss of calcium in the urine, which includes some lost from our bones.
- *The Omega-6 series of EFAs* are found in sunflower and corn oil – and margarine made from them – almonds, sesame and pumpkin seeds. These help maintain healthy skin and influence the risk of heart disease. They also seem to help in the absorption of calcium from the diet.

Recent dietary evidence from the UK shows that intakes of these essential fatty acids, though generally adequate, show great variation from person to person, and that the body's ability to make full use of them declines sharply with age.

In addition to this, smoking, alcohol, a poor diet and some conditions such as eczema and diabetes, disturb the metabolism of these essential fats and can lead to deficiency states.

It appears that a number of connected minor nutritional deficiencies have resulted in many of us being at increased risk of osteoporosis from middle-age onwards.

- The best sources of calcium are dairy products, white bread, boney fish and hard water.
- Vitamin D may be obtained from sunlight, fortified cereals, margarine, butter and eggs.

- Regular exercise is an excellent way of helping to increase the uptake of calcium by bones.
- To help achieve a healthy calcium balance in the body, it is best to eat a broadly based healthy diet, limiting the intake of sugar, convenience foods, salt, alcohol and excessive amounts of animal protein.
- Daily supplements of Efacal (see page 353) provide additional calcium and essential fatty acids which are necessary for healthy bones.

Oestrogen

An important part of oestrogen's role is to maintain bone mass and help with the constant process of bone remodelling. When oestrogen levels are optimum our bones are constantly regenerating but when levels fall calcium is no longer directed to our bones and the net result is bone loss. Bone mass is at its peak during the early thirties, and from then on it declines, with an annual bone loss rate of approximately one per cent per year. However, for most women the bone loss increases at around the time of the menopause, and for up to ten years afterwards, with a further loss of two to three per cent per year. By the age of 70, approximately one-third of bone mass will be lost.

Women who experience an early menopause, or who stop menstruating because of excessive dieting or exercise, will have depressed levels of oestrogen, and as a result will be at greater risk of osteoporosis.

What your doctor can do

Interest in osteoporosis has increased considerably during the last decade because of the more widespread use of detection methods. The density of bones can now be measured by scanning the hips and the vertebrae of the spinal column. There are a number of tests available that help to determine the degree of bone loss or fracture risk.

Ordinary x-rays are used to detect existing fractures, but a measure of bone mineral density, using a specialised form of x-ray, is needed to measure bone mass and to monitor the results of treatment. In principle, for women at risk measures of bone mineral density are available in the UK on the National Health, but as the technology is relatively new, some areas of the country may not, as yet, be well served with the appropriate scanning machines. Bone density measurement is also available in the private sector, and costs vary per scan, depending upon the type of scan. Those with a high risk, or with established osteoporosis, should be scanned at regular intervals, of between one and two years.

Simple blood and urine tests are being developed to help identify those who are likely to be 'fast bone losers'. This will not replace bone mineral density scanning, but may prove to be a useful screening test. The blood tests are for calcium and bone chemistry; blood and urine tests are for hormones.

There are a number of very different treatments available for those with osteoporosis. Your own doctor will need to assess which of these options is the most appropriate for you. Those undergoing treatment from their doctor or specialist will need to be monitored, as no treatment is universally effective or free from side-effects.

Hormone Replacement Therapy

Although until recently HRT was thought to have been the great bone saver, and indeed after ten years it seems that women taking HRT have a considerably greater bone mass than women who have not, this does not appear to be sustained in the longer term. After 20 years of taking HRT it seems that there is a tailing off effect, and the women who took HRT may only have a three per cent greater bone mass than women who for their own reasons did not. The usage of HRT in the first ten or more years of the menopause is associated with a significant reduction in the hip fracture rate in women. However, up to two-thirds of women who take HRT come off it within the first nine months because of side-effects or dissatisfaction. (See the chapter on The Menopause, page 298).

For women with an early menopause (before the age of 45) and for some of the others in the high risk groups (see page 304), it is probably advisable to discuss with your doctor the risks and benefits of taking HRT. Those women who start their menopause in their mid-40s onwards will be well advised to help themselves to better bone health, certainly if they are unable or unwilling to tolerate HRT. Indeed, research shows us that there are many tools which will help us to preserve our own bone mass.

June's story

June Harmen was a 38-year-old mother of three-grown up children who was keen to stop taking HRT even though she had found she had osteoporosis.

'I served in the police force for many years, and was 5 feet, 5 inches tall on my inception. Following a prolapse I had a hysterectomy and although my ovaries were intact, my doctor prescribed HRT in the form of Premarin.

I persevered with the HRT for a few years, but was put off by the awful side-effects of nausea, depression and weight gain. I put on 7.3 kg (16 lb) which took me from a trim size 12 to a large size 14. But I was afraid to stop taking the HRT as I noticed from comparing height with other family members that I had lost 2 inches in height. Additionally I knew that my mother had lost 6 inches off her height, and my father had osteoporosis after long-term use of steroids.

I eventually came off HRT because I felt so awful, and the night sweats and flushes that followed were flattening. My skin became very dry and the condition of my hair had deteriorated. One year later I read a magazine article about the Women's Nutritional Advisory Service's holistic approach to the menopause, and as the case history in the article sounded just like me I decided to book an appointment at their clinic.

During my consultation a programme of diet, exercise, relaxation and nutritional supplements was worked out, and I got started straightaway. I adjusted to the programme quite quickly and soon noticed that I was feeling better in myself. Within two months the flushes calmed down, my libido started to return, and I generally felt more positive.

A year on I have gone from strength to strength. I feel well, I no longer suffer with symptoms of the menopause, and the condition of my skin and hair has improved. I have continued to take the multi-vitamins and the Efacal the WNAS suggested and am managing my health myself. I never did have a bone-density scan so I have nothing to compare, but I haven't lost any more height and I feel more agile than I have for years.'

Calcium supplements with Etidronate or Alendronate

Etidronate (Didronel PMO) and Alendronate (Fosamax) are two synthetic compounds based on phosphorous which combine with calcium in the bones and help to prevent its loss. They reduce bone loss in the spine, and in the case of Fosamax, in the hip and the forearm. Fracture rates may also be reduced. These treatments are usually combined with calcium or a calcium-rich diet. They are available on prescription and need to be taken for a two to three year period in order to reduce established osteoporosis.

Calcium supplements alone

At a dose of 1,000 mg per day by itself these are mildly effective for some men and women with osteoporosis, and have been shown to reduce hip fracture risk by 25 per cent. It is a cheap, simple and safe treatment, but nowhere near as effective as HRT. Calcium absorption varies greatly from person to person, and is influenced by many dietary factors (see page 346).

Calcium supplements with vitamin D

These are a useful treatment for the very old and those with poor sunlight exposure. Low levels seem common in elderly Europeans, especially if they are housebound. Although vitamin D is necessary for the absorption of calcium from the diet, most of us synthesise enough from sunlight.

Giving strong vitamin D supplements to those who are not deficient can actually cause bone loss due to excess stimulation of the bone-dissolving cells. Supplements containing vitamin D should therefore be taken with caution unless there is a proven deficiency.

Calcitonin

This is a hormonal treatment given by injection, which can be quite effective. This hormone influences the movement of calcium around the body. It is not a sex hormone. Its inconvenience limits its popularity.

What you can do

Do not underestimate the benefits of self-help measures. Each of the diet and lifestyle changes will, by themselves, make little difference in the short term, but over a period of years are likely to be of substantial benefit. Many of the measures will help not just osteoporosis, but also help reduce the risk of heart disease and stroke. What you have to do is:

- change and improve your diet
- take regular weight bearing exercise
- make lifestyle changes
- consider taking nutritional supplements
- see your doctor if you are a high risk case to discuss assessment and other treatments.

Dietary and lifestyle tips

New research shows that it is important to consume a regular amount of plant oestrogens, called phytoestrogens. These allow us to top up on naturally occurring oestrogen on a daily basis, and include:

- soya beans and soya bean products like flour, tofu and soya milk
- golden linseeds, sunflower, pumpkin and sesame seeds
- alfalfa, lentils, chickpeas
- the herb red clover.

It is well established that Japanese women, who already eat a diet particularly rich in plant oestrogen in the form of isoflavones, have far fewer problems with bone loss. On average they consume between 50–100 mg of isoflavones per day, compared to 3g in the UK. At the WNAS we recommend a glass of 'So Good' each day, a soya drink that provides approximately 25 mg of isoflavones. Organic golden linseeds with breakfast cereal, and soya milk, and at least one or two further servings of phytoestrogen rich food through the day, will maintain your blood levels.

There are now also isoflavone rich supplements which have been shown in clinical trials to regenerate bone. Ipriflavone, the daidzein based product is used exclusively in Europe and a trial on a very new product made from formononetin, from the red clover plant, recently showed four per cent bone regeneration in six months. Overall the studies seem to show that it effectively helps to improve bone density at a dose of 600 mg per day combined with 1000mg of calcium. However, a recent study concluded that it covers the count of white blood cells which are an important part of our immune function. In the UK it is now being marketed as an over-the-counter supplement distributed by Solgar, and is available in most health-food shops.

The herb red clover is a particularly important phytoestrogen as it contains the four dietary isoflavones that are present in typical diets of Eastern, Latin American and Mediterranean communities, which are absent from the typical UK diet. Novogen red clover is an advanced food supplement developed specifically for women over 45, providing 40mg of dietary isoflavones per tablet. We use this at the WNAS in conjunction with a phytoestrogen rich diet. One study showed that taking 40mg of Novogen red clover for one year suppressed the loss of spine bone mineral density compared to placebo. The newest bone support supplement from Novogen is Rimostil. Rimostil has been formulated using a specific combination of isoflavones for the pevention and treatment of osteoporosis. In a recent clinical trial on 50 women over six months, there were highly significant increases in bone density ranging from 2.9 per cent to 4.1 per cent.

- Concentrate on eating foods rich in calcium (see page 487).
- For those women around the time of the menopause and beyond, consume foods that contain naturally occurring oestrogens.
- Make sure your diet contains a variety of foods rich in essential fatty acids (see page 489).
- Limit your consumption of alcohol to a maximum of three to four drinks each week.
- If you smoke, try to cut down gradually or, better still, give up altogether.
- Consume foods rich in Vitamin D if you do not get much sunlight exposure. They include dairy products, margarine, semi-skimmed milk, reduced fat cheese, or fortified cereals like Cornflakes and Rice Krispies.
- Try the menus on page 482.

General health tips

- Avoid excessive consumption of sugar and foods rich in sugar such as fizzy drinks, sweets, cakes and biscuits. Such foods are low in essential nutrients, especially calcium, and high in calories.
- Reduce your intake of salt, both added to cooking and at the table and avoid salty foods like bacon and kippers.
- Eat vegetables and salads daily.
- Eat at least two servings of fresh fruit per day.

- Limit your intake of saturated animal fats by consuming leaner cuts of meat, reduced-fat dairy products, and avoiding fried foods. This is particularly relevant if you are overweight.
- Reduce your intake of tea, coffee, cola and chocolate which all contain caffeine, and use alternatives now available in most supermarkets and health-food shops.

Regenerating lost bone?

A diet rich in essential nutrients and regular exercise can affect bone mass, and so too can a relatively new supplement called Efacal, a specially formulated product produced by Efamol. A number of studies suggest that combining calcium with EFAs from evening primrose oil and marine fish oil may be an effective way of treating osteoporosis. A recently published study, conducted by Dr Kruger and her colleagues from the University of Pretoria, South Africa, tested the effect of these oils on calcium balance in a group of women with osteoporosis. After a four-month trial period there were a number of changes which suggested increased absorption of calcium from the diet and increased uptake of calcium by the bone. Efacal has been shown to:

- improve the uptake of calcium from diet through the gut wall
- decrease the amount of calcium lost through the urine
- help direct calcium to sites of deposition in the bone and may thus help prevent the bone-thinning process. It is effectively the stamp on the envelope that makes delivery far more likely.

Each capsule of Efacal contains 400 mg of Efamol pure evening primrose oil, 44 mg of marine fish oil and 100 mg of calcium. Those at risk of osteoporosis should take four capsules every day with the evening meal. For preventative purposes, four capsules should be taken every day for an initial twelve-week period, followed by a daily dose of two capsules per day.

Exercise

Exercise is a valuable tool at all stages of life to promote good health, and is an acknowledged way of helping to protect against heart disease and to help keep bones strong. Plenty of exercise in childhood, including sport at school, helps to build up a high peak bone-mass.

From the time bones reach their peak mass, which is approximately in the mid-30s, the destiny of bone health for many rests in their own hands. It is influenced by diet, as you have seen, and also by lifestyle. At the time of the menopause, when women are most at risk of bone loss, exercise must become a vital part of the everyday schedule. Research has shown that weight-bearing exercise, in other words anything that involves putting weight through your bones, helps to stimulate the regeneration of bone tissue by reducing calcium loss.

The consensus from studies is that you need to exercise moderately three or four times each week, for 30–45 minutes each time, so long as you do not suffer with cardiovascular disease. The pay off, apart from helping to strengthen your bones, will be that within twelve weeks you can expect to feel more energetic, cope with stress more effectively, sleep better, have increased resistance to infection and feel a lot better generally.

Anything that involves putting pressure on your bones is classed as weight bearing. Examples are:

- jogging
- brisk walking
- playing racquet sports
- lifting weights
- a workout
- skipping
- press-ups
- squeezing tennis balls

Walking helps to preserve the hips and the spine, but hand and wrist exercises, which consist of gripping and rotating, are necessary to strengthen the wrist bones. The disabled, the bedbound – even if it is only for a few weeks – and the housebound are very much at risk, as are astronauts because of the weightlessness.

However, too much exercise can be damaging. It is now known that young female athletes, gymnasts and ballet dancers are high-risk groups for osteoporosis. Their intensive training and low body weight often prevent them from menstruating, resulting in lowered levels of oestrogen, which subsequently affects their bone mass.

It is important that those who exercise vigorously have an adequate and nutritious diet in order to maintain their body weight. Failure to do so will further increase the risk of osteoporosis. Some performance athletes and young ballet dancers may need nutritional supplements in order to ensure dietary adequacy.

Avoid smoking and alcohol

Smoking and drinking alcohol to excess are two of the easiest ways of increasing your risk of osteoporosis.

- Women who stop smoking and drinking at the time of the menopause may reduce their hip fracture rate by as much as 40 per cent.
- Both smoking and drinking alcohol have a broad spectrum, anti-nutrient effect, and accelerate the loss of nutrients.
- Smokers and those consuming lots of alcohol usually have different diets and different essential fatty acid levels too, but it's never too late to stop!

See also: The menopause, What's wrong with present-day diet and lifestyle?, Thyroid disease, Prevent osteoporosis, sample high calcium menu, References, Recommended reading (*Cruising Through the Menopause, The WNAS Guide to Better Bones*).

Painful Ovulation

Painful ovulation, or *Mittelschmerz*, as it is also known, is quite common and isn't usually severe. The pain is usually on one side of the abdomen and in many cases only lasts a few hours. Slight mid-cycle spotting may also accompany the pain.

Mittelschmerz, literally 'middle pain', can occur in women of all ages. At its most severe, it can feel like a needle-piercing pain combined with severe cramp, as if someone is squeezing your insides, and this can last for several days. The pain often starts as a gnawing sensation with an ache in the groin, which then builds up to a crescendo.

First, let us look at the process of ovulation. It's a natural process that takes place in any fertile woman. It's the body's way of preparing for pregnancy, and it occurs once a month. An ovum or egg is produced by a follicle in the ovary approximately halfway through a regular menstrual cycle. The common signs of ovulation include an increase in body temperature, and changes in the amount and constituency of cervical mucus.

When an egg grows each month it develops inside a small cyst. By the time it is ready to be released, it will have reached about 2.5 cm (1 inch) in diameter. If you are examined on an ultrasound scan immediately prior to ovulation, the cyst would show up on the ovary, and this would be entirely normal. When the cyst ruptures, the fluid from it leaks into the abdominal cavity. Often some blood will escape from the cyst as well, and this too spills into the abdomen. Under normal circumstances the body deals with these fluids through its natural wastage system. Both the fluid, and the blood, are capable of irritating the lining of the abdominal cavity and it is this irritation that causes the *Mittelschmerz* pain in some women.

Why some women suffer ovulation pain and others don't remains a mystery to doctors. Sometimes the ovulation pain signals the beginning of the unpleasant symptoms of premenstrual syndrome, but ovulation pains can just as easily occur in women who do not suffer with PMS. In some cases women suffer with ovulation pain for several days, followed by nearly two weeks of awful PMS symptoms which takes them into a heavy and painful period. This only leaves them with one normal week per month in which to recover!

If you suffer with excruciating pain mid-cycle, and it occurs on a regular basis, you should consult your doctor to ensure that there is nothing more sinister involved. It's a good idea to chart your symptoms to ensure that they do occur mid-cycle, and are not being confused with a grumbling appendix, for example, or another abdominal problem.

As these cycles differ from month to month, the pains may start by themselves, or they may begin after childbirth, but then again they can occur for the first time after childbirth. So there is no hard or fast pattern.

What your doctor can do

- Examine you to determine whether the pain is related to ovulation or something entirely different, like an inflamed appendix or bowel. As everything is so close together it is sometimes difficult to tell, unless you chart your symptoms over a few months, to confirm a mid-cycle pattern.
- Most doctors will recommend the contraceptive pill as a solution, as this usually prevents the body from ovulating. When this happens, the cyst that causes the pain when it erupts isn't able to develop, and as a result the *Mittelschmerz* doesn't occur. So the Pill may be a good solution if you are looking for contraception as well, and if it suits you.

At the Women's Nutritional Advisory Service, we have been treating women with period-related problems since 1984. Initially, we set out to help women over their premenstrual problems but as an added bonus we discovered that we were also helping to lighten and regulate periods as well as helping to overcome period pains and mid-cycle ovulation pains.

Low levels of nutrients, particularly magnesium, iron and B vitamins, can affect brain chemistry, and thus the ability to deal with ovulation and the muscle contractions of the uterus. Pregnancy and breast-feeding place substantially greater nutritional demands on women's bodies, and often, when women are under-educated about foods that are rich in the important nutrients, these nutrients are not replaced.

We know from experience that by improving diet, taking specific nutritional supplements and exercising, you stand every chance of overcoming menstrual symptoms, including mid-cycle ovulation pain.

What you can do

- Try to reduce the number of teas and coffees you drink to no more than a total of four per day. Try decaffeinated varieties and the herbal alternatives. One particular herbal tea, which is a tea lookalike, called Rooibosch Eleven O'Clock, has been shown to decrease muscle spasm, so may well be worth trying.
- Have a salad and three portions each of fruit and vegetables daily. Include green leafy vegetables like broccoli, cabbage or spinach as these are potentially high in magnesium.
- Cut down on sweets, cakes, biscuits and chocolate and eat more wholesome snacks instead, like nuts and raisins, Ryvita and spreads, or fresh fruit and yoghurts.
- Avoid animal fat and use lean cuts of meat.
- Reduce your alcohol consumption to no more than three or four glasses of wine or the equivalent per week.

- When the pain occurs, place a heat pack or hot water bottle over your abdomen, and try to rest, lying face down on your tummy, for 10–15 minutes.
- As well as making dietary changes you may be helped by taking some specific vitamins and minerals which are rich in magnesium. Optivite, a multi-vitamin and mineral preparation which has been through four properly conducted clinical trials for premenstrual syndrome, is useful in regulating other period problems.
- You may also need to take some extra magnesium supplements around mid-cycle.
- Regular exercise is helpful throughout the cycle as it will help to keep your muscles toned.
- Yoga and other methods of relaxation are a useful tool, especially around the time of ovulation, as they will help you to relax.
- Massage is another effective way of helping to reduce muscle spasm. Try the self-massage using aromatherapy oils described on page 31.

Complementary therapies

Acupuncture and cranial osteopathy would be top of our list of therapies to try, both of which are good ways of unblocking the energy channels. Herbal and homeopathic remedies would be worth a try too. If you are self-medicating you could try Colocynth, Naja, Lycopodium or Palladium, all of which are homeopathic remedies. Herbal medicine prepared by a qualified practitioner would also be worth trying. If you would like to consult an expert, you will find the addresses of the relevant associations in the Useful addresses list.

See also: Standard references.

Palpitations

The term palpitations is used to describe rapid or irregular heartbeats. They are felt as a thumping or fluttering sensation in the chest and may last just for a few moments or persist for hours or days depending upon their cause. Associated symptoms include shortness of breath, giddiness or sudden blackout, chest pain or an urgent desire to pass water. The heart has its own clock which keeps it beating at around 70 beats per minute. An impulse is generated at the top part of the heart called the atrium and this is spread to the other parts of the heart by a conducting system which is distinct from the muscles of the heart. The pacemaker or its conducting system may be at fault.

What causes them?

- ischaemic heart disease
- disorders of the heart pacemaker system itself
- disease of the valves of the heart
- an overactive thyroid gland
- infection
- side-effects to drug therapy
- nutritional problems
- alcohol excess
- caffeine sensitivity

What your doctor can do

- Assess the type of palpitation and its possible cause. This always needs an ECG electrical heart tracing, blood tests and often specialist examinations if they are severe.
- Treat the palpitations with a variety of drugs. Occasionally this means using powerful drugs with significant side-effects. These may be minimised by some of the self-help measures.
- Treat any underlying heart problem or other cause.
- For some types of palpitations, treatment with aspirin or another anti-clotting drug is needed as there can be an associated risk of a stroke.

What you can do

- Avoid alcohol.
- Avoid caffeine (see page 6) mainly in tea, coffee, cola-based drinks and some painkillers.
- Exercise regularly if possible and appropriate. This can help to establish a more normal heart rhythm and over-ride the tendency for certain types of palpitations.
- Try and cut short an attack of rapid heartbeat with the following manoeuvres:
  - Lie down, take a deep breath in, pinch your nose, close your mouth and try to breathe out but do not let any air pass.
  - Massage the mid-point at the front of the neck at the level of the Adam's apple. This is where nerves that control heart rate and blood pressure are situated.
  - Close your eyes and press quite firmly with your fingers on them.
    These measures all help to send a certain signal to the heart which can help switch off certain types of usually non-serious palpitations.

- Supplements of vitamin B and magnesium might be helpful. A strong B complex and about 30 mg per day of magnesium would be appropriate. Check with your doctor first before trying this. It should be combined with The Very Nutritious Diet (see page 437). You will need to follow this routine for three to four months before any real benefit can be seen, but the result is unlikely to be powerful enough to control palpitations of a serious nature.

See also: Standard references.

Pancreatic Disease

The pancreas is a large gland situated just below the stomach, and has two main functions. The bulk of the gland is involved in producing digestive enzymes needed for the breakdown of fats, and its other responsibility is the production of the hormone insulin.

What are the symptoms?

Poor function of the pancreas causes diarrhoea due to the poor absorption of fats. The stools are typically pale, offensive smelling and associated with abdominal bloating and wind. Abdominal pain usually occurs at some stage, and can be severe; typically it is situated in the upper abdomen and may pass through to the back.

What causes it?

The main causes are:

- alcohol excess
- in association with gallstones
- following certain infections including mumps virus
- in association with a variety of rare conditions
- after radiation therapy for cancer

What your doctor can do

- If possible, remove the cause.
- Give digestive enzymes to replace those usually provided by the pancreas.
- Consider surgery if the structure of the pancreas is very distorted.

What you can do

- Do not drink alcohol.
- Do not smoke cigarettes – they reduce pancreatic function.
- Follow the recommendations for The Very Nutritious Diet (see page 437).
- Eat little and often, avoiding very fatty foods. Regular snacks between meals of fruit with small amounts of nuts, bread with small amounts of nut or seed spreads, or milk-based beverages should be tried.
- Nutritional supplements are often needed. Multivitamins with vitamins A and D are likely to be an appropriate supplement. Supplements of zinc and selenium may also be necessary. Vitamin C may help relieve the pain from this condition.

Pelvic Pain

Pain in the pelvis can vary from fleeting mild discomfort to severe gripping pains that take your breath away. These can prevent you from taking another step, and they can wreck the quality of your life. The pain may pass up into the abdomen or up into the buttocks and down into the legs. There are a variety of underlying causes for the pain, some of which are more serious than others:

- the presence of fibroids
- cysts on the ovaries
- infected Fallopian tubes
- endometriosis or adenomyosis (endometriosis growing within the muscular coat of the womb)
- an ectopic pregnancy
- pelvic inflammatory disease
- appendicitis or other non-gynaecological condition.

We have covered the conditions that cause pelvic pain that we can influence with self-help measures. They are listed in alphabetical order. See *fibroids, endometriosis, pelvic inflammatory disease, ovarian cysts* and *polycystic ovaries.*

FIBROIDS

Between 20 and 25 per cent of women over the age of 35 have fibroids. They are benign (non-cancerous) tumours or fibrous lumps, which grow in the muscle lining of the uterus wall, and are the commonest reason why women experience regular heavy periods. One-third of women with fibroids bleed so heavily that they become anaemic (see page 60). The fibroids are composed of a combination of smooth muscle and connective tissue. Their size can vary from that of a small pea to that of a large orange, or even larger, which would greatly increase the volume of the uterus.

Fibroids grow slowly, and can cause heavy bleeding, back pain, pelvic pain and, when large, place pressure on nearby organs or structures like the bladder, bowel or rectum. When there is pressure on the bowel constipation can occur, and when pressure is placed on the rectal or pelvic veins, haemorrhoids or varicose veins in the legs can develop. Only very rarely do they develop into cancer.

What are the symptoms?

- long heavy periods
- infertility
- pressure in the abdomen which may press on other organs like the bowel, and cause constipation, or the bladder and cause frequent urination
- swollen abdomen
- backache

Fibroids can occasionally cause problems in pregnancy. A fibroid may grow in a place which blocks the exit of the baby thereby resulting in a difficult labour or creating a situation where a caesarean section is required. Also, there is a greater than normal chance of the baby lying in an abnormal position in the womb and of heavy bleeding after birth.

What causes them?

- Fibroids are thought to depend on oestrogen, as they do not occur prior to puberty and become smaller after the menopause. Just why they occur in some women and not others is not fully understood.
- There is a higher incidence of fibroids amongst obese women who have above average levels of growth hormone and blood glucose.
- It is thought that genetic factors may also play a part in the predisposition, as black women in the USA, for example, are three to nine times more likely to develop fibroids than their white counterparts.
- Fibroids are also more common in women who have not been pregnant or have small families.

What your doctor can do

- Eliminate the possibility of pregnancy by testing your urine and examining you.

- Perform a cervical smear to eliminate the possibility of cancer of the cervix.
- Give routine blood tests to check for anaemia, any underlying infection or sinister growth.
- Prescribe a supplement of iron (to be taken with fruit juice) if you are anaemic.
- Give a vaginal ultrasound to check the appearance of the uterus and other related structures. This is easy to perform and is an excellent test.
- Refer you to a gynaecologist for a laporoscopy, a minor investigative operation that, with the use of a laporascope inserted through the abdominal wall, examines the pelvic structures.
- The surgeon may suggest removing the fibroids if they are potentially troublesome, and this procedure is called myomectomy. Laser therapy is sometimes used also these days.

In the main, small fibroids are not troublesome, and are best left alone. If they do become large, and there is fear of them pressing on a nearby organ or blocking the cervix or the Fallopian tubes they will need to be removed. Women with fibroids are often advised to have a hysterectomy. If you receive this advice, and you are not too troubled by your symptoms, then you should certainly question it, (see page 243).

What you can do

- Waiting to see whether the fibroids cause symptoms that affect the quality of your life is a reasonable policy. If not, they are probably best kept away from the surgeon's knife.
- In theory a diet that prevents oestrogen surges may help to control fibroids. Concentrate on eating a high-fibre, low saturated fat and low sugar diet (see Eating for Health, page 437).
- Avoid or severely limit meat and dairy products unless they are organic. These foods contain an abundance of synthetic hormones and antibiotics. Dairy products are also a primary source of arachidonic acid – the precursor to the pro-inflammatory series-2 prostaglandins. The high saturated fat content of many dairy products is a risk factor for excess oestrogen levels in the body.
- New research shows that it is important to consume regular amount of plant oestrogens, called phytoestrogens. They have a modulating effect on our body's oestrogen, raising levels if they are too low and conversely lowering them when there are signs of 'oestrogen dominance'. Phytoestrogens predominate in soya beans and soya bean products like flour, tofu and soya milk, golden linseeds and the herb red clover (tablets, or sprouted seeds).

- Increase your intake of fibre in the form of wholegrains and fresh fruit and vegetables, especially if you suffer with constipation. Fibre promotes oestrogen excretion.
- Women with fibroids should avoid alcohol entirely or consume it in small amounts. Alcohol is stressful to the liver and can affect the liver's ability to metabolise hormones efficiently. Alcohol also depletes the body's B-complex vitamins and minerals such as magnesium.
- Sugar, like alcohol, depletes the body's B-complex vitamins and minerals, which can impair hormone metabolism in the liver and can worsen muscle tension and irritability as well as nervous tension and anxiety.
- Essential fatty acids (EFAs) are beneficial in the treatment of fibroids particularly where menstrual cramps are severe. EFAs are converted into anti-inflammatory hormone-like substances called prostaglandins. These prostaglandins have muscle-relaxant and blood vessel relaxant properties that can significantly reduce muscle cramps and tension. The best sources of EFAs are sunflower oil, safflower oil, walnut oil, raw flaxseed oil, pumpkin seed oil and oily fish such as pilchards, mackerel and sardines.
- Lose weight if you need to as well.
- The B vitamins and magnesium may also help to regulate oestrogen metabolism, so you could try supplements of these. Any response to these treatments is likely to take months if not years. So be patient!

Complementary therapies

Herbal medicine may have quite a bit to offer. It will take an experienced herbal practitioner to work out the right prescription. Homeopathic remedies are worth a try, and so too is acupuncture.

ENDOMETRIOSIS

Endometriosis, where the tissue forming the lining of the womb grows outside the womb, around other organs, is the most common cause of chronic pain in women of child-bearing age. The pain nearly always coincides with the menstrual period, and may also be experienced at the time of ovulation, approximately mid-cycle. The pain can also be triggered by sexual intercourse, a bowel motion or emptying the bladder, and sometimes causes spotting between periods.

The extraneous endometrial cells (womb lining) not only grow outside the uterus, but they also mimic the function of the endometrium, in that they have a monthly bleed. In mild cases the blood is reabsorbed by the body, but in more severe cases cysts form, which then weep and cause pelvic irritation. The length of time a woman suffers varies from person to person. Some women only suffer for a few months, whilst others suffer all their menstruating lives. It is often better during pregnancy, which is why becoming pregnant may be offered as the solution.

Endometriosis can be very painful, restricting your lifestyle and physical abilities. It is associated with infertility, but it seems that many sufferers do manage to conceive without too much difficulty. Reports of just how common this condition are varied probably because it is difficult to assess precisely. The diagnosis has to be made during a laporoscopy, a telescopic look into the abdominal cavity, which is not something most well women would undergo just to pass the time of day! Therefore, it is impossible to assess how many women without symptoms may or may not be suffering to some degree. The current medical view is that some women are born with a predisposition to endometriosis.

The symptoms are:

- period-like cramp pains which may be quite severe
- heavy bleeding
- inability to conceive
- painful intercourse.

What your doctor can do

To some degree the cause of endometriosis is still somewhat of a mystery, and the choices doctors have at their disposal are limited to drugs and surgery.

- Eliminate the possibility that anything other than endometriosis could be causing the pain, by taking a careful history, examining you and doing routine blood screening. Infection causing PID (pelvic inflammatory disease) must be excluded.
- Drugs such as progestogens and Danazol are able to cause the endometrial tissue to shrink. They work by blocking the action of oestrogen, which seems to be an important factor in the multiplication of endometrial cells. The treatment would need to be continued over several months, and would only mask symptoms. Most of the drugs used do have a list of side-effects, so it is often a question of making a choice between existing symptoms or the drug-induced symptoms. The success rate using drug therapy is in the region of 40 per cent.
- More powerful drugs called gonadotrophic releasing hormone agonists. These hormone suppressing agents switch off the whole menstrual cycle, producing an artificial menopause. They are very effective, but can only be used in severe cases and for a limited period of time. Hot flushes and osteoporosis are inevitable side effects.
- A skilled surgeon may be able to remove the endometrial cells and cysts from the unwanted places in the pelvic cavity by laporoscopy. Laser treatment seems to be equally good at destroying these unwanted

cells as the scalpel. The success rate following surgery is in the region of 80 per cent, double that for drug therapy, but surgery is not without risks.

What you can do

There is no clear benefit from the many branches of complementary therapy, although it is always worth trying new options as research evolves. The nutritional guidelines are very similar to those for fibroids (see page 360).

- Try following a diet high in fibre and low in animal fat, as this may prevent oestrogen surges (see page 446).
- Eating unsalted nuts and seeds contain beneficial essential fatty acids to relieve the pain and inflammation.
- Take supplements of multi-vitamins and minerals, with extra magnesium (300 mg) and evening primrose oil with marine fish oil, for their hormone-regulating and anti-inflammatory potential. Efamol marine fish oil is the purest form, containing *no* trace of heavy metals. Efamol is one of the only brands authorised by Greenpeace for its purity.
- Take a supplement of zinc, a mineral necessary for correct metabolism of essential fatty acids and conversion into hormone-like prostaglandins. Three types of prostaglandin exist – series one, two and three. Series one and three have powerful anti-inflammatory properties, while series two, derived from arachidonic acid potentiate inflammation. Zinc deficiency results in impaired prostaglandin one and three synthesis, therefore increasing inflammation and pain associated with endometriosis.
- Reduce consumption of wheat and bran which contain phytic acid. Phytic acid binds with zinc, inhibiting its absorption.
- Take the amino acid DLPA which is thought to relieve the pain associated with endometriosis. DLPA works by inhibiting the enzymes which normally rapidly inactivate the natural pain-killing endorphins produced by the brain.
- Eat organic foods where possible. Some research has shown a link between pesticides such as dioxin and PCBs which are toxic to the immune system and interfere with hormones.
- Limit meat and dairy products unless they are low fat and preferably organic. These foods contain an abundance of synthetic hormones and antibiotics. Dairy products are also a primary source of arachidonic acid – the precursor to the pro-inflammatory series 2 prostaglandins. The high saturated fat content of many dairy products is a risk factor for excess oestrogen levels in the body.

PELVIC INFLAMMATORY DISEASE

This is a term used to describe inflammation caused by micro-organisms to any of the female organs, including the Fallopian tubes, ovaries, vagina, cervix, endometrium or uterus. The discomfort it causes can vary from none or very little, to in extreme cases substantial pain and a life-threatening situation. It often causes scarring around the organs, and repeated episodes can cause irreversible damage to the Fallopian tubes, a major cause of infertility.

Pelvic inflammatory disease (PID) is common. It is estimated that 10 per cent of women up to the age of 45 have experienced it, and in three out of four of the cases it affects women who are under 25. There are two separate organisms that have been isolated, *Neisseria gonorrhoeae* and *Chlamydia trachomatis*, present in 80 per cent of the cases of PID in women under 25. This clearly means that this condition is sexually trans-mitted. It is most common in promiscuous women who smoke, drink or take recreationsl drugs.

What are the symptoms?

- dull continuous pelvic pain varying from mild to severe
- fever or chills with flu-like symptoms
- increased or changed vaginal discharge in two-thirds of cases (meaning that in one-third of cases there may be no discharge and very few symptoms)
- bleeding between periods, or spotting
- painful periods
- backache
- painful intercourse
- infertility

What your doctor can do

- Exclude the possibility of any other acute problem like an ectopic preg-nancy, where the embryo grows in the Fallopian tube, or appendicitis, through physical examination, urine and blood tests.
- Question you about your sexual behaviour to determine whether you are a likely candidate for PID.
- Perform a cervical smear to determine what sort of organism is growing.
- Treat you with any one of a number of antibiotics, depending on the organism.
- Insist that anyone with whom you have had recent sexual contact be screened too.
- In severe cases where an abscess has developed emergency surgery may be necessary.

As one in four women with proven pelvic inflammatory disease will suffer from either infertility, ectopic pregnancy or chronic pelvic pain as a result of PID, it is vital that treatment be started as soon as it is diagnosed. Remember, in extreme cases PID is a life-threatening condition.

What you can do

- Take the medication prescribed by your doctor religiously.
- Make sure your partner is screened.
- Use a condom.
- If the infection is not clearing with the antibiotics, try taking strong multi-vitamins and mineral, plus 30 mg of zinc per day, for between three and six months.
- Follow the recommendations for The Very Nutritious Diet on page 437.

Complementary therapies

This is one of the times when there is no substitute for a drug. By all means try homeopathic remedies and herbs, but do not rely on them.

OVARIAN CYSTS

An ovarian cyst is a balloon-like structure with a thin wall of cells or fibrous material which contains a liquid jelly-like material. Normally, at the time of ovulation the follicle containing an egg is designed to burst so that the egg can be released. Sometimes, instead, the follicle continues to grow, accumulating fluid and other tissue, and like the ovary itself, it becomes oestrogen producing. Ovarian cysts vary in size, from pea-sized to the size of large oranges, or larger. Some cysts disperse themselves, but others linger on and eventually become surrounded by ovarian tissue.

Single small cysts on the ovaries come and go, usually without being noticed. A large cyst, however, will cause the abdomen to swell, and can be felt on external examination. The majority of cysts are benign (non-cancerous) but approximately five per cent of cysts do become malignant, and your chances of having a malignant cyst increase with age. When a large cyst is present it usually disrupts the menstrual cycle in some way. Apart from the swelling of the abdomen, which could be mistaken for the result of eating a little too much good food, you may notice a change in your menstrual pattern. Either periods become irregular, or disappear completely, and when the cyst is large it is likely that it will put pressure on organs and structures in the vicinity, causing further discomfort, and in the case of the bladder, a desire to urinate frequently.

What your doctor can do

- Feel your abdomen externally, and give you an internal examination. An ultrasound scan will confirm whether one or more cysts are present.
- If the cyst or cysts are small, a wait and see policy may be adopted, in the hope that they disperse themselves anyway. If a large cyst is detected, you will be referred to a surgeon, with a view to having the it dispersed or surgically removed.
- If the cyst is found to be malignant, and it is thought that the cells may have penetrated other structures, it is likely that the Fallopian tube and ovary it is attached to will be removed also as a precautionary measure.

What you can do

- Follow a high fibre and low animal fat diet, as this will help to control oestrogen surges, (see page 446).
- Keep your weight in the normal range, as women who are overweight are more prone to ovarian cysts.
- Possibly take daily supplements of multi-vitamins and magnesium, together with evening primrose oil and marine fish oil. These nutrients have the potential to influence the ovary's response to hormonal signals from the pituitary.
- Introduce naturally occurring plant oestrogens, better known as phytoestrogens into your diet. Phytoestrogen rich foods are predominantly soya, linseeds and pulses (see Phytoestrogen Rich Menu page 480). These compounds have a modulating effect on the body's own supply of oestrogen which is useful for treating any type of hormonal imbalance.
- Take a phytoestrogen rich supplement like Novogen red clover. This provides 40mg of isoflavones which can be taken in conjunction with a phytoestrogen rich diet to help balance hormone levels.
- Take the herbal supplement agnus castus which has been used for centuries for its ability to regulate the menstrual cycle and hormone levels.

Complementary therapies

Herbal medicine and homeopathic remedies are worth a try. See a qualified practitioner, as well as consulting your doctor.

POLYCYSTIC OVARIES

This is a syndrome in its own right, and is characterised by a necklace-like structure of at least ten cysts surrounding each ovary. On an ultrasound scan the ovaries would appear on average to be three times the size of normal. This syndrome was originally associated with women who were of child-bearing age but whose periods had ceased, with an over-growth of hair in unwanted places, and with a tendency to be consider-ably overweight, known as Stein-Leventhal syndrome.

It is now thought that up to 90 per cent of women with infrequent periods and 30 per cent of women whose periods have ceased prema-turely have this syndrome. It has also been suggested that as many as 20 per cent of the normal population have mild polycystic ovarian disease, which can be detected by ultrasound, although in women whose periods are regular it is thought to be in the region of only seven per cent.

What causes it?

- There is undoubtedly an hormonal disturbance in women with poly-cystic ovaries, with an excess of LH (luteinising hormone) from the pituitary and androgens (male hormones).
- The development of obesity is thought to be a precipitating factor.
- Medical conditions where there is an over-production of other hormones may stimulate the ovaries to develop this condition.
- Binge-eating as in bulimia nervosa (see page 184) has also been found to be associated with polycystic ovaries. In one study, published in *The Lancet*, it was discovered that it was rare for bulimics to have a normal ovarian picture on ultrasound. It is thought that the fluctuating levels of the hormone insulin, brought about because of the bingeing, may also stimulate the underlying tendency to polycystic ovaries.

What your doctor can do

- Examine you physically to determine whether there is any other under-lying problem.
- Arrange for you to have an ultrasound scan.
- Suggest that you lose weight, if you are overweight.
- Prescribe the oral contraceptive pill or other hormonal therapy depending on whether you are hoping to conceive or not.
- In severe cases surgery is performed. The current favoured approach is laser or diathermy during a laparoscopy, which aims to pepper the ovarian surface, and is less likely to cause adhesions (fibrous tissues that sticks to other organs).

What you can do

- Lose weight if you are overweight by following The Simple Weight Loss Diet on page 452. This is vital. One study from St Mary's

Hospital in London revealed that even modest weight loss from a low-fat high-fibre diet can correct the hormonal abnormalities, reduce the hirsutism and improve the chances of conceiving. Don't worry if you do not reach an ideal weight. A 6–7 kg (one stone) weight loss can produce a real change in body chemistry.

- Possibly cutting down on wheat (bread, cakes, biscuits and pasta) and relying upon rice, green vegetables and fish, might help hormonal balance.
- Reduce or completely avoid dairy products and use alternatives made from soya, rice, oats and nuts. Follow the Sample phytoestrogen-rich menu on page 480.
- Severely limit your intake of sugar as women with PCOS have a higher risk of developing adult onset diabetes.
- Take a good quality B-complex providing between 50–100mg per tablet. B vitamins are essential for the metabolism of oestrogen in the liver. Magnesium can also be taken in conjunction with the B-complex to help the process.
- Take a supplement of the herb agnus castus which is used successfully in balancing female hormones. The berries contain a wide range of active compounds, including flavonoids.

See also: References.

Peptic Ulcers

Ulcers in the stomach and duodenum are referred to as peptic ulcers. In both conditions there is a break in the important protective lining of the stomach, or the first part of the duodenum. Once breached, the acid from the stomach, the digestive juices and bile from the liver can all irritate the exposed tissues and contribute to the development of a chronic peptic ulcer.

For much of the twentieth century the treatment consisted of dietary change, a variety of antacid medications and surgery. The last ten years has seen nothing short of a revolution in the treatment of peptic ulcers which precipitated a breakthrough in identifying their cause. This work was led by a young gastroenterologist, Dr Barry Marshall, from Perth in Western Australia. As a consequence, highly effective treatment programmes have been developed making surgical treatment nearly a thing of the past.

What are the symptoms?

The symptoms of a peptic ulcer are shared by many other common digestive problems including irritable bowel syndrome and gallstones.

Typically there is pain in the upper abdomen, which may be worse after eating, or worse when the person is hungry. Loss of appetite and weight are more a feature of ulceration in the stomach. Either type of ulcer may bleed with the person vomiting bright red or processed blood. Alternatively processed dark or blackish blood will be passed in the stool. Occasionally the whole illness is silent until the ulcer actually perforates when severe abdominal pain is experienced.

What causes them?

The research of Dr Barry Marshall led to the discovery that peptic ulcers are virtually always associated with the presence of the bacterium *Helicobacter pylori*. The eradication with antibiotics and other drugs leads to resolution of the ulcer and, unlike many other treatments, there is a greatly reduced chance of the ulcer recurring! Approximately 80 per cent of gastric ulcers are complicated by the presence of this bacterium. The infection is often acquired in childhood and may lie dormant for years. Its presence is also associated with a number of other less common types of inflammation of the stomach.

However, important though Helicobacter might be, it is not the only factor and the other long understood one is acid production by the stomach. Very high levels occur in association with duodenal ulcers, and moderately elevated levels with gastric ulceration. If no acid is produced then, ulceration of this type is not a problem. A number of factors either stimulate acid production or damage the protective layer of cells and mucus lining the stomach and duodenum.

- Smoking, alcohol and, to a lesser extent coffee and soft drinks are all associated factors.
- Lower socio-economic status is also a risk factor, and this may simply reflect standards of hygiene or intake of essential nutrients.
- Ulcer-causing drugs like anti-arthritis drugs, aspirin and steroids. They certainly can encourage an existing ulcer to bleed and may contribute slightly to the development of an ulcer in the first place.
- Stress is often blamed, but whilst it may aggravate symptoms it does not cause them.
- Long-term intake of aspirin and other non-steroidal anti-inflammatory (NSAIDs) preparations are associated with a significant increase in the risk of peptic ulcers. The combination of NSAIDs and smoking is particularly harmful.

What your doctor can do

- Assess your symptoms and try to determine the likelihood of there being an ulcer. A chronic ulcer in an older patient requires rather more active treatment.

- Prescribe simple treatment of antacid medicines based upon magnesium or aluminium salts. These may produce rapid relief of pain but the dose often needs to be repeated very frequently. If the symptoms truly subside with this and other simple measures, then it is unlikely that it was a chronic peptic ulcer.
- Arrange for definitive investigations, usually examination of the upper part of the gut by use of a specialised flexible telescope (endoscopy) or a barium meal.
- Test for the presence of *Helicobacter pylori* either from a biopsy at the time of endoscopy, or by a blood test or a new breath test. Its presence alone is not indicative that there is an ulcer present.
- Treat you with powerful antacid medicines called H2 receptor antagonists of which Cimetidine and Ranitidine are two examples (a low dose of the former is now available over the counter from pharmacies in the UK). This treatment is not enough if Helicobacter is present.
- Treat Helicobacter infection with a mixture of antibiotics and H2 receptor antagonist drugs, and sometimes a drug containing bismuth is added.
- Make sure that this germ has been eradicated by repeating the endoscopy or the breath test but not the blood test. This is particularly important if there was a gastric ulcer or if the ulcer had bled.
- Consider surgical treatment for unhealing gastric ulcers or ulcers that have bled repeatedly.

What you can do

Your role is still important, but the advances in medical care have meant that the emphasis on diet for treatment of ulcers has rightly lessened. This doesn't mean you can eat what you like, instead simple sensible measures are worth following, especially in the early stages. Many cases of non-ulcer indigestion may benefit from a change in diet and prevent the need for further investigations.

- Stop smoking as this will greatly improve the response to medical treatment and reduce the chance of recurrence.
- Only consume moderate amounts of alcohol and never on an empty stomach.
- Eat little and often, to minimise the surge of acid with a meal.
- Avoid large amounts of coffee and sugar as there is some evidence that they may stimulate acid production.
- Avoid foods that you feel make it worse. There is too much individual variation, and no set diet is universally successful. It is better to trust your own judgement. Foods to which the odd individual is genuinely

allergic could stimulate the production of acid because of the action of histamine released at the time of an allergic reaction.

- De-stress. If symptoms are severe, some time off work or away may be needed. Take time to consider what lifestyle changes need to be made.
- Chew some liquorice. It contains chemicals that may promote the healing of ulcers. The effect is small and it should not be used by the elderly, those with high blood pressure or kidney problems or fluid retention as it promotes salt and water retention.
- Eating Manuka honey from New Zealand can eradicate *H.pylori* due to its natural antiseptic and antiviral properties. It owes its medicinal properties to the bees feeding on tea tree flowers which are inherently antiseptic. Clinical research has been published in *The Lancet*.
- Aloe vera for its ability to speed healing and reduce pain might be a useful adjunct to the recommended programme.
- Taking a supplement of iron might be necessary to address possible anaemia which occurs with bleeding ulcers. Do not take iron unless anaemia is diagnosed.
- Vitamin A is used to heal and protect the mucous membranes of the stomach and intestines. Take as part of an antioxidant formula containing vitamins C and E for maximum benefit.

Complementary therapies

Again there may be benefit from acupuncture, homeopathy and herbalism, but if you have a proven peptic ulcer make sure you tell your medical specialist what you are doing.

Kay's story

Kay was a happy go lucky 34-year-old play group leader. She really came looking for a diet to help her lose weight. Even though she was only 5ft 3ins, her weight had crept up to 76 kilos, about 18 kilos over her ideal weight. She made light of her other problems which included irregular periods, excessive facial hair growth, fatigue and indigestion. Three years earlier she had been admitted as an emergency because of bleeding from her stomach. Investigation then found that she was bleeding from a duodenal ulcer which had been treated with acid suppressing drugs but not antibiotics.

Clearly she was likely to benefit from a weight-reducing diet but it was likely that there was more than this going on. Blood tests showed a high level of antibodies against the germ *Helicobacter pylori*, suggestive of active or recent infection. There were also mild deficiencies of vitamin B and zinc. Her irregular periods and hair growth were very suggestive of polycystic ovaries.

She began on a weight-reducing low-fat diet, antibiotics for her *Helicobacter* infection and supplements of zinc and multivitamins.

Her 'indigestion' cleared up and she was referred on to a hospital gastroenterologist to make sure that the infection was fully resolved. Falling weight and improved nutritional status may well help her irregular periods but these too may require investigation.

Period Problems

PAINFUL PERIODS

Period pains commonly affect mainly younger women, but not exclusively, as older women may sometimes experience them as well. When periods first begin in early teens, they are usually not painful, but may become so in mid to late teens or later depending upon the reason for the onset of the pain. The development of pain with menstruation is usually taken to indicate the presence of ovulation, the time when the egg is released, within each menstrual cycle.

What causes them?

Period pain or to use the medical term, dysmenorrhoea, most often occurs because of excessive muscle contractions of the uterus with each period.

Four common gynaecological problems may, however, cause the periods to become painful and they include:

- infection of the tubes or ovaries
- fibroids
- endometriosis, where the lining of the womb is found in other tissues such as the wall of the uterus or around the ovaries
- a deficiency of the mineral magnesium, the most commonly deficient nutrient in women of child-bearing age, which is needed for optimum muscle function.

Any woman with excessively painful or heavy periods, in particular if there is pain throughout the month or an irregular menstrual cycle, should see her general practitioner for a gynaecological check-up. A simple examination would normally determine if one of these problems is present.

Often no cause is found and simple dysmenorrhoea is diagnosed. In this situation periods are often painful for the first 24 or 48 hours and perhaps even for the day before the onset of menstruation. Period pains are often felt as mild to severe cramp-like pain or discomfort in the lower abdomen. It can also be felt as low back pain or aching down the legs and, when severe, can be accompanied by giddiness, faintness, nausea and even occasional vomiting. These other symptoms are probably due to the hormonal and chemical changes that occur with menstruation.

Symptoms of premenstrual syndrome such as irritability, mood swings, depression or breast tenderness may also be present, but are not particularly related to the presence of period pains.

Ilana's story

Ilana was a 30-year-old barrister, who had endured severe period pain and vomiting every month for seventeen years.

'It was like someone jerking a knife into my stomach. I'd be doubled over with pain and I'd always have to spend the first day of my period in bed. I experienced nausea and bloating and found it very difficult to function properly at work. I'm a barrister, so I have to be able to think clearly. Taking time off every month was affecting my reputation and career prospects adversely. I had so many symptoms before my period which meant that I was really only normal for seven days each month.

I read about the WNAS and went along to their London clinic. I was asked to follow a very restricted diet initially, which was pretty tough, and to take supplements and to exercise. Within the first month, to my utter amazement I had no pain. The nausea went as well as the bloating, I just couldn't believe it. That was nine years ago, and I haven't had any period problems since. I am able to relax my diet, but I know if I go back to my old ways my symptom will start to return. This programme was a complete cure for me, it totally revolutionised my life. I feel healthy and stable and am extremely grateful to the WNAS.'

What your doctor can do

A variety of treatments already exist that may be helpful, and could be suggested by your doctor when you seek advice.

- *Magnesium check* Measure your red cell magnesium, to see whether you have a deficiency. This is a simple blood test, and should be readily available.
- *Painkillers* Your doctor may recommend the use of certain types of painkillers or hormonal products. Some mild painkillers may not be

very effective for severe pain but a more powerful sort, which are either prescribable *(mefenamic acid-Ponstan)* or are available on the advice of your pharmacist, can be particularly useful. It may be necessary to try a number before finding the most effective one for you.

- *The contraceptive pill* A number of hormonal preparations are available but often the most useful, particularly in young women who require contraception, is to use the oral contraceptive pill. The more modern low dose pills have much fewer side effects than older preparations.
- *Iron* Your doctor can prescribe iron supplements if you are anaemic as well.

What you can do

There are a number of avenues you can explore to help reduce painful periods:

- Physical exercise may sometimes be helpful with a variety of gynaecological problems, and may help your tolerance of pain. Try to exercise three or four times per week. During a painful period try to do some gentle yoga exercises instead of strenuous exercise.
- Heat seems to have a soothing effect. Applying a hot water bottle or a thermal heat pad can be very soothing.
- Changing and improving your diet can help also with minor hormonal abnormalities some of which are thought to underlie such gynaecological problems. Ensuring a well balanced diet without excessive consumption of fatty foods, and with a good intake of fibre from fruit and vegetables may help control hormone metabolism and can reduce some of the excessive hormonal swings that occur during the menstrual cycle.
- Eat a diet rich in EFAs, especially fish oils (see page 489). Women with period pains are known to have a lower intake of these oils, which may have anti-inflammatory, and painkilling properties.
- Some minerals may also be helpful. Magnesium is particularly important in muscle and hormonal functions. Its balance with calcium influences the contraction of uterine muscle and one study suggests that taking supplements may help reduce period pains. Good dietary sources of magnesium include all vegetables, especially green ones, nuts, seeds, beans, peas and lentils. Sugar, sweets, cakes and biscuits are low in most important minerals.
- If your periods are heavy, ensuring a good dietary intake of iron is also important, and this is found in red meat, fish, chicken, eggs, nuts, seeds and vegetarian protein.

Magnesium supplements can be obtained from health-food shops. At the WNAS we tend to use magnesium amino acid chelate. A magnesium rich multi-vitamin, multi-mineral supplement might also be helpful, but too much magnesium may cause loose stools.

Remember if your period pains do not respond to these self help measures or painkillers you must consult with your general practitioner or family planning clinic.

Complementary therapies

When period pain is due to muscular spasm, acupuncture and cranial osteopathy will be obvious choices as they both help to free up pockets of blocked energy in the body. Herbal and homeopathic remedies are also worth a try. If the pain is caused by an infection, this will need to be dealt with by conventional medicine. However, complementary therapy will help to boost the immune system which increases your resistance to infection in the long-term. Often when nutritional deficiencies have been addressed, particularly low magnesium levels, and the muscles are functioning normally, the period pains subside. It may therefore be worthwhile following the advice given in this chapter for a few months before seeking further advice.

HEAVY PERIODS

The average blood loss for each menstrual period is approximately 35 ml, or just over two tablespoons. A heavy period, or menorrhagia as it is technically known, constitutes a loss of 80 ml (just over five tablespoons) of blood loss per period, which is considerably more than average. It is enormously difficult to assess the actual loss of blood during a period. Even studies that counted the number of sanitary towels or tampons that women get through were inaccurate, as it was discovered that women change after collecting differing amounts of blood.

Generally women find that their periods get heavier as they grow older, particularly those who have had children. Flooding can occur in the years leading up to the menopause, resulting in soiled top clothes, as well as underwear. Apart from the sheer embarrassment and hassle of dealing with heavy periods, they can also result in iron deficiency anaemia.

What causes them?

Excessive blood loss at period time is a problem for approximately 10 per cent of menstruating women. Once again there are many possible underlying causes:

- Approaching the menopause, the lining of the uterus can become thicker, resulting in heavier blood loss.
- The presence of fibroids in the uterus can increase the flow of a period.

- A recently fitted IUD can result in heavy periods, which usually settle down after the first few months.
- A hormonal imbalance in the body.
- According to our experience, heavy periods can be caused sometimes by nutritional deficiencies.
- An early miscarriage. Sometimes a woman may conceive without realising, but because it is an unviable pregnancy the body terminates it, in the form of what appears to be a very heavy period.

Alison's story

Alison was a 36-year-old proprietor of a fashion business and mother of three who had experienced irregular, heavy and painful periods all her life.

'My periods had always been irregular heavy or painful, but they became even worse afer I gave birth to my third child. I hated taking painkillers and dreaded the thought of each period. As I was unable to function for several days each month I couldn't keep my mind on my work. I was embarrassed to go out of the house in case I flooded. My GP suggested a hysterectomy, which I wanted to avoid if possible.

I read about the WNAS in Prima *magazine and in desperation contacted them for help. I went on an elimination diet, which involved cutting out certain foods and then gradually re-introducing them to see if I had a bad reaction to them. I discovered that what upset me most were things I ate a lot of, such as wholemeal bread and muesli, and drinking fresh coffee. I was also advised to exercise and to take Optivite, a magnesium-rich multivitamin and mineral supplement, and Efamol evening primrose oil.*

Within four months of following this regime my periods were back to normal, in fact better than they had been for years. No more heavy bleeding and clots, and regular – I could hardly believe it. That was six years ago and my periods have remained regular. I still follow a modified version of my programme and feel extremely well generally. I don't think my success was due to any one thing – but a combination of diet, supplements and increased exercise that worked. I am very grateful to the WNAS for their help as is my husband who says "I am more like my old self again, the girl he married 24 years ago".'

What your doctor can do

If your periods become unmanageably heavy, or you have a sudden episode of flooding you should consult your doctor for advice. After taking a history of the problem, your doctor will:

- Examine you to determine whether there are any fibroids present or any other physical abnormalities – in which case you would then be referred to a gynaecologist who would decide whether you needed minor surgery.
- Take some blood for a serum ferritin test to check whether your iron stores are in fact low, in which case you would need a course of iron.
- Remove your IUD, if you have one, to see whether that alters the flow.
- Prescribe hormone pills to reduce the flow. The first choice for a younger woman might be the oral contraceptive pill, failing that, Duphaston, a progestogen preparation; and if that fails to work, then Danazol, which has considerable side-effects.
- Prescribe tranexamic acid a drug that helps excessive bleeding. It can be more effective than hormones.
- Suggest a hysterectomy, which should be regarded as a last resort (see page 243).

What you can do

- Eat plenty of green leafy vegetables, red meat (organic/additive-free), free-range eggs and other foods rich in iron.
- Take a good strong multi-vitamin and mineral supplement, with extra B vitamins and magnesium
- Take at least 500mg of vitamin C with bioflavanoids together with an iron supplement to enhance its absorption.
- Avoid too much wheat and bran which contain phytic acid, a compound which inhibits iron absorption.
- Rest when the flow is heavy, and avoid important social engagements until the bleeding has reduced.

Complementary therapies

Try herbal medicine or homeopathy. If your periods are exceedingly heavy, it is better to consult an expert rather than attempting to self-treat.

IRREGULAR OR ABSENT PERIODS

Women were designed to have regular periods, somewhere between every 23 and 35 days, which end a cycle or 'failed conception'. Each month the body should release eggs whose job it is to find a sperm to merge with. When this fails, a period arrives, approximately some two weeks later. After the first year, periods usually establish a pattern, which become the normal cycle, and for many this continues until they reach their menopause. Others experience irregular periods, or an absence of periods altogether, which means they are not releasing eggs (see Painful Ovulation page 355).

What causes them?

The medical term for an absence of periods is amenorrhoea, and there are two types. Primary amenorrhoea is when no period ever arrives, which is rare, and secondary amenorrhoea, is when periods have 'disappeared' for in excess of four cycles. Primary amenorrhoea may be associated with late puberty or a defect in the hormone and reproductive system, and there is little that can be done to correct that. There are many underlying causes of secondary amenorrhoea though, most of which can be addressed. Your periods can become irregular or disappear because of:

- Pregnancy and breast-feeding – but this is perfectly normal. Very often when fully breast-feeding, periods will not return for between six months to a year.
- Sudden weight loss due to any illness, including the slimmers' disease, anorexia nervosa.
- Over-exercising. Athletes and ballet dancers often develop amenor-rhea, and as a result, decreased oestrogen levels, which greatly increase their chances of developing osteoporosis later in life.
- Episodes of extreme stress, e.g. bereavement or divorce.
- Undetected and therefore untreated thyroid disease.
- Anaemia and monitored deficiencies, especially of vitamin B.
- Long-term medication.

Susan's story

Susan was the first woman in Britain to break 70 minutes for the half marathon, in 1988. She is a well known Olympic marathon and cross country runner who, with her twin sister, has been training since the age of 20. Her periods stopped for ten years as her diet did not meet her energy requirements.

'Both my sister and I have discovered that we were at risk of having osteoporosis. When we began our training long-term damage didn't really seem relevant to us then. We felt fit and healthy and had the chance of going to the Olympics. At that time it would have been hard to persuade us about a possible risk in 30 years time.

I was conscious that I was a little on the plump side for a runner, and as I ran better when I was lighter I paid far too much attention to dieting. Looking back I realise that I was not eating an adequate diet to meet my energy output, and was certainly not consuming anything like enough calcium in my diet. I'm 5ft 4 in tall, and at one point weighed as little as 46.8 kg (7st. 5lbs). My weight was so low that my periods stopped for ten years, which I now know would have reduced my oestrogen levels, and increased my chances of getting osteoporosis. I used to eat fruit only for breakfast, a scone for lunch and a slice of quiche and salad with fruit for my evening meal.

I sometimes felt pretty weak, and I became very susceptible to injury. In my career I have experienced three stress fractures in my legs, with a fourth suspected. Because of this record the British Olympic Association included both myself and my twin sister in a bone-scanning survey that they were conducting. We were both found to be at risk of osteoporosis and put on a course of HRT and calcium. My sister came off HRT after the first course, but I stuck it out for six or eight months before giving up. I felt bloated, moody and my running was impaired whilst on the HRT, but once off it my running performance improved again.

I was due to compete in the Commonwealth Games in Auckland in 1990 but had to pull out because of a stress fracture, and at that point I realised that I would have to call a halt to my running career.

I got married in 1991 to Geoff who is also an international marathon runner and after eating a better diet, my periods returned and we managed to produce twins. I am delighted to say that a recent test showed that my bone mass has improved and I no longer have signs of osteoporosis.

If I had my time again I would undoubtedly have eaten more sensibly, and I would not encourage a young female athlete to diet as we did.

I still run 40 miles per week, and work as a PE teacher in Nottingham. I have improved my diet, and I now take Efecal with the hope that I can maintain my new bone mass.'

What your doctor can do

If your periods haven't arrived by the age of sixteen or seventeen it is time to ask your doctor for some advice. You will need to be investigated by your doctor initially, and subsequently by an endocrinologist.

If you had established periods, but they have since disappeared there are a number of things your doctor can do:

- Check to see whether you are pregnant.
- If you are taking prescribed drugs – assess your programme to see whether they are interrupting your cycle.
- Take blood to check your thyroid and iron levels.
- Assess the function of your pituitary gland, which is responsible for hormone function.
- Refer you for gynaecological investigation to check that your ovaries are functioning, and that there are no other obvious problems.

What you can do

- Follow the recommendations for A Very Nutritious Diet on page 437.
- Take regular vitamin and mineral supplements.
- Introduce naturally occurring plant oestrogens, better known as phytoestrogens into your diet. Phytoestrogen rich foods are predominantly soya, linseeds and pulses (see Phytoestrogen-rich menu page 480). These compounds have a modulating effect on the body's own supply of oestrogen which is useful for treating any type of menstrual irregularities.
- Take a phytoestrogen-rich supplement like Novogen red clover. This provides 40mg of isoflavones which can be taken in conjunction with a phytoestrogen rich diet to help balance hormones.
- Take the herbal supplement agnus castus which has been used for centuries for its ability to regulate the menstrual cycle. The first major clinical study on the use of agnus castus was published in 1954 showing positive results on women with menstrual irregularities and even amenorrhea. It is the fruit of the agnus castus which contains essential oils, glycosides and flavonoids.
- Get some help with sorting out any stressful situations that face you or counselling if you are bereaved or recently separated or divorced.
- If you are an athlete, a professional dancer or an exercise addict, work hard to ensure that you are meeting your calorie requirements.
- If your weight is low for your height and frame, actively work to increase your weight to the optimum range.

Complementary therapies

Many complementary therapies would be worth investigating. Consult a qualified homeopath or medical herbalist, as they will certainly have numerous remedies for you to try. A burst of acupuncture wouldn't go amiss, as acupuncture is very good at unblocking the energy channels in the body.

See also: Standard references and Recommended reading.

Peripheral Vascular Disease

Just as the blood vessels supplying the heart muscle can become narrowed, so can the main arteries to the legs. The blood vessels in the upper limbs are almost never affected in this way; consequently all the symptoms relate to below the waistline. ·

What are the symptoms?

The first symptom is usually pain in the calf on exercise. The pain is often severe, causes the sufferer to stop walking or to walk with a limp, and clears after a few minutes' rest. This clinical picture is called intermittent claudication (limping). Cold feet, changes to the skin colour, loss of hairs on the legs and in men loss of the ability to have an erection are other features.

What causes it?

Essentially much the same factors as for ischaemic heart disease and atherosclerosis apply. Smoking, an elevated blood cholesterol and diabetes are the three most important and treatable factors. Increasing age is also important too.

What your doctor can do

Anyone presenting with intermittent leg pains on walking, that clears with rest, should be assessed for the main risk factors for atherosclerosis.

Examination of the legs and abdomen will give a good idea of the severity of the disease. Those with severe symptoms, absent pulses in the feet, and younger patients may need specialist assessment. Surprisingly accurate assessment of the degree of atherosclerotic narrowing can be made from measuring the blood pressure levels in the leg, and the from the use of an ultrasound pulse detector.

In those in whom major disease is suspected then specialist x-rays to look at the blood vessels can be undertaken. From this the appropriateness of surgical correction can be ascertained.

Drug treatments are not very effective at all. More important is control of elevated blood fats, both cholesterol and triglycerides. These latter can contribute to atherosclerosis and are more important in peripheral vascular disease than in coronary artery disease. Being overweight, drinking alcohol or consuming sugar to excess, or being diabetic raises this type of fat greatly. Combined drug and dietary treatment is known to control the elevated fats and can even reverse the atherosclerotic process if followed assiduously.

What you can do

- Stop smoking completely.
- Walk, walk, walk! Painful though exercise might be, it helps to keep open the existing blood vessels. Daily walks to the limit of exercise tolerance are mandatory.
- Lose weight if you are overweight.

- Follow The Very Nutritious Diet (see page 437), keeping the total fat content very low.
- Take supplements of vitamin E, at least 300 IU per day. These are prescribable on the National Health in the UK and are of proven benefit even though in coronary heart disease their benefit is uncertain.
- Other supplements might be helpful but this is not certain. Multivitamins, anti-oxidants such as vitamin C and selenium and the trace element chromium look like the best bets.

Complementary therapies

Acupuncture and herbalism might be able to encourage the opening up of blood vessels. Worth a try, but don't rely on them.

See also: Standard references.

Preconception

When a couple decide to have a family they are taking on one of the most important jobs in the world, so they must be in good health to ensure a healthy baby.

The ova, female eggs, and sperm may be adversely affected by inadequate diet, and by social and environmental factors. The egg is at its most vulnerable for about 100 days leading up to ovulation, the time when it is released, and sperms are also particularly vulnerable for approximately 116 days before they mature. So eating well, having a wholesome lifestyle and environment will contribute to the health of the next generation. It's an awesome task, and one that requires careful planning *at least four months* before conception.

What your doctor can do

- Check your serum ferritin levels if you suffer with fatigue, have pale skin and heavy periods. This will determine whether you have low iron stores.
- Check to see whether you are up-to-date with your rubella immunisations. It is important to be immune to German measles because it can cause so much irreversible damage to an unborn child if contracted in the first few weeks of pregnancy.
- Arrange for you to have a thorough check up to ensure:
  - your blood pressure is in the normal range
  - you are free of diabetes
  - you have no pelvic problems
  - you have no vaginal or bladder infections

- ○ you are not an HIV carrier
- ○ you do not have any sexually transmitted disease.
- Remove an IUD if you have one. This needs to be done at least six months before you plan to conceive. An IUD can also increase the risk of vaginal infection.
- Advise on medication. Ideally you should not be taking any medication during pregnancy that is not absolutely necessary. If you are taking prescribed drugs, discuss the situation with your doctor to see whether there is any need for you to reduce your medication or to switch to an alternative prior to trying for a baby.
- Prescribe supplements that contain folic acid and vitamin B 12 to help prevent neural tube defects (see page 386).

What you can do

Here are some simple dietary recommendations which should be followed in order to help achieve an adequate intake of all the essential nutrients. This is especially important in the preconceptual phase and in the first twelve weeks of pregnancy as it determines the growth and development of your baby.

- Eat three regular meals a day. Doing so will give you the best chance of obtaining a balanced intake of all essential nutrients. Do not miss meals.
- Eat one cooked main meal per day. Cooked meat, fish or vegetable based meals will again allow a good intake of essential nutrients, especially protein.
- Eat at least one portion (120g/4oz) of meat or fish or vegetarian protein, such as beans, peas or lentils. Many convenience or prepared meals are low in protein, vitamins and minerals.
- Ensure a good intake of foods rich in folic acid, including green leafy vegetables, fortified breakfast cereals, oranges and orange juice, eggs, almonds and sweetcorn. You can eat cooked liver once a month if you wish until you are pregnant, when you should stop.
- Enjoy good sources of calcium, including dairy products, milk (whole, skimmed or semi-skimmed) and cheese, but avoid soft cheese and cottage cheese. Soft cheese may contain the infecting organism Listeria, and cottage cheese is low in protein and B vitamins.
- Eat at least three portions of fruit per day, and two portions of green leafy vegetables or green salad per day. This is in line with the latest recommendations for healthy eating for the general population, and will help maintain a good intake of fibre, vitamins and minerals.
- Eat two or three slices of wholemeal bread per day. White bread may be acceptable if the rest of the diet is well balanced. Some will need

more bread than others, and those on weight-reducing diets may need to consume less.

- Use good quality vegetable oils, which are high in essential fatty acids, especially sunflower, safflower, rapeseed and walnut. Olive oil is not rich in essential fatty acids. Use margarines based on these oils, e.g. sunflower, or you can use a small amount of butter. Again cut down on these if you need to lose weight.
- Eat from a selection of foods rich in essential fatty acids. These include oily fish like mackerel, herring, salmon, pilchards and sardines, and walnuts, almonds, hazelnuts, pecans (peanuts are not so nutritious in this respect) and beans, especially pinto beans.
- Trim the skin and fat from meat and poultry. These tend to be high in the less helpful saturated fats, and most of the environmental toxins, if present, will be found in the fatty portions of them.
- Get your partner to follow the same dietary recommendations. The health of the father-to-be can also be a factor in the health of your future offspring.

Current thinking on nutritional supplements

Many multi-vitamins from chemists are not suitable for the preconceptual phase as they contain animal vitamin A (retinol) and inadequate amounts of folic acid (not enough to prevent neural tube defects). However, in recent years, research demonstrating the need for extra folic acid and vitamin B12 during the preconceptual phase, and the first trimester of pregnancy, has resulted in a number of new products arriving on the shelves.

- Folic acid alone, at a strength of 400 mcg, is now widely available, and is recommended to be taken by all women prior to conception. The research shows that when this is taken with vitamin B12, the protection against developing a neural tube defect is even greater.
- A much higher dose of folic acid, 4 mg, is recommended for those women who have already given birth to a child with a neural tube defect and wish to conceive again.
- Pregnavite-Forte is NHS preparation designed for women who have already given birth to a child with a neural tube defect.

A preconceptual programme

- If you have been taking the contraceptive pill you will need to stop six months before you plan to conceive. The pill can interfere with essential vitamin and mineral levels.
- Use natural methods of contraception during your preconceptual programme. Getting to know your body and learning to recognise when you are ovulating will help you in the long term to know when it is right to conceive.

- Follow the diet plan outlined above for at least four months before conception, and get your partner to follow a similar diet, perhaps eating extra quantities if he is larger than you.
- Take care to avoid all the foods and drinks which have been shown to impede the absorption of good nutrients or might harm your chances of a healthy baby (see page 390).
- Do not consume any alcohol. This is probably the best advice, though it is obviously hard for some to follow. You should not drink from about day ten of your cycle until when your period begins, when your egg is at its most vulnerable. Ideally both you and your partner should avoid drinking alcohol. At most, consume no more than three units per week.
- You should spend at least four months in a smoke-free environment. That means that neither you nor your partner should be smoking, and you should avoid smoky atmospheres.
- Take a multi-vitamin and mineral supplement that contains 400 mcg of folic acid and vitamin B12 but not vitamin A (as retinol). The pharmacy or health-food shop will be able to show you the range of products now available.
- If either you or your partner are concerned about your nutritional status, you could contact one of the organisations listed in the Women's Health section of the Appendix to arrange for appropriate blood tests.
- Take three or four good sessions of exercise per week, and try to get outdoors as often as possible, especially when it is sunny.
- If either you or your partner use street drugs you will need to stop, either with the support of each other if it's a social habit, or with the help of a clinic if you are addicted.
- Avoid chemicals wherever possible. You should:
  - use lead-free petrol
  - use ecologically safe cleaning creams at home
  - avoid using aerosols
  - avoid using any chemicals if you are a keen gardener or grow vegetables
  - eat organic food where possible
  - avoid sitting for too long in front of a VDU on a regular basis
  - not use copper or aluminium saucepans
  - only use the microwave for reheating or defrosting
  - keep away from busy main roads – if you live on one try to move
  - not spray pets with chemicals to prevent fleas
  - avoid paint which contains lead, and should not sleep in a freshly painted room
  - not use a sunbed whilst you are pregnant
  - use a hot water bottle to heat your bed rather than an electric blanket
  - sort out areas of stress in your personal and work life before you conceive.

Once you have conceived, you will need to continue with a healthy regime throughout your pregnancy. Refer to Pregnancy (see below), for extra help and advice. Additionally, we now know that the type of diet our babies are fed during the first year of life will also play a major role in determining their long-term health prospects, so adopting a sound weaning plan thereafter is advisable.

See also: What's wrong with present-day diet and lifestyle?, Nutrition is the key to health, References, Recommended reading (*Healthy Parents, Healthy Baby*).

Pregnancy

The effect that diet, environment and lifestyle before and during pregnancy have on our unborn children should never be underestimated. Research shows quite clearly that we can 'programme' the health of a baby and influence its growth and development, at least four months before it is even conceived (see Preconception, page 384), and during the first three to four months of pregnancy. We can affect the shape and size of the baby, the health of its important little organs, its intelligence in later life, and even its fingerprints!

Examples of how our diet and lifestyle can influence the unborn are many.

- Babies who are small for their dates are likely to have high blood pressure in later life and have a different fingerprint pattern to normal weight babies.
- Low birth-weight babies are seven times more likely to develop blood sugar problems or get diabetes than babies whose weight is in the normal range.
- Impaired lung growth during the developmental stages and early infant life, due to inadequate nutrition and environmental conditions, point to potential abnormal lung function and increased chances of suffering bronchitis, asthma and chronic chest infections.

There is enough new evidence to convince even the most sceptical amongst us that diet and environmental factors influence the well-being of the unborn child not only in infancy, but also in adult life.

From the time of conception, each minute bodily system has its own timetable for development, and the supply of essential nutrients and timing of contact with a toxin, will determine the type of damage that results. According to relatively recent research data, babies who are undernourished in the first four weeks of development stand a much higher chance of developing heart disease, a major cause of death in middle age, and brain disorders, present from birth, which show up later in life in one in eight adults.

Low birth-weight babies, those born at term who weigh under 2.5 kg (5.5 lbs), if they survive, suffer higher rates of childhood illness, and stand a greater chance of being mentally retarded, of suffering from cerebral palsy, behaviour disorders, impaired vision or deafness.

Dietary requirements

Despite the fact that many of us feel incredibly hungry during pregnancy, our actual requirement for extra calories does not increase significantly in the first six months, and only by an additional 10-20 per cent during the last three months of pregnancy. What does increase is our need for good quality, nutrient-dense foods, which are rich in folic acid, vitamin B12, EFAs, and the mineral zinc and iron in particular (see below).

We experience the largest demand for nutrients during pregnancy and breast-feeding. Besides looking after yourself, you have the needs of a growing baby to meet, as well as the increased tissue of the uterus, placenta and blood. All this new tissue requires more calories, proteins, vitamins and minerals.

It is normal to gain nearly 12.5 kg (27–28 lb) during pregnancy, but weight gain can vary depending on individual metabolic rate. Some women hardly notice any change in appetite, whilst others feel like they are eating for an army! Studies show that women who gain in excess of 13.5 kg (30 lb) during pregnancy have significantly more healthy babies. Slim women, who only experience a small weight gain, can have babies with a low birth weight. You should be eating enough to gain weight at the rate of 225–450g (1/2–1 lb) per week, unless you are overweight.

- Folic acid deficiency and vitamin B12 insufficiency are now clearly linked to neural tube defects.
- Zinc deficiency during pregnancy has been linked with low birth weight, under 2.5 kg (5.5 lb).
- Vitamin A is another nutrient linked to growth, and in fact it has long been recommended by the Department of Health in the UK, that all pregnant and breastfeeding mothers take supplements of vitamin A as beta-carotene the non-animal source (not as retinol) as well as vitamins D and C, in order to build up vitamin stores that can then be passed across the placenta.
- Essential fatty acids (EFAs) are vital for growth and development of the baby, particularly for the brain and the central nervous system. Recent research suggests that a deficiency of these long-chain polyunsaturated fatty acids in the tissues of growing babies results in low birth weight,

which may have life-long implications. We now know too that adequate intakes of EFAs in the new-born infant seem to influence vision and subsequent intelligence.

Babies born after an apparently normal pregnancy often have borderline levels of EFAs, as do premature babies. Breast milk, from a well-nourished mother, is a good source of EFAs, which probably explains why some breast-fed infants make better progress than bottle-fed ones. Trials feeding Efamol Marine (a combination of evening primrose and marine fish oils) to pregnant women during the final three months of pregnancy have produced raised EFA levels in newborn babies. Good sources of essential fatty acids can be found on page 489.

Sadly, many of these important medical facts, which undoubtedly affect the welfare of our unborn children, are kept almost as trade secrets. The health and well-being of your growing baby is undoubtedly in your hands and, with a little knowledge, there are many positive steps that you can take to ensure your baby has the best possible chance in life.

What your doctor can do

- Give regular checks to ensure that the growth of the baby is on target, and that you are in good health.
- Prescribe iron supplements, should your levels drop below the normal range.
- Offer screening facilities for prospective mums who are either at risk or over 35 years of age.
- Refer you to a specialist if there are any concerns during your pregnancy.

What you can do

- *Eat a wide variety of nutritious foods* The best are those rich in protein, such as lean meat (preferably additive-free or organic), fish, free-range chicken, nuts, seeds, peas, beans and lentils. Foods that are particularly nutritious and should be consumed regularly through pregnancy are:
  ○ lean meat
  ○ eggs, preferably free-range
  ○ all green vegetables
  ○ wheatgerm
  ○ nuts
  ○ wholemeal bread (up to three slices per day)
  ○ fortified breakfast cereal.

- *Include vegetable rather than animal fats* Use polyunsaturated margarines and cold-pressed oils, rather than animal fats which are high in saturated fats and low in essential nutrients. Beware of seemingly healthy vegetable fats that contain hydrogenated vegetable oils. These fats have been chemically altered to make them stable at room temperature, and have the same adverse effects as saturated fat. Trim any visible fat from meat or poultry and don't eat the skin.

- *Eat plenty of foods containing calcium and other good nutrients* Dairy products such as milk, yoghurt and cheese are all important sources of calcium. So too are the small bony fish like whitebait, sprats and sardines and nuts, seeds and green vegetables. Aim for 300-600 ml (1/2-1 pint) of milk and yoghurt per day, and 175–225 g (6–8 oz) of cheese per week.

- *Feast on organic salad, vegetables and fruit* Aim to eat a salad daily, plus three portions of vegetables, including one green leafy vegetable, and at least two portions of fruit each day. These are important sources of vitamins, minerals and fibre.

- *Don't use pregnancy as an excuse to pig out on sweet food* Many women develop cravings for sweet foods during pregnancy, and use their lost waistline as an excuse to indulge. Sweet food, like puddings, cake or chocolate are permissible, but only in addition to nutritious food. Sweet foods are normally a very low source of good nutrients, and should never replace wholesome food. As long as you are not overweight to start with, have your treats after meals.

- *Increase fruit juice, and reduce tea* It is vital to make the most of all the dietary iron during pregnancy, as your growing baby will be steadily stocking up on iron to last through the first few months of life. Drinking tea, which contains tannin that binds with iron from vegetable protein, will reduce the amount of iron that you are able to absorb by about half. Choosing citrus fruit juices, like orange or grapefruit, which are rich in vitamin C, you will approximately double the iron that is available to both you and your baby. Other foods and drinks rich in vitamin C are listed on page 486.

- *Use tea and coffee substitutes* You will see from the list of alternatives on page 7 that there are many different varieties to try. It is worth noting that Rooibosch/Redbush Tea, which is a caffeine-free tea lookalike, has shown positive results in South African trials on babies with colic. It contains a mild muscle relaxant. Raspberry tea could be consumed before delivery as it is thought to relax the perineum.

- Raspberry leaf tea helps with uterine contractions. It is available loose and in tea bag form. Consumption should be limited to one cup a day.

- Morning sickness can be alleviated by chewing on crystallised ginger or drinking an infusion of root ginger in boiling water.

- *There's nothing better than regular exercise* Sticking to a regular exercise routine during pregnancy will help to keep you feeling healthy and will tone your body for the delivery. The endorphin release which results from exercise (see page 32) not only raises your mood, but also that of your baby. Research has shown that endorphins cross the placenta, and the baby is therefore able to share your sense of well-being!
- *Continue with all the relevant steps in the Preconceptual Programme* (See page 386). Avoid alcohol, cigarettes, street drugs plus environmental chemicals and hazards.

Potential dangers during pregnancy

There are a number of bugs which can be very dangerous, particularly during pregnancy. Avoid them and the foods that might harbour them at all costs.

Listeriosis

Even in a mild form, listeriosis can cause miscarriage, severe illness in a newborn baby, or a still birth. It presents as a flu-like illness that is caused by the *Listeria monocytogenes* bug, found in some common foods. It is therefore imperative to avoid:

- Roquefort, Stilton and other blue-veined cheeses.
- Unpasteurised cheese such as Camembert and Brie or dairy products including goat and sheep's products.
- Liver pâté of any type.
- Cook-chill meals. These are ready-cooked, and kept cold, but not frozen, and are designed to be eaten cold or reheated at home. Preferably avoid them altogether, or cook them until they are piping hot to kill off the listeria.
- Undercooked meat of any description.
- Pre-prepared salads.
- Soft ice-cream from a machine.
- Food that is past its best-before date.

Salmonella

This is a bacteria responsible for more food poisoning than any other, and manifests itself in sickness and diarrhoea. Poultry and eggs are probably the most common foods to be contaminated with Salmonella, but thorough cooking often eliminates it.

- Don't eat anything that contains raw or uncooked egg, and don't forget less obvious foods like mousse and mayonnaise.
- Only eat eggs that have been cooked so thoroughly that the egg yolk is hard.

- Always wash your hands thoroughly if you have been touching raw meat, especially poultry.
- Don't let raw meat come into contact with any other food. This includes any spillage that may occur in the fridge.
- Use a special board to prepare meat and poultry, kept only for that purpose. Scrub it very thoroughly with hot water after use, and do the same with any surface touched.
- Cook all meat and poultry thoroughly so that the bacteria are destroyed.

Toxoplasmosis

This is again a flu-like illness, which is caused by an infection by the bug called *Toxoplasma gondii*, sometimes found in raw meat, especially lamb, and also in cat faeces. As it can affect the unborn child it is important to take precautions.

- Never eat undercooked or raw meat.
- Wash your hands thoroughly after preparing meats.
- Wash all food preparation surfaces with very hot water or bleach.
- Clean and scrub all vegetables thoroughly to ensure that all soil and dirt is removed. If cats have soiled the earth, food can be contaminated.
- Don't let your cat have kittens at the time you plan to be pregnant, as kittens carry toxoplasmosis.
- Clear up cat mess with boiling water or bleach.

Unpasteurised milk

Milk that has not been heat-treated may contain bugs that are harmful to health. Avoid 'green top' unpasteurised, or any milk that has not been heat-treated, from the time you start to plan your baby, until you have finished breast-feeding.

Current thinking on nutritional supplements

There is broad medical agreement that supplements containing 400 mcg of folic acid and possibly vitamin B12 should be taken for four months prior to conception, until the end of the twelfth week of pregnancy, in order to prevent neural tube defects. However, opinions vary about what to do after that.

If you are eating an exceptionally healthy diet, which includes organic produce, and drinking very little tea, coffee or alcohol, then the chances are that you will be getting many of the nutrients that you and your baby need. However, if you have a poor appetite, have an unplanned pregnancy, or have not been eating very well, then as a precaution it would be advisable to take a multi-vitamin and mineral supplement, without animal vitamin A (retinol), each day anyway. It is far better to err on the side of caution.

Additionally, recent research shows that it may be advisable for some women to take supplements of evening primrose oil and marine fish oil for the last three months of pregnancy and during breast feeding. Another study on breast-feeding mothers using Efamol evening primrose oil from between two to eight months of feeding, showed improved levels of essential fatty acids at a time when the natural supply in the milk would be tailing off.

The mineral zinc plays a fundamental role in the health of the foetus. Zinc is also useful to reduce the risk and of stretch marks and speed healing. According to Dr Neil Ward at the University of Surrey, deficiencies of zinc have been linked to low birth weight babies with a smaller head circumference.

Knowing that you can influence the health prospects of your new child may be rather daunting. There are countless rewards, though, to be had if you prepare your body for pregnancy and look after yourself to the best of your ability whilst pregnant. Creating a new little person is such a miracle, it's important to ensure that you are well enough to savour it, and that you do all in your power to enhance the miracle rather than damage it inadvertently.

See also: References and Recommended reading (*Healthy Parents, Healthy Baby*).

Premenstrual Syndrome (PMS)

Premenstrual syndrome, or PMS as it is more commonly known, is a collection of symptoms that occur up to two weeks before the menstrual period and tail off as bleeding begins. For many women it brings with it fear, misery and incapacitation. Sufferers often describe it as the Jekyll and Hyde Syndrome, which comes upon them relentlessly at a similar time each month.

One of the difficulties of PMS is that it is not a syndrome which shows up under the microscope. Furthermore, despite the fact that women have been suffering for centuries, to this day doctors are unable to agree on the cause. Whilst some schools of thought class it as a hormone imbalance, others feel that it is associated with brain chemical metabolism, or indeed is actually all in the mind!

The WNAS have spent many years researching premenstrual syndrome, and our conclusions show that although all of these hypotheses are partially correct, the underlying factor is related to nutritional and lifestyle inadequacies which, once corrected, result in relief from symptoms within a matter of months for over 90 per cent of sufferers.

What are the symptoms?

The symptoms of PMS are always cyclic, and there are of some 150 variations. The most common 'mental' symptoms include:

- anxiety
- irritability
- mood swings
- nervous tension

- depression
- confusion
- forgetfulness
- crying and loss of libido.

Some of the most common physical symptoms include:

- breast tenderness
- headaches

- cravings for sweet food
- abdominal bloating and fatigue.

According to one WNAS survey 73 per cent of women of child-bearing age suffer with PMS, and over half of all sufferers have experienced suicidal feelings at some time premenstrually. In addition many women report feeling violent and aggressive during their premenstrual phase, lashing out physically, and verbally abusing their partners and children. Productivity at work is effected by as many as five days per month, and working sufferers often organise their calendar around this monthly nightmare.

Judy's story

Judy was a 36-year-old mother of two who had been working part-time as a secretary until she was knocked sideways by her uncontrollable premenstrual syndrome.

'I didn't suffer from PMS until my second child was born. Even then I didn't realise what the problem was. I knew that PMS could cause bloating and breast tenderness but I thought the other symptoms were in my head – I thought I was going mad.

I'm normally a calm person but for two or three days a month I became a madwoman – especially at night when I couldn't sleep. I'd scream, swear, smash milk bottles and slam doors. My physical strength was frightening. I'd rip towels apart, and once I tied a nylon comb into a knot. I felt my brain was going to burst. I'd even punch and kick my husband, Robert, when he was asleep. I tried to slash my wrists and, when I took an overdose of tranquillisers, I bit right through Robert's thumb as he was trying to get them out of my mouth.

I just couldn't control my emotions. I'd pinch myself until I was bruised, cut my skin with glass and bang my head against the wall, then spend hours crying. I felt ugly and worthless, convinced my husband didn't love me. But he didn't know what to do with me. Confused he'd just sit and stare into space while I was ranting.

When I yelled the kids huddled in bed together, crying – sometimes my husband had to take them out at night to get them away from me. Then when my son Steven was eleven he developed pains in his stomach and a twitch in his eye. He was referred to a paediatrician and eventually to a child psychiatrist. During the fifth visit Steven announced 'I'm scared Mummy's going to kill herself, or leave me!' I felt awful. I thought 'I've done this to him'. I knew then I needed help.

By chance, a few days later I read about a woman with PMS who'd stabbed her husband and for the first time I realised just how extreme PMS could be. When I read she was cured by diet I was disappointed – I'd tried the popular remedies like evening primrose oil and vitamin B6 and they hadn't helped. I didn't see a doctor as I didn't want to admit I wasn't in control but Robert urged me to try the diet so I contacted the WNAS. They told me I was one of the worst cases they'd had. I had every symptom of PMS.

They put me on a diet of fresh fruit and veg, meat, fish, corn and rice, plus nutritional supplements. I could drink only mineral water or herbal tea. It was tough but worth it. At the end of the third month I wrote in my diary: 'No PMS!' I was finally free after ten years of hell.

I began re-introducing foods to check my reaction and that's when I found caffeine had been the culprit. I used to drink 6–8 cups of coffee a day and I craved chocolate before a period.

I haven't had PMS since. I feel I've been reborn – the diet saved my marriage and my kids. We're all so close now, but I really believe if I hadn't had help Brian would have left with the kids and I'm sure I'd have committed suicide. PMS would have killed me one way or another. I've taken up amateur dramatics again. I'm now writing a book about my experiences in the hope it'll save other women from the same nightmare.'

What causes it?

A hormonal cycle requiring production of oestrogen and progesterone by the ovaries is necessary for the development of PMS. However, contrary to early theories, there is rarely a lack of either of these two hormones in the average PMS sufferer.

Research has shown us that over 50 per cent of women with PMS have low levels of magnesium, which is a mineral vital for normal brain chemical metabolism, hormone function and smooth-muscle control (the uterus and the gut are both smooth muscles). Other nutrients like B vitamins, zinc and essential fatty acids may also be in short supply.

Women often go through episodes in their lives that place extra nutritional demand on their bodies. Pregnancy and breast-feeding are two classic examples, where Mother Nature has deemed that the baby is served with nutrients first in order to develop and the mum is second in the queue. Therefore symptoms of PMS commonly get worse after pregnancy or weaning, or indeed may occur for the first time in a mother who is suffering with nutritional depletion.

Our bodies have very specific nutritional requirements. Just as our cars would not run well lacking oil or petrol, the brain will not be able to send out correct messages, and hormones will not be produced in adequate amounts at the appropriate time of the cycle, when levels of important nutrients are at a low ebb.

The WNAS programme, which successfully helps the majority of women over their PMS, is designed to redress the balance, by putting back into the body what time and nature have taken out. In the short term it will undoubtedly involve making certain dietary sacrifices until nutritional levels have been restored and symptoms abated, but the general consensus is that the medium- to long-term plan is immensely enjoyable.

In addition to making dietary adjustments, the WNAS programme consists of taking regular exercise, and scientifically based supplements (at least in the short term) that act as a nutritional prop.

What your doctor can do

Although many experts now believe that the nutritional approach to PMS is the best first-line treatment, the majority of doctors remain uneducated. According to a WNAS survey, 92 per cent of general practitioners have little or no nutritional training. Therefore what is on offer from your doctor is likely to be more drug or hormone oriented.

Hormone treatments

Many of the hormone treatments for PMS were designed on the premise that this syndrome was associated with a lack of a particular hormone, but research over the last decade had shown that this is not so. However, when artificial hormones either abolish or suppress normal hormone function it is likely that they may influence PMS symptoms. Whilst some hormone treatments may suppress symptoms, they do not address the root cause and thus alleviate symptoms in the long term. Additionally, most hormone treatments produce significant side effects, presenting the sufferer with additional hurdles.

398 THE NATURAL HEALTH BIBLE

Progesterone

This is one of the two main hormones produced by the ovaries, and is used by many doctors as a pessary inserted into the vagina. It was once one of the commonest medical treatments for PMS, and yet only one of many studies on progesterone suppositories has shown only a small benefit in PMS.

Synthetic progesterone

Known as progestogens, this is taken by mouth and has been shown to have modest success in two out of four clinical trials.

Oestrogen implants

These are inserted under the skin of the abdomen by a small surgical procedure and are sometimes considered for older women with PMS. Implants are not without side-effects, however, and in cases where these occur women have to wait for the implant to wear off, which can further add to their existing burden of symptoms. For women who still have their uterus, the hormone progesterone must also be taken in conjunction with oestrogen in order to prevent the risk of cancer of the uterus. Implants are best reserved for older women with PMS symptoms who are also approaching the menopause.

Hormone injections

These are now on offer to some women, but once again they can often precipitate side-effects which a woman has to live with until the effect of the injection wears off, usually three months at least.

Other hormone-related products

Danazol and Bromocriptine are powerful agents that are not suitable for long-term use. Danazol, for example, suppresses ovulation and may bring side-effects of hair growth and deepening of the voice.

The oral contraceptive

This can improve PMS symptoms in some, but in others it makes matters worse or has no effect at all. Perhaps a useful treatment for mild PMS in younger women.

Diuretics

Water pills have been popular treatments in the past. However, many of the older preparations lead to loss of important minerals that may already be in short supply. Spironolactone, a newer type of diuretic has been shown to be moderately helpful with water retention, but is not recommended by the manufacturers for long-term use in younger women. The good news, however, is that most of the symptoms of fluid retention respond to dietary adjustments anyway, especially salt restriction, within a few months.

Anti-depressants

These are not regarded as appropriate treatment for PMS, but some of the newer preparations may be helpful for severely depressed or suicidal women. Studies show that Prozac (Fluoxetine) has been shown to help PMS depression but it is not effective in every case.

Vitamin B6

Pyridoxine is prescribed by some doctors, but has not been shown to be consistently effective in clinical trials. PMS is a multi-factoral condition that is unlikely to respond to one single nutrient in the long-term.

Efamast

Evening primrose oil, has been shown to be effective in clinical trials for premenstrual breast tenderness, and it is available on prescription from your doctor. It needs to be taken every day of the cycle at a dose of between 6-8 capsules per day, for at least four months.

What you can do

Here are some simple dietary recommendations:

- Never miss a meal. You will need to eat little and often in order to maintain optimum blood sugar levels, and to keep a constant supply of good nutrients flowing through to the brain and the nervous system.
- In your premenstrual week, your calorie requirements increase by up to 500 additional calories per day. In order to avoid dips in blood sugar, and temptation to eat chocolate or other processed sweet food, you will need to eat both a mid-morning and a mid-afternoon snack as well as your breakfast, lunch and dinner. (See Menu for PMS on page 474.)
- Ensure you have a daily salad, three portions of vegetables – including one green leafy vegetable, which is particularly rich in magnesium and iron – and at least three portions of fruit per day.
- Aim to eat three portions of oily fish per week – mackerel, herring, salmon, pilchards and sardines are all good examples. These can be eaten fresh, or tinned for convenience, with a salad at lunch-time.
- If you follow a vegetarian diet ensure you eat plenty of vegetarian protein each day: unsalted nuts, seeds, beans, lentils, peas, brown rice, soya bean products and sprouted beans.
- Eat some protein with your lunch and again with your dinner: chicken, fish, lean meat, low-fat cheese, eggs or a vegetarian protein.
- Avoid caffeine in the form of tea, coffee, cola or chocolate and choco-

late drinks. Do not drink more than two decaffeinated drinks per day as they contain other chemicals called methylxanthines that can aggravate other symptoms. Use alternatives like Rooibosch/Redbush Tea, which is a tea lookalike, other herbal teas or coffee substitutes like Barley Cup, and Dandelion Coffee (see page 7).

- Sodium salt and salty food should be avoided as salt tends to drag fluid into the cells and can make you feel bloated. You can use a potassium-rich salt substitute like Lo Salt in small amounts, or fresh herbs, garlic, ginger, spices and black pepper to flavour your food.

- Instead of eating foods that contain a large amount of sugar like cakes, biscuits, puddings, chocolate and sweets, aim to eat intrinsically sweet foods, like dried or fresh fruit, nuts and seeds, as these are much more nutritious. The PMS diet is not a weight-loss diet, and so it is acceptable to eat wholesome cakes and biscuits. You will find a selection of menus and recipes in *The Beat PMS Cookbook*, details of which can be found on page 493.

- Keep your dairy consumption down to the equivalent of milk in your cereal, milk in your drinks and one other serving of dairy per day, like yoghurt or cheese.

- Concentrate on eating a diet rich in the minerals magnesium, iron, zinc and chromium, and vitamins B, C, E and essential fatty acids. For details about rich sources of these nutrients refer to the Nutritional Content of Foods on page 483.

- Take the herbal supplement agnus castus which has been used for centuries for its ability to regulate the menstrual cycle and balance hormone levels. The first major clinical study on the use of agnus castus was published in 1954 showing positive results on women with menstrual irregularities and even amenorrhoea. It is the fruit of the agnus castus which contains essential oils, glycosides and flavonoids.

Constipation, abnormal wind and bloating

It is best to avoid products that contain phytic acid such as wheat and bran and, in some extreme cases, oats, barley and rye, for an initial period of at least six weeks. If you suffer with constipation take two tablespoons of golden linseeds with your breakfast cereals each day. You may also need to take some additional supplements of magnesium, preferably in the form of magnesium amino acid chelate – up to 800 mg per day. Magnesium needs to be taken to gut tolerance level as eventually it will cause diarrhoea. See chapters on constipation, abdominal wind and bloating, plus refer to the menu for irritable bowel syndrome on page 472.

Migraine headaches

Women commonly experience cyclical migraine headaches, which are sometimes associated with diet. Root or crystallised ginger taken as the headache begins often helps to relieve symptoms. There are also a number of foods associated with migraine headaches which you can read about under that heading.

Other conditions

Thrush, Fatigue, Craving for Sweet Food, Acne, Eczema, Loss of Libido and Panic attacks often occur premenstrually. Details of how to overcome these problems can be found in the relevant chapters. A suggested menu for PMS can be found on page 474, menu for fatigue is on page 472, menu for sugar craving is on page 476, and the menu for acne is on page 470.

Exercise

You will need to do three or four sessions of exercise per week, to the point of breathlessness. Following aerobic exercise, when the heart increases its number of beats per minute, the brain releases chemicals called endorphins, which raise mood, energy levels and influence the hormones positively.

Cycling, swimming, brisk walking, jogging, skipping, racquet sports, gym work or a workout are all suitable forms of exercise. Choose the sort of exercise you will enjoy and make yourself an exercise schedule that fits in with your lifestyle. If you cannot easily get out of the house to exercise, try using an exercise video at home. We recommend the YMCA 'Y' Plan videos which are scientifically based, and present twelve minute blocks of exercise to get you started. Details of these can be found on page 509.

Nutritional supplements

In the short term at least, until the symptoms are well under control, it is likely that you will need to take some nutritional supplements to speed up your recovery. There are a few scientifically based supplements which we recommend at the WNAS which have been through properly conducted clinical trials.

- *Optivite* This is a multi-vitamin and mineral supplement that has been through four properly conducted clinical trials. It has been shown to influence both brain chemicals and hormones, and is the general recommended supplement for PMS. Severe sufferers will need to take between 4–6 tablets per day, every day of the cycle. The dose should ideally be split between breakfast and lunch.
- *Normoglycaemia* A supplement rich in B vitamins, magnesium and the mineral chromium, all of which have been shown to be necessary for normal blood sugar control. It was formulated by the WNAS some eight years ago, and has been a very useful short-term tool in helping to overcome cravings for sweet food premenstrually. It needs to be

taken at a dose of between 1–2 tablets, before breakfast and/or lunch, every day of the cycle for at least the first two cycles.

- *Efamol evening primrose oil* has has been shown to be extremely effective in helping to alleviate premenstrual breast tenderness and eczema. It is the only form of evening primrose oil that has been subjected to extensive research and is recommended by the WNAS as part of their programme at a dose of between 6–8 x 500 mg capsules per day. Once again the dose should be split between breakfast and lunch, and should be taken for at least a four-month course.

Complementary therapies

Herbal medicine may be useful in helping to normalise hormone levels. Herbs such as black cohosh, damainana, raspberry leaf, vitex agnus castus, wild yam and dong quai are all used to correct hormone levels. Herbal 'tranquillisers' like Quiet Life or Valerina Night, a combination of soothing herbs, may help to reduce symptoms of anxiety, irritability and nervous tension.

Cranial osteopathy is a particularly good method of getting your body into correct balance. Tension in the neck and back, or trauma following childbirth, can prevent the body from functioning normally. If you have had a neck or back injury or feel this is a weak area it may be worth having a consultation with a cranial osteopath. Unlike ordinary osteopathy, this form of treatment is extremely gentle and relaxing. To find the address of your nearest practitioner, contact the European School of Osteopathy (see page 515).

Acupuncture and acupressure are two valuable ways of helping to return your body to normal function (see pages 36 & 37). These traditional Chinese methods can be used at two levels: self-help with acupressure which involves finger pressure, or acupuncture, with needles, which should be administered by a qualified practitioner. Acupuncture is particularly valuable for stubborn, chronic and severe problems. For details of your nearest qualified practitioner contact the British Acupuncture Council (see page 513).

Massage is a lovely way of helping to relax your mind and body, and is easily accessible and inexpensive. You could either treat yourself to a massage, or persuade your partner or a friend to volunteer their hands, or you could literally reach many parts yourself. Aromatherapy massage oil makes the massage extra soothing. Try using a combination of ylang-ylang, clary sage and neroli.

A combined programme of diet, exercise and scientifically based nutritional supplement has been shown to be the most effective approach to overcoming symptoms of PMS. Following these recommendations is likely to help you over your PMS and to leave you feeling better generally than you have felt for some time.

Further information about the WNAS programme for PMS can be found in our books *No More PMS!*, and *Beat PMS Cookbook*. Details of these and other books can be found on the suggested reading list on page 493.

Eleanor's story

Eleanor was a 32-year-old wife and mother of two who worked as a nanny in Surrey. Her PMS began after the birth of her second daughter, and the final straw came when she was found screaming and naked in the road in the middle of the night by her husband. She was unable to control her behaviour before her period and as a result her relationship with her husband and children was severely threatened.

'I felt as if an alien had taken over my body each month, as I struggled to control my raging temper and mood swings. I was a real Jekyll and Hyde. I am usually pretty laid back and sociable, but about ten days before my period I'd turn into a 'hag from hell' and refuse to go out of the house. I was also plagued by headaches and water retention.

I'd snap and shout at my husband and the children for no real reason. I began throwing plates and clenching my fists with the children, and wrote off a car. I was lucky I didn't kill myself, but things got so bad I did seriously contemplate suicide.

My husband read an article about the WNAS and phoned them in desperation. I reluctantly went with him to a consultation at their clinic, during which time a programme was tailor-made for me. I changed my diet, took supplements of Optivite and regular exercise, and within three months my symptoms completely disappeared. At first I was wary as I was sure it was a fluke, but to our utter delight I have remained symptom free. PMS is gone and I've got my family back.'

See also: Depression, Breast problems, Food cravings, What's wrong with present-day diet and lifestyle?, Nutrition is the key to health, Menu for PMS, Menu for breast tenderness, References and Recommended reading *(No More PMS!)*.

Prostate Disorders

The prostate is a gland at the base of the bladder which performs a number of functions. Its main function is to contribute secretions that assist in the ability of semen to fertilise an egg. It also produces chemicals with anti-bacterial properties and helps to minimise the risk of men developing urinary tract infections. The gland itself can occasionally become infected, increase in size with age causing outflow obstruction to the bladder and may also become cancerous.

There has been considerable progress in the treatment of prostatic related problems over the last 30 years due to earlier detection and more effective treatments.

URINARY AND PROSTATIC INFECTION

What are the symptoms?

Urinary tract infections are much less common in men than women. The symptoms are similar, with pain on passing urine and frequency.

What causes it?

In young men, the most common cause is usually urethritis with an infection caused by sexually transmitted organisms. These individuals are best referred on to a genito-urinary medicine clinic and require treatment with antibiotics, sometimes for prolonged periods of time.

What your doctor can do

- Any male developing a simple bacterial urinary tract infection requires examination for associated prostatic disease and antibiotic treatment.
- Usually an x-ray of the kidneys needs to be performed to exclude any anatomical abnormality or kidney malformation.
- Bacterial prostatitis produces symptoms of a urinary tract infection together with pain at the base of the penis. Urine samples, sometimes taken after prostatic massage will help identify the organism and treatment with antibiotics is usually for several weeks and sometimes several months.

What you can do

- In order to prevent the bacterial flora in your gut from being upset, take a course of high strength acidophilus daily whilst you are taking the antibiotics.
- Take the antibiotics conscientiously, especially if they are for a prolonged period.
- Avoid alcohol completely whilst the condition persists.

- Eat a nutritious healthy diet. See page 437.
- Consider taking supplements of zinc – 20 to 30 mgms daily and a strong multivitamin supplement to help boost resistance to infection.
- Limit intake of tea and coffee as occasionally this will aggravate the symptoms of urinary frequency. See page 7 for suggested alternatives.
- Take cranberry juice or cranberry juice extract on a regular basis.
- If sexually transmitted urethritis is confirmed, use a condom to protect your partner.

PROSTATIC ENLARGEMENT

What is it?

Prostatic enlargement is a very common problem, the main risk factor for which is age with well over 50 per cent of men experiencing some problem during the course of their life. As the prostate gland enlarges, it compresses the urethra – the outlet tube which passes through its substance and also pushes up on the base of the bladder. This produces symptoms of outflow obstruction, poor flow, dribbling and incomplete emptying and other symptoms of frequency, urgency, sometimes with incontinence and a need to pass water at night (nocturia).

Many sufferers put up with these symptoms, particularly in the early stages but would usually report to their doctor, particularly if there is any degree of incontinence or severe difficulty passing water. Acute retention recurs when the prostatic enlargement has completely obstructed the flow of urine which then needs to be relieved with the passage of a catheter – a fine tube.

Who gets it?

- Those increasing in age – affecting up to 90 per cent of men aged 85 and above.
- Those living in western and developed societies are much more at risk for prostate enlargement compared with those living in South East Asia.

What your doctor can do

- Examine you to see if the prostate is enlarged or whether the bladder is not emptying properly. In severely affected individuals, damage to the kidneys can occur with a rise in blood pressure. A urine test to look for infection and the presence of blood is also important.

- Men with severe symptoms, blood in the urine, a urinary infection or at risk for prostate cancer should be referred.
- Drug treatment with drugs termed alpha-blockers may help to reduce symptoms. A trial of these drugs for two weeks will help determine those who are likely to respond and may then be continued for several years.
- Referral for surgery, usually performed through a telescope passed along the length of the penis, can be highly effective but it is not without risks. Mild incontinence, erectile dysfunction and retrograde ejaculation are all known as significant complications, though more modern techniques have reduced the frequency of these problems.

What you can do

- Limit fluid intake if you are drinking excessively and, in particular, limit intakes of tea, coffee and alcohol, all of which have diuretic effects.
- Try eating foods with potential effects to reduce prostatic enlargement or prostatic symptoms. These include soya products which are rich in isoflavones that block the stimulatory effects of testosterone upon prostate tissue. Pumpkin seeds have been through a successful trial to reduce urinary symptoms due to prostatic enlargement. Try sprinkling these on your breakfast cereal or consuming them as a snack. Other good dietary sources include lentils, seeds, chick peas and beans.
- Phytoestrogen products are worth considering. Trinovin is an extract of red clover which contains four potentially important isoflavones – genistein, biochanin, daidzein and formononetin – all of which may potentially influence prostate health.
- Saw palmetto has also been used with some success in helping prostate related symptoms. Extract from this palm-like plant, native to North America, has been popular and it too contains phytoestrogen chemicals which inhibit the potential adverse effects of testosterone upon the growth and enlargement of the prostate gland.
- Extract of rye grass has also been used with some success in the treatment of prostate related disorders.

PROSTATE CANCER

Cancer of the prostate is the third leading cause of cancer deaths in men in the UK. Early detection is vital to its successful treatment and this has been aided by the development of the blood test PSA (Prostate Specific Antigen). There has been much debate in the last few years as to whether this would be a useful test to perform in the general population, to screen for the early detection of cancer of the prostate. As yet no recommendation for this test to be used has been made. However, refinements of the test may lead to greater usefulness and thus it may become appropriate for men aged 50 or 60 years or older to then be screened.

Symptoms of prostate cancer

These are usually symptoms of prostate enlargement but they may be complicated by the presence of blood in the urine or blood in seminal fluid, pain typically at the base of the penis or on urination. Other symptoms relating to the cancer may occur if it has spread to the liver or bones.

What your doctor can do

- Early referral to a specialist centre is of course vital. Treatment involves a number of approaches including radiotherapy, use of potent drugs to block the action of testosterone and occasionally castration – removal of the testicles. Modern drug treatments have become increasingly effective so that radical surgery is not required.
- Surgical treatment to remove cancerous tissue may also be required but if the cancer is early and is not producing symptoms of outflow obstruction then this may not be necessary.

What you can do

- Consume a diet rich in phytoestrogens from foods such as soya and linseeds together with supplements of red clover. These phytoestrogens may in theory inhibit the growth of cancerous tissue in the same way that they may also inhibit the growth of breast cancer. Refer to the phytoestrogen-rich menu on page 480. Aim to have three servings of phytoestrogen-rich food or drink each day. For example sprinkle linseeds and pumpkin seeds on your cereal and use soya milk. Later in the day have a soya fruit milk drink or a glass of soya milk and have a soya milk dessert after dinner or a slice of cake or fruit loaf made with soya flour. For further suggested menus and recipes see *The Phyto Factor*, details on page 494.
- Also consume a diet rich in fruit and vegetables as there may be other plant derived products that generally inhibit the growth of this and other cancers.

See also: Standard references.

Psoriasis

Psoriasis is a common, often chronic, skin complaint where red patches of variable size are covered with fine scales. The patches, which are well demarcated, are found most commonly on the trunk or concentrated over the elbows and knees. Other areas that can be affected are the scalp, which becomes very scaly, shedding large amounts of dandruff, and the nails which may be thickened with scales at their edge or pitted by minute craters. The face is rarely affected. Very often the disease varies from month to month with spontaneous remissions occurring. Some patients develop an associated arthritis. The effected skin is very active, growing at ten times the rate of normal skin and can contain a very high concentration of chemicals that are produced in situations where there is a lot of inflammation. Just what triggers this change is uncertain.

Who gets it?

Psoriasis effects two per cent of the white population, and is less common in populations originating near the equator. Some forms of the rash may develop in childhood, especially the form that looks like a series of raindrops.

What causes it?

- It may follow an infection such as a sore throat.
- It can run in families, and is more common in smokers, especially when it affects the palms or soles of the feet.
- Deficiencies of folic acid, selenium, possibly zinc and sometimes calcium are known to occur, especially if the skin involvement is widespread and severe.

What your doctor can do

A number of different medicines seem to help, although certain drugs can worsen psoriasis. Long-term use is usually the order of the day.

- Creams based on coal tar, like Dithranol, are smelly but effective.
- Steroid creams and ointments can be used but are often limited if the psoriasis is widespread.
- Calcipotriol cream and ointment are derived from vitamin D and are quite effective at reducing the inflammation and scaling of psoriasis. They cause less irritation and are less smelly than some of the tar preparations.
- Phototherapy with ultraviolet light is highly effective. UVA light is used

and the patient is given a dose of a medicine called apsoralen that sensitises the skin to light. The treatment is thus often called PUVA.

- Shampoos usually based on tar preparations are useful for excessive scalp scaling. Sometimes an anti-fungal shampoo (Nizoral) is worth trying, and oral antifungal agents are sometimes effective too.
- A powerful vitamin A derived drug, Etretrinate, is occasionally used.
- Powerful anti-inflammatory drugs or immune-altering drugs are now used for severe cases.

What you can do

- *Stop smoking* This can worsen psoriasis.
- *Sunbathe* This is helpful in up to 75 per cent of patients. Some sun-beds may be helpful too (check with your specialist) and how about a trip to the Dead Sea where the combination of sun, low humidity, mud and mineral salt applications can be effective.
- *Eat a diet rich in essential fatty acids* These fats influence skin quality and inflammation. A high intake of the Omega-3 essential fatty acids is known to help psoriasis. Follow The High EFA Diet on page 446. If you are overweight then you will need to lose weight as well for this to be effective.
- *Take supplements of fish oils* Usually 4–6 high-strength fish oil capsules will suffice. It is the content of EPA (eicosapentaenoic acid) and DHA (docosahexaenoic acid) that you are interested in. Taking an EFA supplement is useful because in psoriasis there is often faulty utilisation of these essential fats.
- *Vitamin A* has been scientifically proven to slow down the rate of keratinisation (the process of skin cell growth and development) which is important in the treatment of psoriasis.
- *Vitamin B-complex* is necessary for normal cell division.
- *Take a supplement of acidophillus* to improve colon health as the skin and digestive system are intrinsically related.
- *Try avoiding wheat, oat, barley and rye foods* A recent report noted that 10 per cent of those with psoriasis may have evidence of sensitivity to these types of cereals. Generally exclusion diets do not seem to work well for psoriasis in the way that they do for eczema, but it might be worth trying to exclude these cereals for six to eight weeks to see if this helps.
- *Try taking supplements of multi-vitamins, zinc and selenium* The first two may influence skin quality, and the requirement of all three may well be increased in long-standing widespread psoriasis. Zinc at a dose of 30 mg per day might be particularly useful for psoriasis effecting the palms and soles, and is known to help the arthritis associated with this skin condition.

Complementary therapies

Homeopathy and herbalism are perhaps the two most worth considering. These therapies can be comfortably combined with both conventional and nutritional approaches.

See also: Standard references.

Raynaud's Disease and Poor Circulation

Sometimes poor circulation is due not to furring up of the arteries but to a reversible spasm of the muscles in their wall. Typically this happens in the hands and feet. These extremities change colour, become cold and tingle. The skin follows a sequence of pale then blue then a dusky red. This phenomenon was first described by a French physician Raynaud in the nineteenth century.

Who gets it?

Typically young women are affected. Both hands are usually involved and there are a number of triggering factors and sometimes causative diseases. Some researchers have associated this problem with irritable bowel syndrome and migraine, two conditions where spasm of muscles in the gut wall and the blood vessels of the head may play a part.

What causes it?

Common trigger factors include:

- cold weather
- emotional upset
- trauma
- smoking a cigarette.

Sometimes the condition is associated with other illnesses such as arthritis, skin diseases, pressure on nerves in the neck (following use of vibrating equipment, chain saws, for instance), in association with an increased stickiness of the blood which may sometimes follow an infection.

What your doctor can do

- Mainly examine you for some of the rare underlying causes.
- Prescribe a vasodilating drug, but they are not usually very effective.

What you can do

- Wear gloves. Obvious but effective.
- Wear a silk scarf around your neck.
- Regular physical exercise may improve cold tolerance.
- Stop smoking.
- Try some nutritional supplements. None is of proven value but the following might help:
  - Fish oils and plenty of oily fish in the diet.
  - Supplements of magnesium might help. They could in theory reduce the tendency to spasm of the blood vessels.
  - Supplements of nicotinic acid up to 300 mg per day; try it as 100 mg three times a day. This form of vitamin B3 can cause a flush reaction so always take it after food rather than on an empty stomach.
- Take a supplement of co-enzyme Q10 to improve tissue circulation.
- The herb gingko biloba appears to function by increasing the blood supply to the brain and throughout the body's network of blood vessels that supply blood and oxygen to the organs. In addition, it also has an anti-clotting action, preventing the blood platelets from clumping together. It is becoming an increasingly popular treatment for Raynaud's. However, it may contraindicate with some anti-coagulant medication so check with your GP before introducing the herb.
- Ginger is an age-old remedy for improving circulation, so incorporate it into your cooking or perhaps chew on crystallised ginger. Ginger infusions are simple to prepare by placing some root ginger into a mug of boiling water and adding a little honey to sweeten.
- Garlic is renowned for its circulatory benefits. However, supplements are often prefered to eating whole cloves of garlic!
- Combined supplements are now available which contain ginger, garlic and ginkgo biloba, but as with most complementary therapies, improvement is likely to be seen after approximately three months, so do persevere.

See also: Standard references.

Stress

More than half the adult population claims to be suffering with stress to some degree. It's not only the high flying executives that are suffering, but also exhausted mothers, the unemployed and the homeless. And it's not just nineties hype either. A paper published recently in the *British Medical Journal* confirmed that women who developed breast cancer were far more likely to have experienced bereavement, redundancy, homelessness, violent crime or family crises within the past five years than their healthy counterparts. We also know from a study of Danish bus drivers that those who faced the worst traffic died earlier than their colleagues who drove country routes.

There is scientific evidence linking stress to certain diseases, perhaps not as a cause, but certainly as an underlying factor, although the nature of the link between stress and disease is not fully understood. These stress-related disorders include:

- High blood pressure
- Headaches
- Facial pain
- Irritable Bowel Syndrome
- Ulcerative colitis
- Stomach ulcers
- Infections
- Rheumatoid arthritis
- Anorexia nervosa
- Asthma
- Period problems, including irregular periods and PMS.

There is a fine line between stress and distress. Professor Hans Selye, the founder of modern research into stress described it as 'the rate of wear and tear on the body'. He distinguished between good and bad stress. Good stress can be reasonably healthy as it stretches us to capacity and keeps us on our toes. Dealing with challenges as they present themselves is good for our morale. However, when we get the point of overload the stress becomes bad. The product of modern-day lifestyle is that it leaves many of us feeling overwhelmed and under-par. If these conditions continue for anything other than a short period of time, it can take its toll on our health.

What are the symptoms?

The rational ones amongst us do not usually take on our 'case load' all at once, we don't ask to be overwhelmed, it just grows on us gradually. We collect our responsibilities as we go along. Perhaps we have been coasting along quite successfully, then a promotion comes along which demands more from us, and at the same time a close relative gets sick, or our partner gets made redundant, and then we find we are pregnant again and so on. Additionally, when asked to commit to a project some of us have not learned to say 'no'. And so we soldier on as martyrs, believing that we can manage somehow, until one day our body sends out the warning. Whilst this scenario is occurring we are snacking instead of eating properly and not doing much in the way of exercise or relaxation.

The most common symptoms of stress include:

- Disturbed sleep and early morning waking
- Insomnia
- Panic attacks
- Palpitations
- Headaches
- Loss of appetite
- Compulsive eating
- Desire to increase consumption of alcohol
- Excessive smoking
- Fatigue
- Irrational thoughts
- Minor illnesses.

The first warning for some of us could be a bout of 'flu, or the onset of headaches. Alternatively our digestive system or our energy levels could be affected. Were we to re-evaluate our runaway lifestyle at this point, and invest time in getting our body back into shape, we might well be able to circumvent the health crisis brewing. Invariably, in our blind state, we get up from our sick bed, and go into the ring for the next round.

Many of us feel that we have to soldier on, no matter what. There does not seem to be an obvious alternative. And so we continue, until our body says 'no'. We all have both physical and mental limits, and the body can only tolerate so much abuse. It is a vicious circle. Because we feel so awful, usual tasks are more demanding, and looking after ourselves becomes even less likely. When something goes wrong with the car the warning light goes on, and when the computer doesn't like the conditions it makes a noise or puts up a message, but our poor body fails to communicate its troubles. Most of us wouldn't recognise the body's signal anyway until the writing was on the wall.

We don't necessarily have a nervous breakdown, but we develop a weakness in some area of our body as a result of an immune system dysfunction. Some of us develop migraine headaches, other get recurrent thrush, irritable bowel syndrome, panic attacks, depression, chronic fatigue or a nervous rash. The unlucky minority will simply have a fatal heart attack or develop a serious medical condition. New research reported in *The Lancet* show that people who bottle up their emotions are more likely to die early, and in particular to have heart attacks.

The adrenal glands are responsible for maintaining the balance of many bodily functions by secreting several important hormones. An abnormal adrenal response, either deficient or excessive hormone secretion, significantly alters an individual's response to stress. Often the adrenal glands become exhausted as a result of the constant demands put on them. Various nutrients and herbal substances can be very useful in supporting and enhancing adrenal function, particularly during times of stress. Vitamin C, vitamin B6, zinc, magnesium and vitamin B5 are essential nutrients for the manufacture of adrenal hormones, and if the body is under constant stress, these nutrients are rapidly depleted.

What your doctor can do

- Eliminate the possibility of any underlying cause to your symptoms by giving you a physical examination, and performing routine tests to check your iron levels, thyroid function, plus checking for underlying infection or early diabetes.
- Suggest some counselling to help you sort out the stressful situations you face.
- If you are suffering with panic attacks your doctor may prescribe a low dose of beta blockers to help you cope with anxiety symptoms.
- Alternatively you may be offered tranquillisers, but these should not be taken for longer than a few weeks.

Whilst all this has been going on it is likely that many of us will have become regular visitors to our doctors surgery, and have begun taking the 'appropriate' medication. So we are now treating the symptoms, and at best suppressing them. You might even get labelled as 'neurotic' if you are really persistent. What we actually should be doing at this point is looking seriously for the root cause of the problem and addressing it. Whilst some doctors are enlightened and may question you about your troubles or refer you for counselling, they are used to dishing out 'a pill for an ill'. They do not usually have the time in their short consultation to really find out what underlies your symptoms.

What you can do

Many of us have the ability to cope with near tragedy or disaster, and it is not until it is over, and the dust has settled, that we feel it is safe to 'fall apart'. With hindsight, the warning signals were all there and we could have reversed the situation had we come to our senses in time.

Here are some tips to help you next time!

- Eat regular wholesome meals and have a supply of nutritious snacks. Don't fall into the trap of missing meals and eating junk food or chocolate instead. Follow the recommendation for The Very Nutritious Diet on page 437.
- Concentrate on a diet rich in magnesium and vitamins B and C to support the adrenals. Good sources include wholegrains, fresh fruit and vegetables, low-fat dairy produce and lean poultry and meat.

- Panax ginseng has been used for centuries as a tonic, due to its ability to enhance adrenal gland function and improve reactions against a variety of stresses. Ginseng is described as an adaptogen which means it has a unique ability to normalise bodily functions.
- There are also plenty of foods that should be avoided, such as 'simple', highly refined carbohydrates and sugar, which can affect mental symptoms by causing blood sugar abnormalities and triggering stress.
- Excessive alcohol consumption can also exacerbate stress as it substantially decreases the ability of the body to extract nutrients from the food we eat.
- Make sure you have some sacred time for yourself. Time to think, and time to switch off from your responsibilities.
- Tell your family how you feel, and ask for their support whilst you get yourself sorted out.
- If your stress comes from work, discuss with colleagues how you can make changes, or if you are self-employed you will need to re-evaluate.
- Try to get away, even if it's only for a few days. Sometimes we can see things more clearly from a distance.
- Learn not to take on too much – if you feel fully committed learn to say 'no'.
- Prioritise your responsibilities and see if you can off-load or delegate some of the lesser important tasks.
- Take time each week to exercise – you should be doing three or four sessions of exercise per week, even if its just skipping or a workout to a video at home.
- Make time each day to relax formally – you will need fifteen minutes, with no interruptions. Really switching off is an art, you may need some instruction or to read a book on the subject.
- Get your partner or a close friend to give you a massage, preferably using some relaxing aromatherapy oils like geranium or lavender.
- Watch an entertaining film or make time to read a good book.
- Make sure you laugh occasionally. Laughter is so good for us, and yet when we get absorbed with problems in life we forget about our sense of humour.
- If you can't see a solution to your current stresses find someone to talk it through with, or get some professional help (don't forget Useful addresses on page 512).

Complementary therapies

When the symptoms you are experiencing are related to stressful events in life, the most effective thing to do is handle the stress – but it is not always that simple or instantaneous. As well as following the recommendations suggested here there are several complementary therapies that would be helpful. Massage and any method of relaxation would be good to incorporate into your lifestyle on a regular basis. Acupuncture will help to boost your immune system so that you feel more able to cope, and cranial osteopathy may help to ease the tension that has built up in your body as a result of being stressed.

There are homeopathic remedies to try, or even the Bach Rescue remedy to help you cope with stressful moments. There are also some very effective herbal tranquillisers like Valerina Day and Valerina Night which can be taken when needed, and do not have any addictive properties. However, herbal products do not have an immediate benefit, so you need to persevere if you want to see results.

Bernice's story

Bernice was a 34-year-old mother of two who, despite her apparently normal life, was at breaking point through stress.

'My husband, who is a conservative, high-powered, executive said I should have been able to "pull myself together" but I was unable to. He wouldn't discuss my upset over the termination I had had after the birth of our last child, or the problems we were experiencing with our sex life, which was non-existent. I was so anxious and tearful, I honestly don't know how I got through each day. Everything seemed too much, I couldn't even bring myself to answer the telephone when it rang. The most frightening thing of all, which I didn't bring myself to tell anyone, was that I kept seeing "little people" out the corner of my eyes. I knew they weren't there, but they seemed so real. I really thought I was going insane.

Formerly I was such an organised and rational person. I have a very idealistic brain in my head and usually like things to be just so. I used to entertain a lot and loved doing activities with my two children. I have many friends and lots of close family, but I couldn't cope with seeing them as I felt antisocial. One minute I'd feel violent and aggressive, and then I'd think morbid thoughts about dying. I also had chronic back pain and as well as the sleeping pills I took regularly, most days I took at least eight painkillers, which made me very constipated.

My doctor suggested that I got in touch with the Women's Nutritional Advisory Service, and in sheer desperation I did. My diet was overhauled, I was sent off to the cranial osteopath, and took Optivite and Efamol. Once my back was feeling better I started to exercise gently and was able to stop taking all the painkillers and sleeping pills. I found the WNAS programme hard to stick to for the first few weeks but was so determined to give it my best as I honestly felt this was the last resort for me.

It did get easier and within a month I was feeling considerably better. Miraculously the osteopath sorted out my back problem, so that I no longer suffered constant pain. My constipation cleared up and the "little men" disappeared thank goodness. After following the programme for three months my symptoms had vanished, and my husband felt that his wife had returned. I was relieved too. I hate to think what might have happened to me and to my family if I had not been pointed in the right direction when I was at such a low ebb.'

See also: Standard references.

Thyroid Disease

The thyroid is a gland in the neck which produces the hormone thyroxine that essentially controls the metabolic rate of all cells throughout the body. A fall in the production of thyroxine leads to an underactive thyroid, also termed hypothyroidism. An excessive production produces an increase in metabolic rate and is termed hyperthyroidism.

What are the symptoms?

Symptoms of hyperthyroidism include:

- weight loss
- rapid pulse rate
- palpitations
- fine tremor of the hands
- increased sweating
- intolerance to heat
- increased appetite.

Symptoms of hypothyroisism may cause:

- fatigue
- muscular aches and pains
- weight gain
- intolerance to cold
- slow pulse rate
- an elevation in blood pressure
- dry skin
- hair loss and a variety of other changes if the disease is prolonged
- changes in facial appearance, especially puffiness which may be noticed by friends and relatives.

Who gets it?

Thyroid disease is common and often runs in families. It can be associated with diabetes, rheumatoid arthritis and pernicious anaemia and either an under- or over-active thyroid gland can affect over one per cent of the adult population. These disturbances occur more easily in women than they do in men. In women of child-bearing age menstrual disturbance, including premenstrual syndrome, may occasionally be due to an under-active thyroid.

What causes it?

- Antibodies against the thyroid gland are a common cause of an under-active thyroid gland and they also may lead to over-stimulation of the thyroid. This is termed auto-immune thyroiditis. This can be detected by blood tests which are different to the measurements of the actual level of thyroid hormone.
- An over-active 'nodule' in the thyroid.
- A virus infection which may produce a temporary rise in the production of thyroid hormone. This is often associated with painful swelling of the thyroid gland.
- Radiation treatment for an overactive thyroid gland. The thyroid may become under-active many years later.

What your doctor can do

- Tests for thyroid function are very sensitive and will easily detect an over- or under-active thyroid gland.
- Tests for thyroid antibodies will help decide on the cause and best treatment available.
- Treatment for an over-active thyroid involves:
  - drugs to control the level of thyroid hormone
  - surgical removal of part of the thyroid, or
  - use of radio-active iodine to partially destroy part of the thyroid gland.
- Treatment for an under-active thyroid gland involves giving replacement thyroid hormones usually as thyroxine, and occasionally as triodothyronine.
- Continual blood tests to monitor progress of treatment are vital. Complicated patients may require the services of a thyroid specialist. This is especially true for those with an over-active thyroid.

What you can do

- Be a good patient. This is one situation in medicine where standard medical treatment produces excellent results.
- Do not take kelp or other forms of iodine. These do not boost or lower thyroid function and may disturb the test that your doctor wishes to do. Iodine is often put into slimming pills and cellulite pills which should not be taken by anyone on thyroid medication.
- Research does show that goitregens found in cabbage, broccoli, mustard greens, radishes, horseradishes, turnips interfere with thyroid hormones. Other foods are soya beans, peanuts and millet. Cooking does destroy some of the goitrogenic activity, but caution should still be taken. However, it should be noted that exceptionally large quantities of these foods would need to be eaten to cause any interaction.
- Natural sources of iodine predominating in sea vegetables, including wakame, dulse, arame, nori, and kombu provide nourishment for the thyroid.
- Vitamins E and A, together with the mineral zinc are necessary for the manufacture of thyroid hormones. Zinc is also necessary for the conversion of beta-carotene into vitamin A. This conversion process is often compromised in the hypothyroid patient.
- There are natural thyroid formulas which claim to support thyroid function, but are often contraindicated with thyroxine medication.
- If you are not making satisfactory progress, let your doctor know. Especially in the treatment of an under-active thyroid, hypothyroidism, the adjustment of the dosage of thyroid hormone depends upon not only your thyroid hormone tests, but how you feel.

Complementary therapies
Don't even think about it!

See also: Diabetes, Rheumatoid arthritis, Anaemia, Standard references.

Tonsillitis

The tonsils are swellings formed by white cells, blood vessels and supporting tissues, which are situated at the back of the mouth on either side. They are essentially lymph glands of the mouth, and are there to fight infection. Sometimes they become badly infected themselves either by a virus or a bacterium called *Streptococcus*. These infections can also occur even after the tonsils have been removed. Infected tonsils are common in childhood and should be treated as Influenza (see page 262) although a number will require treatment with antibiotics, most commonly penicillin, if bacterial infection is suspected. Sometimes the tonsils remain enlarged though they are not always infected.

Removal by operation is appropriate for enlarged, repeatedly infected tonsils. If they are not infected, but just large, they can still cause problems of pressure in the throat, discomfort on swallowing, and snoring! (Snoring is also related to being overweight, high blood pressure, alcohol consumption or other distortions of the upper airway).

What you can do

For enlarged, repeatedly infected tonsils, treat as for recurrent infections (see page 262). For those who have enlarged non-infected tonsils it may sometimes be worthwhile trying The Simple Exclusion Diet (see page 460). Sensitivity to dairy products seems to be the most likely situation in such cases, and avoidance for as little as a week may make a noticeable difference. You can also follow the advice about supplements given in the chapter on Influenza, recurrent coughs, colds and sore throats (see page 262). To relieve the pain gargling with aspirin is quite effective.

See also: Standard references.

Ulcerative Colitis

Ulcerative colitis is a chronic non-infective disease, producing inflammation of the lining of the colon and the rectum. It is a relatively common disorder with about five to ten new cases per 100,000 of the population per year. Adults aged 20 to 40 years are especially vulnerable, but children, including infants, may be affected.

What are the symptoms?

Diarrhoea with blood and mucus are typical symptoms. Abdominal pain and weight loss are not as commonplace as they are in Crohn's disease. Often the symptoms start gradually but may be of sudden onset. Sometimes constipation is a feature if the disease is confined to the rectum; this is termed proctitis. In more severe cases there may be inflammation in other organs, causing arthritis, mouth ulcers, liver problems, eye pains and skin rashes.

What causes it?

As with Crohn's disease, there appears to be a mixture of genetic and environmental factors. The genetic element seems to be smaller than that for Crohn's disease. Some 10–20 per cent of sufferers have a near relative also with the disease. It is more common in some Jewish communities around the world. The possible environmental factors include:

- *Infection* The bacteria in the colon are continually changing, and some relatively normal bacteria, present in the colon of those with colitis, have the potential to produce chemicals that could damage the lining of the colon. Whether they actually cause colitis is not clear.
- *Allergy or intolerance to foods* This is possible in a minority of adults. Cow's milk appears the most likely culprit. Intolerances to wheat, yeast and other foods are a possibility too (see page 422). In infantile colitis, food allergy is in fact the rule.
- *Sulphur in the diet* There is some recent evidence that sulphur in the diet together with other factors lead to the production of hydrogen sulphide (bad eggs) gas in the colon. This is a highly toxic compound and is particularly noxious to the cells lining the wall of the colon. It interferes with their energy metabolism. A diet low in sulphur – which is found mainly in beer, wine, bread, preserved meats (salami and sausages) and any other food containing sulphite preservative (E220–227) – should be excluded especially if you suffer with smelly wind.
- *An intolerance to some strong vitamins* A side-effect of high-dose vitamin E in infants is colitis. We have seen a few patients experience abdominal pain with passage of blood in the stools after taking either vitamin E or a strong multi-vitamin preparation containing it. This is rare though.
- *Not smoking cigarettes or being an ex-smoker* This is one of the great oddities in medicine. Several studies show that smokers are protected against ulcerative colitis. Ex-smokers, however, have a particularly high incidence. For them we cannot recommend re-starting cigarettes, but nicotine patches may be a possible therapy. We await further research on this.
- *Following use of painkillers* These do not cause colitis but they may account for its aggravation. This applies to paracetamol and anti-arthritic drugs. Occasionally there may be marked sensitivity to aspirin and food containing salicylates. Such patients are made much worse if they take aspirin or are given a drug often used in colitis called sulphasalazine. If this makes the bowel condition worse, then a low salicylate diet is worth a try. This can occasionally lead to a complete resolution. Such a diet is complicated and requires expert management as many fruits, vegetables and spices need to be avoided.

What your doctor can do

- Assess the extent of the disease using a barium enema x-ray or colonoscopy (examination of the large bowel with a flexible telescope).
- Assess the severity of the disease from blood tests, frequency of bowel movements, the presence of blood in the stool and if there is a fever.
- Exclude the presence of any bowel infection, including home-grown as well as tropical infection.
- Prescribe drug treatment with:
  - Steroid by mouth, or in the form of an enema for those with disease confined to the last part of the bowel. Steroids are useful for controlling a flare up, but have no benefit as a maintenance therapy, so every attempt should be made to withdraw them from the patient once the disease is controlled.
  - Anti-inflammatory drug based on 5-aminosalicylic acid (sulphasalazine and related compounds). Again this comes as tablets or as an enema and is useful for maintenance therapy.
- Suggest hospital treatment which may involve blood transfusions and fluids and specialised feeding intravenously.
- Recommend surgical treatment to remove a diseased colon or part of it. Cancer can develop in the colon usually after fifteen years of disease. Regular examinations of the whole of the colon are recommended for many patients with colitis, even if their disease is quiet.

What you can do

In theory there should be a diet or diets for colitis, but this has not really proved to be the case. There are a number of possibilities to consider though it is probably best to discuss these with your specialist first.

- A diet free of cow's milk products and lactose is perhaps worth most sufferers trying at some stage. Calcium supplements are necessary if followed long-term.
- Ask your doctor about a low salicylate diet for those made worse by drug treatment or if there is a history of aspirin sensitivity (see Asthma and Rhinitis pages 89 and 226).
- A diet avoiding foods that commonly irritate the gut which include coffee, wholemeal bread, bran and other wholegrain products, sweetcorn, beans and other high-fibre foods. It may be useful to avoid these foods during an attack and when in remission. Even when the disease is not active, the bowel habit is often erratic, and this may respond to the avoidance of these or other foods.
- A diet low in sulphur containing foods could work if there is a lot of foul-smelling wind due to hydrogen sulphide. These sorts of compounds are found at a high level in those with active disease and

the drug 5-aminosalicylic acid inhibits their production. It may therefore be prudent to avoid the main sulphur-containing foods which are: sulphite preservatives E220–227, wine and beer, bread, eggs and dried fruit.

- Take supplements if there has been significant weight loss, or you need to follow a restricted diet. The following may be needed:
  - iron, if there is anaemia from blood loss
  - multi-vitamin and multi-mineral, if there is weight loss
  - folic acid, if on 5-aminosalicylate
  - calcium, if on a dairy-free diet long term
  - fish oils may help to reduce the inflammation slightly, and may reduce the need for steroids. They are perhaps worth considering if there is an associated arthritis and you cannot take anti-arthritic drugs.
- Take a probiotic supplement providing 'friendly' bacteria to repopulate the colon. Acidophillus or bifido bacteria are the most frequently used probiotics.
- Vitamin A is necessary for healing of the gut lining and its antioxidant properties protect the mucous membranes from free radical damage.
- Take L-glutamine, an important amino acid for healing the gut lining and is the primary metabolic fuel for growth and replication of intestinal cells.

Complementary therapies

There is a real possibility that some herbal preparations might influence the degree of inflammation in the colon. Expert advice from a qualified herbalist is needed.

See also: Standard references.

Urticaria

Urticaria is an itchy skin rash, characterised by short-lived, sometimes severe, swellings called weals. It may occur as a one-off episode, or several episodes may happen over the course of a few weeks. Sometimes it is chronic, lasting for three or more months with the eruption appearing suddenly, then disappearing and changing from day to day. In these instances there is a strong need to try and identify the cause. The rash and irritation are due to the release of histamine and other chemicals into the skin. Allergies often play a part but are by no means the only cause. A severe form, where there are large deep swellings which may effect the lip, tongue or airways is called angio-oedema, may occasionally be life-threatening.

What causes it?

There are many possibilities to consider and often in one-off episodes no clear cause may be identified.

- A food allergy. Egg white, fish, tomatoes and cows' milk are known possibilities.
- A food intolerance reaction. This can happen with strawberries, artificial colours (Tartrazine E 102 and Sunset Yellow E 110), the preservative benzoate (commonly found in fizzy drinks), salicylates in food and shellfish.
- Reaction to a drug. Antibiotics, aspirin (a salicylate) and, rarely, others are all possibilities.
- Contact allergies to housedust and animal fur, saliva and, rarely, semen.
- Genetic factors, as this condition may run in families.
- Exercise can be a trigger, and this may interact with other triggers, especially foods.
- Exposure to cold and occasionally heat.
- Pressure may trigger localised urticaria.
- Infection, especially hidden parasitic infection causing chronic urticaria.
- Candida infection is another known, albeit rare, trigger.
- Insect bite or sting, jellyfish sting and, of course, stinging nettles.
- In association with various diseases.

What your doctor can do

Investigations are necessary only for those with chronic urticaria (lasting three months or more), if the reactions are very severe or if there is a family history. Usually the likely trigger is decided from the history and an awareness of the events and circumstances preceding repeated attacks. Allergy tests are not very helpful but may uncover a food allergy or sensitivity to *candida albicans* (thrush*)*.

Treatment, as a rule, is by use of one of several antihistamines. Many of these are now available without prescription. Their use is limited by drowsiness which is the main side-effect and by their inability to control all of the reaction. Many chemicals other than histamine are released in a reaction and thus antihistamines do not always control the reaction. Other drugs with antihistamine-like effects can be used, and adrenaline by injection is needed for the severe life-threatening reactions.

What you can do

- Try and find the cause. Make a list of all activities, food and drink consumed, and any medicines or other pills (including vitamins) consumed in the 24 hours before an attack. Collect several of these and go and discuss them with your doctor.

- Exclude common likely triggers such as all drugs, aspirin, foods containing artificial colouring agents, beverages containing benzoates, foods rich in yeast and yeast-derived beverages (all forms of alcohol except those that are filtered e.g. gin and vodka).
- Take some supplements. Vitamin C at a dose of 1g twice a day can halve the level of histamine in the blood after two weeks. So it may be useful for those with chronic urticaria. It probably won't replace a good antihistamine in the short term.
- Magnesium helps to stabilise the allergy cells called mast cells that release histamine and other chemicals. Supplements of this mineral at a dose of 300–400 mg per day combined with The Very Nutritious Diet (see page 437) might reduce the intensity of the rash after two or more months. Zinc may also help in a similar fashion (supplements of 10–20 mg) and vitamin B6, pyridoxine, is needed by the body's own enzymes that break-down and detoxify histamine.
- Be patient. It sounds terrible but many resolve spontaneously disappearing as mysteriously as they came.

Complementary therapies

Again homeopathy is perhaps the most promising. Homeopathic preparations of bee sting and stinging nettle are available and are worthy of use for symptomatic relief at least.

Veronica's story

For twelve years Veronica, a 37-year-old teacher, had experienced recurrent itchy red swellings on her face. Urticaria had been diagnosed but no cause had been found, though she herself was suspicious that there were a number of dietary triggers. In fact she felt better when following a high-protein, high-dairy product diet. Her rash had been so severe that she had used steroids in the past but had stopped these.

A few simple skin allergy tests did not reveal any obvious potential triggers. It therefore seemed possible that she had a degree of salicylate sensitivity. These compounds are found widely distributed in a number of fruits, vegetables and yeast derived products. She began a low salicylate diet and took supplements of vitamin C and magnesium for their antihistamine effects. Over several months her skin reactions diminished though occasional episodes still occurred for reasons that were not entirely clear. The general conclusion was that she was likely to have a degree of salicylate sensitivity though there is no specific test to confirm this.

See also: Standard references.

Vaginal Problems

VAGINITIS

During the child-bearing years, for most women the vagina is a warm moist place which has a constant supply of secretion, stimulated by the hormone oestrogen. When the vaginal cells stop secreting fluid the vaginal walls and tissue naturally become dry, and sometimes itchy. Sexual intercourse then becomes painful, as there is no natural fluid being produced, possibly placing a strain on a relationship, and wrecking sexual enjoyment.

Vaginitis, or inflammation of the mucous membranes lining the vagina manifests as a burning sensation and/or itching and abnormal vaginal discharge. Vaginitis may be caused by bacterial or fungal infection, age, and irritation from using perfumed soaps and deodorants. Other factors, including poor hygiene and tight clothing can also be triggers.

The use of antibiotics can disturb the body's natural balance, creating an environment in which infectious organisms can thrive.

What your doctor can do

- Prescribe some hormone cream to insert into the vagina.
- Suggest a course of hormone replacement therapy. (Refer to page 298 before making a decision about taking HRT.)

What you can do

- Concentrate on eating a diet rich in naturally occurring, phytoestrogens as these have been shown to bring about the same changes in the lining of the vagina as HRT.
- Follow the recommendations for The Very Nutritious Diet, on page 437, unless you are approaching or going through the menopause, in which case you need to refer to the WNAS Programmes on page 477.
- Use a vaginal lubricant in the short-term like Replens or KY Jelly before attempting to make love.
- As well as vitamins and minerals, it is advisable to take the herbal supplement Novogen red clover. This provides 40mg of isoflavones which can be taken in conjunction with a phytoestrogen rich diet to help balance hormone levels.
- Take a probiotic supplement like acidophillus which contains strains of

'friendly' bacteria. Probiotics are particularly useful if antibiotics have been administered.
- Take garlic in supplement form, as well as increasing your dietary intake for its natural anti-fungal properties.
- Do daily pelvic floor exercises.

Vaginal infections

- Apart from the falling levels of oestrogen at the time of the menopause, causing vaginal dryness, there are three main types of infection that cause vaginitis:
  - *Candida Albicans* – which causes thrush (see page 124)
  - *Trichomonas* – a sexually transmitted infection
  - *Bacterial vaginosis* – which may co-exist with other vaginal and sexually transmitted infections.

TRICHOMONAS VAGINALIS

This is the name of the organism causing this common infection. It is estimated that there are 180 million new cases per year worldwide. In men infection is often without symptoms, however in women, common symptoms include:

- vaginal discharge – which may be yellowish-green and frothy.
- an unpleasant odour.
- swelling and redness of the vaginal walls.
- inflammation of the cervix may also be seen on internal examination which may cause spotting or bleeding between periods. Some women may carry the infection with relatively few symptoms, or it may be associated with other sexually transmitted diseases.

What your doctor can do

- There is good response to a single oral dose of metronidazole – 2 g. Do not drink alcohol whilst taking this medicine.
- Check for other infections.
- Screen your partner.

What you can do

- Ensure your partner either uses a condom, or has been cleared as a carrier of *Trichomonas vaginalis*.
- If your infection is slow to clear, supplements of zinc, 30 mg daily, and a multi-vitamin preparation, may be helpful.

BACTERIAL VAGINOSIS

This was also known as Gardenerella, and is due to an infection with a variety of co-existing organisms. In this condition there is no inflammation of the vagina, hence irritation is normally absent. There is usually a whitish discharge which may have a distinctive fishy smell, due to the presence of ammonia. The odour may be more noticeable after sexual intercourse, because of the chemical effect of semen. Again, many women may have this condition without knowing as there are few symptoms. Recent research has shown that this condition is associated with an increase risk of:

- Having a premature baby.
- Having low birthweight babies.
- Infections during pregnancy, after delivery, following a hysterectomy and after an abortion.

Some women will need to be screened before conceiving, during pregnancy and before planned gynaecological operations. Male partners may be carriers for similar bacteria, but transmission has not been proved.

What your doctor can do

- Prescribe antibiotic treatment, with either metronidazole or clindamycin. Both can now be given as vaginal preparations as well as tablets.
- Screen both you and your partner for sexually transmissible disease.

What you can do

Some women may be predisposed to this type of infection and may be helped by:

- Eating well. Follow the recommendations for The Very Nutritious Diet on page 437.
- Applications of plain live yoghurt into the vagina daily for two or three weeks.
- Take a probiotic supplement like acidophillus which contains strains of 'friendly' bacteria. Probiotics are particularly useful if antibiotics have been administered.
- Reduce your sugar intake by avoiding shop bought cakes and biscuits, sweets and desserts. Sugar contains no nutrients and encourages the overgrowth of bacteria and can exacerbates fungal infection.
- Avoiding alcohol and cigarettes completely.
- Taking supplements of multi-vitamins and zinc.

ALLERGIC VAGINITIS

Believe it or not allergy is a possible cause of vaginal irritation. This should only be considered after infection has been excluded.

Curiously, one of the first reports of this came from a study of migraine in over 90 children. Not only did the headaches often improve following the exclusion of certain foods but ten of the eleven girls in the study who were observed to have a vaginal discharge also noticed that this complaint resolved. Sensitivity to wheat, dairy products and yeast-rich foods, both baker's and brewer's, seem particularly likely. It may therefore be useful to try an exclusion diet (see page 460).

Finally, it is possible to be allergic to your man! A report from America (where else) revealed that some men's semen may have high levels of antibodies which react with the woman's vaginal proteins. Improvement will occur if the woman takes an antihistamine or if her partner uses a condom.

One of the women in this study noticed her vaginitis was worse after her husband drank beer, and allergy to brewer's yeast is not impossible. It may be possible to test for this using a modified skin prick test technique.

Mary's story

Mary had known for years that she had a number of food allergies. Mouth tingling and swelling occurred when she consumed a variety of foods, especially certain fruits and thus she was easily aware of the connection. Curiously one of her sensitivities was to avocado, an unusual but known sensitivity.

Her complaint was – however – of vaginal irritation which she had noticed was worse after intercourse. She had been carefully checked for vaginal infection and this was not the problem. Furthermore, her husband always used a condom and so it seemed unlikely her irritation could be related to his semen.

There is in fact a botanical similarity between rubber and avocado plants, which she was aware of. It was suggested that she might be sensitive to rubber and that she changed to using hypoallergenic condoms which are now widely available. This appeared to improve the problem greatly. Unfortunately her wish to be desensitised to food, especially fruit allergies, could not be fulfilled and it is likely that these will persist for some time.

VAGINISMUS

A minority of women experience this unpleasant condition, which involves spasm of the muscles at the entrance to the vagina. This makes intercourse or even the insertion of a tampon difficult, painful or impossible. In severe cases routine gynaecological examination may even require an anaesthetic.

What causes it?

- Anxiety about intercourse or the possibility of becoming pregnant.
- Following episiotomy – an incision made during labour to widen the birth canal.
- Psychological trauma following rape.
- In association with irritable bowel syndrome.

What your doctor can do

- Discuss the problem and potential trigger factors with you.
- Perform a physical examination.
- Refer you for some counselling.
- Suggest the use of graded dilators which you can gently introduce into the vagina on a daily basis.

What you can do

- Discuss the problem with your partner to generate more understanding.
- Understanding the workings of the sexual organs and how the problem occurs is very important.
- Prolonged foreplay may help to relax the muscles.
- Treat any irritable bowel syndrome (see page 270). Resolving associated constipation is particularly important.
- Take daily supplements of magnesium, between 300–400 mg per day.
- Do pelvic floor exercises at regular intervals throughout the day.
- Make sure you take time out each day, 15–20 minutes at least, to relax properly. Refer to page 29 for some useful tips.

Complementary therapies

Vaginal problems need to be addressed by conventional means initially, and any underlying infection cleared. The strength of complementary therapies is that they are good at helping to boost the immune system, which then makes your resistance to a recurrence that much better.

Massage is particularly relaxing, you could even administer some self-massage to tight muscles with some almond oil, if you suffer with vaginismus. Acupuncture, herbal therapy and homeopathy may or may not be helpful, but they are certainly worth a try if all else fails.

Joanne's story

Joanne was a 54-year-old mother of four who approached the WNAS for help with her menopause problems. She had also experienced vaginal and pubic itching following treatment for erosion of the cervix 29 years previously which still persisted.

'I had an abnormal smear 29 years ago which needed attention. When I went to the hospital for a cauterisation I turned out to be pregnant. I noticed during the pregnancy that I had continuous itching around the pubic area and vagina and assumed that I had picked up some infection in the hospital. My doctor took swabs but could not find any abnormal organism and when the problem continued after the pregnancy it was felt to be hormonal. The doctor suggested it was worse before my period due to a rise in temperature.

Five years ago I saw a dermatologist who suggested it might be a form of eczema although I have never suffered with eczema before. I have had normal smears since that one abnormal episode 29 years ago, so I knew it was nothing sinister.

I read about the work of the WNAS, plus I was recommended to seek their advice about my menopausal problems, as I was experiencing hot flushes, night sweats, palpitations and was generally feeling exhausted. I went along to the clinic and had a very thorough consultation. I left with a detailed plan for a modified diet, exercise and a specific nutritional supplement regime. I did not imagine that the vaginal and pubic symptoms would be influenced by the programme I was given but I am pleased to say that everything has cleared up. I occasionally get a mild version of flushes when I am not practising my relaxation regularly but I feel a million times better, and I'm delighted to say that after 29 years the pubic itching and vaginal discomfort is hopefully a thing of the past.'

See also: Standard references.

Varicose Veins

If you read the section on haemorrhoids (see page 220), which are the equivalent of varicose veins but in the tail end, you will recall that veins contain valves, which shut off to prevent the backflow of blood. When these valves malfunction, a pool of blood collects, weakening the walls of the vessel, which eventually balloon out and appear swollen. The veins at the back of the legs and thighs are more often affected, giving an appearance of a shrivelled bunch of black grapes, and this often runs in families.

Varicose veins can also occur in the vulva during pregnancy which is usually due to the increased weight of the uterus, the size of the baby and the fact that blood vessels relax because of the pregnancy hormone relaxin.

Sometimes the blood in the veins may clot, especially if there is a superficial injury or skin infections which may be associated with the oral contraceptive pill, and with smoking. This leads to further damage to the valves and worsening of the varicose veins.

What are the symptoms?

- aching in the legs, which is worse at the end of the day.
- swelling of the ankles.
- episodes of thrombosis (blood clotting) with further pain and swelling.
- eczema of the overlying skin (called varicose eczema).
- ulceration of the skin, if the varicose veins are severe and long-standing.

Treatment should focus on increasing circulation and strengthening connective tissue.

What your doctor can do

- Recommend support stockings, which are not very sexy, but are effective.
- Inject fluid to shrink the worst of the varicose veins, which takes several weeks to effect.
- Operate to tie off and remove the worst of the veins. Heavy support bandages are worn after the operation and support stockings may be needed subsequently until healing is complete.
- Treat any varicose ulcer, which includes leg elevation to reduce any swelling, a non-stick antiseptic dressing, compression bandage, antibiotics if infected, and possibly low-dose aspirin.

What you can do

- Lose weight if you need to.
- Follow a low-salt diet if ankle swelling is a particular problem (see page 449).
- Take supplements of vitamin C, 1 g twice daily, with bioflavonoids, as these may help to strengthen the vessel walls.
- If you have a varicose ulcer, take supplements of multi-vitamins and zinc, 30 mg per day, which may aid ulcer healing.
- Take a herbal supplement of horse chestnut. Horse chestnut is the second most popular herb prescribed in Germany, greatly outselling

herb extracts such as echinacea and St. John's Wort. Horse chestnut reduces the number and diameter of small pores in the capillary membranes, thus reducing the escape of fluid into the surrounding tissues. This improves blood flow in the veins, and reduces swelling of small veins in the legs.

- Butcher's broom is another herb used to prevent and treat vascular disorders, especially varicose veins and haemorrhoids. It works by reducing vaso-constriction of the blood vessels (narrowing) in the legs.
- Rutin, a bioflavonoid has been popularised for its ability to strengthen capillary walls in the legs. Buckwheat, part of the rhubarb family is a particularly good source of rutin.
- Avoid standing for long periods of time.
- Exercise, in particular, increases circulation and strengthens the action of the venous valves. It helps improve muscle function around the vein, which in turn helps tighten and support the blood vessels.
- Keep your legs elevated whenever possible so that the fluid can drain away from the varicose vein.
- Wear support stockings, don't just keep them in the drawer!

Complementary therapies

Acupuncture, homeopathy, herbal medicine and cranial osteopathy all have something to offer in their own way. Improving the flow of fluid around the body will help to unlock the areas of stagnation. Additionally acupuncture may also be able to help strengthen the walls of the vessels.

See also: Standard references.

Part Three

EATING FOR
HEALTH

The Very Nutritious Diet

Everyone has different needs. Women in particular are likely to be short of certain nutrients at certain times in their lives, which affect not only their metabolic rate, and their hormones, but also their mental and physical well-being. Inadequate nutrition and lack of exercise are two known ways of adversely affecting hormone function and energy levels, and perpetuating common symptoms like moodswings, depression and headaches. The appearance of our skin, the health of our hair and nails, our hormone function and our general sense of well-being are all directly affected by our diet, lifestyle and environment.

There is also plenty of scientific evidence to show that there is a direct link between our hormone function and what we eat. Japanese women, whose diets contain a large amount of soya protein (rich in natural oestrogen) and oily fish (rich in essential fatty acids) have far fewer health problems than women living on a western diet. Women, whose needs change throughout their lives, need to be aware of the real dietary rules that can greatly influence their quality of health and longevity.

Two essential factors in assessing the adequacy of our diet are whether the intake is adequate in amount, and whether the balance is correct. Nowadays lack of intake is not usually the problem. The Very Nutritious Diet has been designed to provide a healthy diet with a good balance of all the important nutrients. The portion sizes should be adjusted according to your appetite and activity level. One major point worth noting about this diet, is that it is supposed to be enjoyable, and can be adapted to individual taste. Use the recommendations as a basic guideline. Additionally, look over the Nutritional Content of Food lists which begin on page 483 for other appealing foods to include into your diet.

Food allowances and cooking instructions

Meat and fish Always use lean cuts and trim the excess fat.
Fried food Use the stir-fry method with a minimum of oil, and keep fried foods to a minimum.
Oils and fats Use polyunsaturated oils e.g. sunflower, rape, walnut and sesame. Polyunsaturated spreads like Flora are preferable to butter. Small amounts of butter can be used on toast or crackers if preferred. Avoid margarine containing hydrogenated oils and trans fatty acids.

Sugar and sweet foods Keep sugar-rich foods to a minimum, and always consume after a wholesome meal. Options for cooking include fructose, concentrated apple juice and small amounts of organic honey.

Bread Try to incorporate a variety of grains into your diet as well as wheat including rye, oats, corn and rice. Health-food shops often stock a good variety of breads.

Bran Avoid bran and foods containing bran completely as it impedes the absorption of good nutrients.

Salt and salty foods Try not to add salt to cooking or at the table especially if fluid retention is a problem as it tends to drag fluid into the cells. We already consume too much salt.

Fruit Preferably fresh, although tinned in fruit juice is permitted. Aim to eat three portions of fresh fruit per day (one bowl of berries = one portion).

Vegetables Aim to consume three portions of fresh vegetables (excluding potatoes) daily including one green leafy vegetable, i.e. cabbage, spinach, broccoli, kale, Brussels sprouts, etc. Where possible have raw vegetables in salads and raw vegetable crudites. Cook in the minimum amount of water, or steam if possible.

Tea and coffee Avoid caffeine and keep decaffeinated to a maximum of four cups per day. Ideally try some of the alternatives listed on page 7.

Milk and yoghurt Aim to use organic milk, preferably semi-skimmed. Try to consume live yoghurt (bio yoghurt). Aim to consume between 400–600 ml (3/4–1 pint) of milk per day.

Cheese A variety of cheeses are permitted – a portion daily if desired.

Eggs Preferably free-range may be consumed daily if desired.

Sample menu

Breakfast options

A substantial bowl of cereal i.e. muesli, oat- or wheat-based, or corn-flakes with added nuts, seeds and dried fruit plus a portion of chopped fresh fruit, bio yoghurt and semi-skimmed milk
or
A bowl of porridge and a large egg, boiled, scrambled or as an omelette, with sautéed or grilled mushrooms and tomatoes
and, or
One slice of toast with polyunsaturated spread and sugar-free jam or marmalade

Mid-morning snack
See opposite

Lunch options

A salad with meat, poultry, fish, egg, cheese, beans or nuts

A salad with jacket potato with filling e.g. tuna and sweetcorn, baked beans or cheese

or

A bowl of soup, ideally home-made, vegetable-based with either peas, beans, lentils fish or meat

or

Sandwich containing lean meat, fish, chicken, egg, cheese, etc

or

Pasta with tomato and meat or fish sauce with salad

Mid-afternoon snack

See below

Dinner option

A portion of lean meat, poultry, fish or vegetarian protein weighing approximately 175–225 g (6–8oz). Three portions of vegetables or salad

Root vegetables, rice and pasta are an optional extra, followed by a fresh fruit dessert

Snacks and desserts

Choose from:

Fresh fruit
A combination of dried fruit, nuts and seeds
Bio yogurt with fruit and nuts
Raw vegetables with dips like hummus, taramasalata or guacamole
Fruit, nut and oat bar/flapjack
Cheese and biscuits
Scone with sugar free spread
Yoghurt and fruit
Baked apple stuffed with dried fruit

Beverages

Choose from:

Moderate amounts of tea and coffee – ideally no more that two or three cups or mugs per day

Limited amounts of decaffeinated drinks, as these contain other chemicals – no more than two or three cups or mugs per day

Unlimited amounts of herbal teas and coffee substitutes – see the Caffeine-free Diet suggestions on pages 440–441.

Unlimited amounts of fresh fruit juice, water (preferably filtered) or a combination of the two

Instead of cola-based drinks or lemonade, regular consumption of the healthy varieties of fruit juice and fizzy water, like Amé, Appletise, and Irish Spring. These days most of the supermarkets have their own brand of healthy drinks on offer. Try several until you find the ones that suit your taste.

Basic dietary guidelines

- Eat three proper meals a day.
- Always start the day with breakfast – it is the most important meal of the day.
- Plan your meals ahead, preferably a week in advance, so that when you go shopping you can make sure you purchase the correct ingredients.
- Eat wholesome snacks between meals to keep your blood sugar constant particularly in your premenstrual week if you are still menstruating.
- Avoid convenience foods and junk food which are high in sugar, salt or fat.
- Go shopping at least twice a week to buy fresh fruit and vegetables.
- Don't go shopping on an empty stomach as you may end up buying the wrong foods. Take a list with you and try to stick with it.
- Arrange to eat with family and friends as often as possible.
- Savour your food as you eat, and chew it well.

The Caffeine-free Diet

It is particularly important for people suffering with nervous tension, mood swings, irritability, headaches, breast tenderness or insomnia to avoid caffeine. Many alternatives are listed below but beware the withdrawal symptoms. In the first week of avoiding caffeine people often experience extra symptoms of headaches, anxiety, irritability, mood swings, insomnia and sometimes fatigue. These symptoms will pass within the space of a few days to a week, so do persist.

Follow the instructions for The Very Nutritious Diet but avoid caffeine in the form of tea, coffee, drinking chocolate, cola-based drinks and other products containing chocolate. Read labels carefully, as painkillers often contain caffeine. Look out for alternative products to tea and coffee and other drinks which are available from the supermarket and the health-food shop.

Herb teas There are a wide variety of choices of fruit teas like raspberry and ginseng, lemon verbena, mixed berry teas, etc. on the market, and very often they are sold in single sachets so that you can buy and try without being committed to a whole box of tea bags.

Rooibosch/Redbush Herbal *tea* lookalike. A very tea-like alternative to tea when made with milk but contains no caffeine, very little tannin and a mild muscle relaxant. There are a number of other teas available in the health-food shop that fit into this category.

Coffee There are many caffeine-free coffee alternatives such as – Barley Cup, Caro, NoCaf, and Dandelion Coffee. The latter comes in two varieties: the instant in a jar which is sweet; and the dandelion root which can be ground in a coffee grinder and stored in a jar. This is best used through a coffee filter or strainer either over a cup or through a coffee filter machine. It makes a very strong malted drink.

Fizzy drinks There are many sparkling drinks available to take the place of cola-based drinks and other fizzy drinks that contain caffeine. Most supermarkets do their own brand as well as leading makes like Appletise, Irish Spring, Amé, Aqua Libra, etc.

Chocolate The bad news is there are no real alternatives although some people find carob acceptable and this can be purchased in the health-food shop. Fresh fruit or dried fruits, unsalted nuts and seeds, which are intrinsically sweet, are a much more nutritious alternative. Organic chocolate in moderation is the best option if you need to satisfy your sweet tooth.

The Dairy-free Diet

The Dairy-free Diet is particularly indicated for people with allergies, eczema and asthma. Irritable bowel symptoms can be aggravated by dairy products as can skin problems, catarrh and arthritis.

Follow the instructions for The Very Nutritious Diet with the following modifications.

Milk There are numerous varieties of soya 'milk' available, some more palatable than others. The Tesco soya 'milk' has been popular with most WNAS patients and Granose is a good brand to try. Also try nut 'milk' including hazelnut and almond, rice 'milk' and oat 'milk' if permitted.

Butter Use sunflower or soya spreads instead.

Oil Use sunflower, safflower, or rapeseed for cooking and oils like sesame, walnut, and olive oil for dressing salads.

Yoghurt There are some very acceptable soya yoghurts on the market now.

Ice cream Use sorbet or soya ice cream like Ice Dream, which is made from natural ingredients and is very palatable, or Carob Ices, which are the equivalent of choc ices.

Cream An acceptable pouring cream substitute is Provamel's Soya Dream

Cheese There is a soya version of cheese which is available from health-food shops. It is reasonably acceptable sliced with crackers. It does not seem to cook at all well, however.

Although soya is a rich source of calcium those following a dairy-free diet should ensure they have an adequate intake. It is advisable to refer to the calcium food list on page 487.

The Gluten-free Diet

Foods containing gluten are most commonly the grains wheat, oats, barley and rye. Whilst those suffering with coeliac disease know that they must avoid gluten, according to recent research there are may pre-coeliacs or gluten-sensitive individuals who also would do well to avoid gluten.

Food allowances and cooking instructions

Avoiding foods that contain gluten is not necessarily as easy as it sounds, for wheat in particular is used as a thickening agent in the form of modified starch in so many types of foods, ranging from yoghurts to sauces. In order to avoid gluten completely you will need to arm yourself with alternatives, and to read food labels carefully before making your purchases. There are plenty of alternatives, it is just a question of knowing what to look for.

Bread

There are now many alternatives to ordinary bread, some of which can be purchased and others which you need to bake yourself. Both chemists and health-food shops usually have some stocks of the alternative grain products; in our experience the chemists are usually the most reasonably priced. Behind the counter in the pharmacy you will usually find a stock of products kept for people with gluten allergy. Ask the pharmacist for help, as they sometimes have to order products on request.

Look out for some of the following products:

- Ener G white or brown rice bread (which toasts nicely).
- Glutafin wheat-free bread and rolls and Glutafin crackers.
- Glutano crackers, part-baked bread and corn wafers are all very acceptable.
- Rice cakes.
- Barkat white and brown rice bread which can be gently warmed or toasted for best results.

- Lifestyle gluten and wheat free-bread and cakes delivered fresh to your home.
- Dr Scharr wheat and gluten-free bread rolls and baguettes.
- Plenî day gluten-free part baked rolls.
- Orgran corn crispbreads plain or paprika flavoured.

Home-made bread It is possible to make something that resembles bread using a combination of rice, corn, potato and gram flour. A new multi-purpose gluten-free flour from Dove's Farm is excellent for making bread and scones.

Pizza base You can make an excellent pizza base with Dove's Farm gluten-free flour mix.

Pasta

Although you will need to avoid the pasta made with wheat, there are many reasonable alternatives you can try. Most of these are available from health-food shops, the Chinese supermarket or the pharmacist.

Glutafin have a range of pasta which is sometimes available in health-food shops, and again can be ordered from the chemist. Mrs Leeper makes corn- and rice-based alternatives to spaghetti that the whole family can enjoy.

Rice noodles are available in a wide variety from Chinese supermarkets. There are wide, flat rice noodles that resemble tagliatelle, spaghetti-like noodles, and the very skinny variety that only need soaking in a covered pan in boiling water for a few minutes. You will probably find that these are cheaper than the alternative pastas available from health-food shops and chemists.

Breakfast cereal

Any rice or corn cereals will be fine, even ordinary Rice Krispies and corn-flakes from the supermarkets. Add some chopped fruit and some crumbled nuts, perhaps a few seeds and a little dried fruit to your cereal to make it a bit more wholesome, or make a muesli using nuts, seeds, rice, corn and dried fruit. There are some alternative mueslis available, but they are usually very expensive for only a small packet.

Home-made cakes

If you enjoy cooking there are plenty of very acceptable biscuits, cakes, pastries, sponges and pancakes you can make using alternative flours. If you have never used any of the alternative flours before it may take you a little time to find the consistency that you like.

Sponge Brown rice flour is probably the best for making a sponge. Make it up to the weight given in the recipe by mixing it with a little ground almond and a raising agent (cream of tartar and bicarbonate of soda).

Soya flour is also good (if it is combined with brown rice or corn flour) because it tops up your daily phytoestrogen intake. Experiment with Dove's Farm Gluten Free Flour. It is a versatile mix which makes light cakes and sponges and can be used in most conventional recipes. Terence Stamp All Purpose Wheat-free Flour is a mixture of barley, rice, millet and maize which works well in cookies, cakes, biscuits and scones.

Raising agents As baking powder contains wheat, you will need to use an alternative. Either use a combination of one part bicarbonate of soda to two parts of cream of tartar, or use Glutafin wheat-free baking powder.

Savoury pancakes These can be made with pure buckwheat flour, which is part of the rhubarb family and tends to be quite heavy, or buckwheat mixed with a little white rice flour, which is very light.

Sweet pancakes These are best made with a combination of brown rice flour, or ground rice and cornflour, purchased from a health-food shop or Chinese supermarket. Use half cornflour and half rice flour to replace the normal quantity of flour in the ordinary pancake recipe.

Breadcrumbs or batter A crisp coating for fish or meat can be made with maize meal, which can be found in health-food shops. Coat the fish or meat with maize meal, then with beaten egg, and once again with maize meal. You can then bake, grill or even fry the food, which should emerge with a crispy coat.

Biscuits There is a variety of biscuits that you can make using brown rice flour, or ground rice, and ground nuts or coconut. If you make plain biscuits you can flavour them with lemon or ginger. Recipes for almond macaroons and coconut biscuits are very acceptable, and at the same time more nutritious than the average biscuit, as they are full of eggs and nuts. It is a good idea to make some and keep them in the freezer, so that you can take a few out when you really feel you need something sweet to eat.

There are many other flours that you can use in your cooking. Gram flour made from chickpeas, potato flour, soya flour, tapioca flour and millet flour are all good examples. Glutafin make flour mixes for bread, pastry and cakes, as do Tru Free, and these are available in some health-food shops. Dove's Farm have brought out a new multi-purpose gluten-free flour mix. It is ideal for making cakes, biscuits and bread and is so simple to use.

Shop-bought cakes and biscuits

Acceptable cakes and biscuits can now be purchased in health-food shops and ordered from most chemists.

Both Glutafin and Glutamo have a range of biscuits, including digestives, and Rite-Diet have a range of biscuits and cakes. The coconut biscuits are the least sweet, and the banana or lemon cakes are worth trying too. Dr Sharr and Plenî day cakes and biscuits are available from selected health-food shops. Lifestyle products manufacture gluten- and wheat-free bread, rolls, cakes and savouries and deliver them to your door!

Snacks

It's nice to have something to crunch on when you are avoiding wheat. There are lots of corn products available, but do remember to read the labels, as some have added wheat. Try corn chips, crisps and wafers, and look in the Mexican section of the supermarket. Also, poppadoms are fine, and little mini spiced poppadoms are nice to nibble on or dip.

Sample menu

Breakfast

Puffed rice, Cornflakes, chopped almonds, sunflower seeds, raisins, chopped apricots, with chopped banana, Bio-yoghurt and semi-skimmed milk

Rooibosch Eleven O'Clock Tea, or decaffeinated tea

Mid-morning snack

Gluten-free bread or crackers with nut butter or fruit spread with a glass of orange juice or milk

Lunch

Jacket potato with protein filling, i.e. fish, poultry, cheese or beans, with mixed salad

or

Home-made soup and salad

or

Fish, meat, poultry, egg, cheese and salad with gluten-free bread or crackers

Decaffeinated coffee or herbal tea

Mid-afternoon snack

Wheat-free cake or biscuits with tea, decaffeinated or herbal tea

or

Raw vegetable crudités with hummus dip and Nachips corn wafers

Dinner

Grilled or steamed fish with spring onions and ginger, courgettes, carrots and mangetout *or*

Chicken or nut and mixed vegetable stir-fry with rice noodles

Fresh fruit salad, fruit mousse or baked apple stuffed with dried fruit and
nuts

Herbal tea or coffee substitute

The High Essential Fatty Acid (EFA) Diet

A diet rich in essential fatty acids (EFAs) is particularly suitable for
patients with cardiovascular disease, peripheral vascular disease, multiple
sclerosis, rheumatoid arthritis and psoriasis.

Follow the directions for The Very Nutritious Diet with the following
modifications.

- Use sunflower margarine.
- Consume plenty of green leafy vegetables daily.
- Use walnut, rapeseed, sunflower and corn oils in your salad
  dressings.
- Consume game meat.
- Consume plenty of fish, such as herring, mackerel, salmon, pilchards
  and sardines.

The High-fibre Diet

This is particularly useful for patients with benign breast disease,
constipation or diverticulosis. Portion sizes according to energy levels
and size.

Food allowances and cooking instructions

Despite the wide use of wholemeal cereal and bran, it is now recognised
that the phytic acid content of these foods may impede the absorption of
good nutrients and can also produce an antibody reaction resulting in
worsening symptoms. Fruit and vegetable fibre are preferable as these
speed up gut transit time, so avoid excessive consumption of food
containing wholewheat, wholegrain pasta and bran.

Concentrate on vegetables, fruit and salad and grains that contain low phytic acid like corn, rice and buckwheat.

Sample menu

Breakfast

Fruit juice, grapefruit or fresh fruit salad
Oat based muesli or oat crunch cereal
  or
Home-made muesli with rice, corn, nuts, seeds, dried fruit with added fruit, bio yoghurt and milk
  or
Brown rice cake, Ryvita or oatcakes with nut butter or low-sugar spread
Decaffeinated tea or coffee or herbal alternative

Mid-morning snack

Raw vegetables with dip
Fresh fruit, dried fruit, nuts and seeds
Oat crunchy bar

Lunch

Vegetable soup including plenty of chopped fresh vegetables, peas, lentils and barley
  or
Jacket potato with baked beans and cheese filling or tuna and sweetcorn
  or
Salad with protein i.e. meat, fish, chicken or vegetarian protein, cheese, egg, nuts, seeds, beans, lentils
  or
Raw vegetable crudité and dips like hummus, taramasalata or guacamole

Mid-afternoon snack

Oat flapjack
Fresh fruit or dried fruit, nuts and seeds

Dinner

Portion of meat, fish, poultry or vegetarian protein
Baked jacket potato
Three portions of vegetables and/or salad
Fresh fruit or fresh fruit dessert like baked apple, fruit salad
Herb tea or decaffeinated tea or coffee

The High-protein Diet

A high-protein diet is particularly indicated for people who have a high energy output like manual workers or athletes, for those suffering with recurrent infection, or recovering from a period of weight loss.

Follow the directions for The Very Nutritious Diet with the following modifications:

- Have some protein at each meal.
- Include unsalted nuts and seeds, or eggs and cheese with your breakfast.
- Increase your protein portion size at your main meal from 175–225 g (6–8oz) to 225–350 g (8–12oz).
- Eat plenty of high-protein snacks like cheese and biscuits, cheese and apple, and nuts and seeds.
- Consume between 600 ml–1.2litres (1–2 pints) milk a day, and include eggs and cheese into your diet on a regular basis.

The Low-salicylate Diet

Salicylates are naturally occurring chemicals found in a wide variety of different foods. A few rare individuals may be sensitive to salicylates and this may cause or aggravate urticaria (nettle rash), asthma and rarely colitis. Such individuals may also be sensitive to aspirin or related pain-killing drugs. Salicylates are not destroyed by cooking.

The main sources of salicylate are fruits, vegetables, spices and yeast-rich foods.

If you follow a low-salicylate diet, avoid the following:

Fruit Only bananas, mango, pomegranate, pawpaw and peeled pears are allowed. Peeled Golden Delicious apples may be tolerated.

Vegetables Avoid carrots, cucumber, onion and peas. All others allowed.

Salads Lettuce and celery allowed. Tomatoes to be avoided.

Nuts All nuts contain salicylates.

Yeast Avoid all foods containing yeast including bread, or fermented beverages, yeast extract and stock cubes and many savoury snacks.

Cereals Maize/sweetcorn contain salicylates. All others including wheat, oats and rice are allowed.

Miscellaneous Avoid tea, coffee, soft drinks and foods containing artificial flavourings.

When extreme salicylate sensitivity is suspected, detailed dietetic advice is usually required.

The Low-salt Diet

The word 'salt' is usually used to refer to sodium chloride (table salt) which has long been used as a natural flavour-enhancer and preservative. Compared with the diets consumed by primitive man, we consume ten to 50 times as much sodium salt and not all of us have had the ability to adapt to making such a change. It is now appreciated that high intakes of sodium salt in some people may cause or aggravate a variety of different conditions, including:

- High blood pressure
- Kidney disease
- Heart failure
- Liver disease
- Fluid retention, especially in women
- Patients on high doses of steroids
- Certain types of asthma.

Benefit may be experienced by many of those troubled by the above conditions if they reduce their sodium intake. Unfortunately, this is not just simply a matter of not adding salt to meals, or not using it in cooking. Some two-thirds of our sodium intake now comes from processed and prepared foods, rather than that which is added to the cooking or at the table.

How to reduce your salt intake

1. **Do not add salt or sodium bicarbonate when cooking foods.** If cooking savoury dishes or vegetables, try adding herbs instead, to help give more flavour.
2. **Do not add salt at the table.** At first, food may taste a little bland or unexciting, without its usual spray of salt. After four to six weeks, your tastebuds should adjust, and food will regain its original flavour, and you may even develop a dislike for salty foods.
3. **Avoid foods rich in sodium salt.** As a rule, all fresh vegetables and fresh fruits are low in sodium and high in its healthy mineral counterpart, potassium. Many processed and prepared foods are rich in sodium. Often they will not give the sodium content, but if on the listed ingredients they include the words 'salt', 'sea-salt' seasoning, they should be avoided completely. Also, some additives, especially monosodium glutamate, sodium benzonte or any other sodium compound means the food should be avoided.
4. **Avoid all foods tinned in 'brine'. Brine is simply salted water.**

The following foods are high in sodium, and should not be consumed as part of a low-sodium diet.

Vegetables   Baked beans, tinned peas, potato crisps, instant potato, salted peanuts, any canned vegetables (unless stated as being salt-free). Fresh vegetables have a low sodium content and can be eaten in abundance.

Meats   Almost all preserved meats, including bacon, ham, gammon, corned beef, sausages, frankfurters, tinned meat and meat sauces, pork pies, sausage meat, sausage rolls, pâté, meat or poultry pies, tongue.

Fish   Tinned, frozen or cooked shellfish, including cockles, shrimps, lobster and crab, unless alive and uncooked. Tinned fish, e.g. tuna, anchovies, salmon (unless stated to be salt-free).

Cheese/ Butter   All types of cheese, salted butter. Foods made with cheese, e.g. pizza.

Bread and grain products   All bread (unless stated to be salt-free). Other wheat products, e.g., naan, rolls, most crackers and savoury biscuits.
Cakes, puddings and desserts may all contain moderate quantities of sodium, and if salt is an ingredient on the packet, they should be avoided.
Breakfast cereals are low in sodium, unless it is stated as an ingredient on the packet. Allbran, Cornflakes and Rice Krispies contain substantial amounts of sodium, and should be avoided. Most mueslis and Shredded Wheat are low in sodium. Nuts and seeds are low in sodium, unless it is added, e.g. salted peanuts.

Condiments   Sauces and pickles should be regarded as being high in sodium, unless it is not listed as an ingredient. Many packet soups and canned soups are also high in sodium, and should all be avoided.

Others   Bovril, Marmite and Oxo cubes and similar savoury products are high in sodium.
Baking powder.
Soft drinks are low in sodium, except tomato juice, unless it is stated to be salt-free.

Sugar and sweet foods   Sugars and sugar products, e.g. toffees, sweets, etc. contain small amounts of sodium, but should not be consumed in anything other than small quantities, as they themselves may enhance fluid retention in some people.
Alcoholic beverages are low in sodium, but again should only be consumed in moderation.

Sample menu

Breakfast

Fruit or fruit juice

Low-salt cereal eg puffed rice, salt-free cornflakes
    or

Home-made muesli using salt-free cornflakes, puffed rice, dried fruit, sunflower seeds, nuts with chopped fresh fruit, bio yoghurt and semi-skimmed milk
    or

1 egg, unsalted with low-sodium bread or crackers, unsalted butter and low- or sugar-free jam or marmalade

Decaffeinated tea or coffee with milk

Mid-morning snack (if desired)

Any unsalted snack from the snack list on page 439.

Lunch

Fruit juice if desired

Salad with low-sodium or home-made salad dressing with unsalted meat, poultry or fish

Potato or rice or pasta cooked without salt

Fresh vegetables

Low-sodium bread or crackers
    or

Home-made soup (salt free)

Mid-afternoon snack (if desired)

Any unsalted snack from the snack list on page 439.

Evening meal

Grapefruit or avocado or home-made unsalted soup

Unsalted meat, fish, chicken or vegetarian protein like nuts, beans or lentils

Three portions of vegetables or salad if desired

Low-sodium bread, roll or crackers

Herb tea or decaffeinated coffee

The Simple
Weight-loss Diet

This Simple Weight-loss Diet aims to achieve three things:

- reduced intake of calories.
- good intake of essential nutrients including protein, vitamins and minerals.
- avoidance or reduction of intake of common foods that are often associated with weight gain and certain health problems.

Food allowances and cooking instructions

Meat and fish Always choose lean meat and trim off excess fat, remove skin, and cook by grilling or baking.

Fried foods Ideally none, or use stir-fry method with the minimum of oil.

Oils and fats Use low-fat polyunsaturated spread, 2 teaspoons per day (e.g. Flora Light), and 1 teaspoon of oil per day (e.g. sunflower or rape seed.

Sugar and sweet foods Ideally none. 1–2 teaspoons of honey per day may be allowed.

Bread Limited to two pieces of bread, white or wholemeal, per day. Use slimmer's bread e.g. Nimble or Slimcea without bran, if available.

Bran Do not eat bran or foods or breakfast cereals containing it.

Pasta One portion of white pasta only.

Salt and salty foods Avoid especially if fluid retention is a problem.

Fruit Preferably fresh. If tinned then drain off the syrup. Eat three pieces of fresh fruit per day. A banana counts as two pieces.

Vegetables Eat fresh vegetables daily. Cook in the minimum of water or steam without salt if possible. Green vegetables – quantity unlimited.

Tea and coffee Allow a total of four cups (2 1/2 mugs) per day of either ordinary or decaffeinated, but preferably Rooibos/Redbush herbal tea lookalike. No sugar allowed.

Milk and yoghurt Use skimmed or semi-skimmed milk and low-fat yoghurt. Allow a total of 300–450 ml (1/2 to 3/4 pint) per day.

Cheese Low-fat or medium-fat cheese only e.g. cottage cheese, Cheddar or Gouda, 75 g (3oz) per week only.

Eggs Allow four per week. Boiled, poached or scrambled, not fried.

Sample menu

Breakfast options

Choose from:

A bowl of cornflakes or Rice Krispies 40 g (1^1/2 oz) and milk with fruit if desired
or
A bowl of porridge without sugar
or
A large egg, boiled or scrambled and bread/toast
or
One rasher of bacon grilled and two tomatoes
or
Sauteed mushrooms 50 g (2oz) and toast or a small egg
or
One piece of toast and low-fat spread and low-sugar marmalade

Lunch options

Choose from:

A baked potato 175 g (6oz), no butter and baked beans, sweetcorn, tuna/ham/chicken 75 g (3oz) with onion/peppers/olives and low-calorie mayonnaise or occasionally cheese
or
A large salad either green or made from cold rice with 75 g (3oz) of chicken breast/lean ham or beef/tinned tuna or mackerel. Use low-calorie mayonnaise or oil-free dressing
or
A bowl of soup ideally home-made vegetable based, with either peas/beans/lentils or approximately 75 g (3oz) lean meat
or
A sandwich, one round, containing lean meat, fish, chicken, egg, cheese etc. and always a lot of salad, e.g. tomato, lettuce, cucumber.

Dinner options

One each of the following:

A protein portion of lean meat, poultry or fish 120–175 g (4–6oz) weight,
Green vegetable or salad portion 225–350 g (8–12oz) weight
Root vegetable, pasta or rice portion (optional) 120–175g (4–6oz) cooked weight
or
Any of the Lunch options provided above

Desserts and snacks
You may have one dessert and two snacks per day

Choose from the following:
A piece of fresh fruit or fruit salad
A low-fat yoghurt, with some fresh fruit or a little dried fruit
Two rice cakes spread with low-sugar jam or a little peanut butter
An apple and a few nuts e.g. almonds, Brazils or walnuts
A little cold rice salad with 25 g (1oz) cold meat and mixed nuts
A bowl of cornflakes or Rice Krispies 25 g (1oz) only and low-fat milk

Basic dietary guidelines

Here are some pointers to eating well, and tips to help you keep to a diet, regardless of its type.

- Eat regularly – have three meals per day.
- Always have breakfast. Missing it may cause you to eat more later.
- Plan your meals for the day or week. Make sure that you can have the right foods in the house or you will end up eating the wrong ones.
- If you are hungry between meals have a snack, a nutritious low-calorie one. Convenience foods are high in fat, sugar and calories.
- Make sure that you have a cooked main meal every day and that this contains plenty of vegetables.
- Enjoy your food and eat your main meal with family or friends where possible. Don't eat it while watching the television.
- Go shopping twice a week to buy fresh fruit and vegetables and never go shopping when you are hungry. Take a list and stick to it.
- Tell your friends that you are on a diet. Some will want to join you, and it will help to stop them leading you astray.
- If necessary have the occasional cheat. A few small pieces of chocolate after a good meal is not the end of the world or the diet.
- Finally, make sure that you do have a very good reason for losing weight. It may be to look better, to feel more comfortable or for a medical reason. In case you don't know, being seriously overweight is strongly linked to heart disease, high blood pressure, strokes, diabetes and even some types of cancer.

The Tunatarian Diet (Vegetarian plus Fish)

A tunatarian diet is particularly indicated for those who wish to avoid red meat and poultry and those directed to a diet rich in essential fatty acids who do not wish to consume meat or poultry.

Follow the directions for The Very Nutritious Diet with the following modifications:

- Replace meat or poultry with fish, beans or eggs.
- Consume fish, beans or eggs every day.
- Eat plenty of nuts, particularly walnuts.
- Consume green leafy vegetables regularly.
- Use walnut, rapeseed, sunflower or safflower seed oil in salad dressings.
- Consume at least three portions of oily fish per week i.e. mackerel, herring, salmon, pilchard or sardines.

The Vegetarian or Vegan Diet

Strictly speaking, a 'vegetarian' should mean someone who eats only vegetable derived foods, but a strict vegetarian is now more usually referred to as a vegan. Vegetarian is usually used to describe somebody who simply avoids meat, fish and poultry, but this can be further sub-divided. Those who consume dairy products as well are known as lacto-vegetarian, and those who consume eggs as well as dairy products are known as ovo-lacto-vegetarian.

Food allowances and cooking instructions

Avoid refined carbohydrates as they are low in essential minerals and vitamins. It is advisable that they should be consumed only in very small quantities by vegetarians and vegans. The intake of essential nutrients, particularly iron and zinc, may be borderline in some vegetarians and vegans and this will only be further hindered by consuming refined carbohydrates.

Ensure an adequate balance of protein in your diet. A major problem with vegetarian and vegan diets is borderline, or poor quality, protein intake. This is particularly true in those who have not taken care to learn the protein-rich foods or the combinations that vegetarians and vegans should eat. Protein-rich foods include nuts, seeds, peas, beans, lentils, wholegrains, brown rice, sprouted beans and soya bean preparations. Vegetarians and vegans should not rely heavily upon any one source of vegetable protein. In particular, they should not rely heavily upon soya protein, as on its own it is not a complete protein.

If you are not a strict vegan, make use of other protein-rich foods. High quality, well-balanced protein is found in eggs which are also rich in iron. One or two eggs can be consumed quite easily per day and would be beneficial.

Good protein combinations
- rice with legumes, sesame or cheese.
- wheat with legumes or mixed nuts and milk or sesame and soya beans.
- corn with legumes.
- mixed nuts with sunflower seeds.
- sesame seeds with beans or mixed nuts and soya beans or mixed nuts and soya beans or wheat and soya beans.

The addition of any first-class protein i.e. milk, or particularly eggs, may substantially enhance the protein value of the vegetable food. Not all members of the legume family are high in protein. Those that are particularly nutritious include mung beans, red kidney beans, haricot beans, butter beans, chick peas, pinto beans, lentils, peas and split peas.

Sprouted beans may be more appetising. Soaking beans for 24 hours and de-husking them may reduce the problem of wind which occurs in some bean eaters.

Avoid foods that block mineral absorption
Many foods contain substances which bind with essential trace minerals and prevent their absorption. Such foods include bran, unleavened wheat – particularly wholewheat as in pastry or when used as a thickening agent – tea, coffee, soft drinks and foods containing phosphate additives. Alcohol also causes increased losses of trace minerals. Iron and zinc absorption may be inhibited by the above foods and drinks. Accordingly such foods should be avoided or consumed in small quantities. It should never be necessary for a vegetarian or vegan to eat bran as there is plenty of fibre in other foods. Tea should not be consumed with a vegetarian meal because of its powerful effect in reducing iron absorption. It is suggested, therefore, that tea consumption should be minimal, particularly in female vegetarians and restricted to two or less cups per day.

Ensure an adequate supply of mineral and vitamin-rich foods. Usually if you are careful to balance the quantities of protein in your diet, and avoid mineral-depleted convenience foods, then your intake of trace minerals would, on the whole, be good. It is strongly recommended that vegetarians and vegans learn which foods are nutritious. The worst possible combination is a poor quality vegetarian diet together with a high intake of sweets, chocolates, and other nutrient-depleted foods.

Vegetarian and vegans in special situations

There are certain situations when a vegetarian or vegan diet may be distinctly inadvisable, or should only be undertaken if one has a very good knowledge of what a healthy vegetarian diet is. Particularly at risk are:

- infants under the age of one year as well as young children.
- the elderly, pregnant or breast-feeding women.
- people who are ill or who have nutritional deficiencies.

Usually medical advice should be sought, in particular to determine whether any additional supplements may be required by people in such situations. Infants, for example, frequently become short of iron on a strict vegetarian or vegan diet. Severe vegan diets may in fact lead to rickets in young children because of lack of vitamin D and calcium in the diet.

The nutritional requirements of pregnant and breast-feeding women must be met, and a poor quality vegetarian diet will often not satisfy the additional needs at these times. The specific advice about nutrient intake and the use of supplements in the preconception phase and pregnancy can be found in the relevant chapters. *See* Preconception (page 384), and Pregnancy (page 388).

The elderly have a declining food intake and so the quality of their dietary intake must be very high in order for them not to develop deficiencies.

While there are certain medical conditions that would benefit from a vegetarian or vegan diet, patients who are ill or who have nutritional deficiencies should seek medical advice before embarking on such a programme.

Food allergy/intolerance and vegetarians/vegans

Food allergies are increasingly common and the major foods that appear to cause trouble are wheat, milk, yeast and soya, many of which may be staple foods in a vegetarian or vegan diet. Thus if your health deteriorates after embarking upon a vegetarian or vegan diet, this may be because of inadequacies in the diet or the presence of food allergies or intolerances. On the other hand, certain aspects of vegetarian or vegan diets may be beneficial for people with food allergies or intolerances, in particular the high consumption of salads and vegetables. If you suspect you may have food allergies refer to the chapter on Allergy on page 58, The Simple Exclusion Diet on page 460, and The Strict Exclusion Diet on page 466.

Vitamin B12

Many experienced vegetarians and vegans appreciate the importance of ensuring adequate vitamin B12 in the diet. The major source of vitamin B12 is meat. Other reasonably good sources include eggs, brewer's yeast and dairy produce. Only strict vegans may need a vitamin B12 supplement. However, anyone who develops vitamin B12 deficiency should receive appropriate investigations to precisely determine the course of their deficiency, and it should not be presumed to be due to dietary inadequacy.

Sample menu

Breakfast

Glass of orange juice
Wheat- or oat-based muesli with additional nuts, seeds, dried fruit, chopped fresh fruit
Toast with nut butter or low-sugar spread or marmalade
Mug of Rooibos/Redbush herbal tea lookalike

Lunch

Salad made with sprouting alfalfa and other mixed salad
Home-made soup or jacket potato with filling
Vegetarian option: cheese or eggs may be added in addition, with a glass of milk
Fresh fruit juice, herb tea or decaffeinated coffee

Dinner

Protein and vegetable combinations such as:
Nut Roast with baked parsnips, carrot and boiled spinach
    or
Tofu and mixed vegetable stir-fry with brown rice
Stir-fry vegetables and nuts or beans
    followed by
Fruit dessert e.g. baked apple, rhubarb crumble or apple pie
Vegetarian option: Cauliflower and broccoli cheese with jacket potato
Fresh fruit mousse followed by herb tea, decaffeinated coffee or fruit juice

NB Pasta should be accompanied by protein as it is not sufficiently nutritious by itself.

Snacks

There are many wholesome vegetarian snacks that can be included into your diet encompassing both sweet and savoury options. Examples are:

oat, fruit and nut flapjacks
dried fruit, nuts and seeds
fresh fruit and soya yoghurt
raw vegetable crudité and dips
nut butter on toast or crackers

Further reading

Diet for a Small Planet Frances Moore Lappe (Valentine Books)
The Reluctant Vegetarian Cookbook Simon Hope (Heinemann)
For further information you may wish to contact the Vegetarian Society, whose address is listed on page 519.

The Yeast-free Diet

This is particularly suitable for thrush sufferers, those with an itchy bottom, bloated abdomen, cracking at the corners of the mouth, excessive wind, cystitis and often depression.

Two or more episodes of thrush and/or any other two symptoms certainly qualify you for the yeast-free diet.

Food allowances and cooking instructions

It is surprising how many foods actually contain yeast, and yeast itself is often used in the food preparation process, in which case it is generally marked on the label of the product. However, yeast is a fungus which grows on food, particularly leftover food, even if well covered. It is also fond of foods with an acid base like citrus fruits and vinegar, and of course foods that contain sugar.

Aim to avoid:

- All foods containing sugar or honey, as yeast thrives in sugary or starchy food.
- All bread, buns, biscuits, cakes, etc.
- Most alcoholic drinks. These often depend on yeast to produce the alcohol, especially beer.
- Citrus fruit, juices – only fresh home-squeezed juice is yeast free.
- Malted cereals, malted drinks.
- Pickles, sauerkraut and chilli peppers.
- Blue cheese (Roquefort etc).

- Mushrooms and mushroom sauce.
- Hamburgers, sausages and cooked meats made with bread or bread-crumbs.
- Yeast extract (miso), Bovril, Marmite, Vegemite.

Follow the instructions for A Very Nutritious Diet whilst avoiding the yeast-based foods and drinks listed.

The Simple Exclusion Diet

The Simple Exclusion Diet is divided into three stages.

In the first four weeks during Stage I, it is very important to eat only the permitted foods. If you introduce other foods you will lose the beneficial effects of the diet and it will be necessary for you to begin again!

In Stage II, also four weeks, you start trying out groups of foods to see whether they push your weight up or produce unwanted symptoms or side-effects.

During the final two-week period you will be eating a diet composed of the foods you have selected through trial and error in the preceding four weeks.

Stage I: Permitted foods

Meat and poultry

For non-vegetarians: all meat, including lamb, beef, pork, chicken, turkey, other poultry and game, and offal, such as liver, kidneys, sweetbreads and hearts, can be eaten if desired. Meat and poultry can be fresh or frozen.

Meat must be lean, with all visible fat trimmed before cooking. Do not eat the skin of chicken or other poultry; it should be removed before or after cooking.

Fish and shellfish

For non-vegetarians: all types are included and they may be fresh or frozen. Do not eat the skin of fish as it is high in fat.

Note: all meat, poultry and fish should be cooked by grilling, dry-roasting, steaming, baking, or stir-frying with low-fat ingredients, e.g. tomatoes or vegetables.

All vegetables

You can and should eat larger amounts of vegetables, especially green ones or salad foods daily. Your allowance will be detailed in the daily menus.

Root vegetables, e.g. potatoes and parsnips, are limited to 120–175g (4–6oz) per day. Beans and peas, which are protein-rich vegetables, are also included in moderate amounts.

Vegetarian proteins

For vegetarians and vegans these proteins are an essential part of the diet. You are allowed all types of nuts, beans, peas, lentils, seeds, corn maize, rice and potatoes. Vegans in particular should have two or three portions per day. Some people experience abdominal bloating and wind with beans, and these should be well soaked and cooked, if necessary de-husked.

Fruits

All fruits are allowed, except dried fruits, glacé fruits, dates, figs, mangoes, and tinned fruits with sugar. Keep tinned fruits without sugar to a minimum also. Aim to consume three portions of fruit per day. Fruit can be either eaten whole or as a fruit salad.

Vegetable oils and vegetable mayonnaise

A small amount of these are allowed daily. You can have up to 2 teaspoons of a low-fat polyunsaturate-rich margarine, such as Flora Light, per day. There are no fried foods on the diet (you didn't really expect them, did you?), but there are some stir-fry dishes and here you just wipe the inside of the pan or wok with a piece of kitchen roll dipped in sunflower or corn oil.

Nuts and seeds

Peanuts, Brazil nuts, almonds, pistachios, cashews, sunflower seeds, and sesame seeds are very nutritious. Nuts and seeds can help to liven up a salad or can be used as a nutritious snack, combined with an apple or another fruit.

Rice and other salads

Brown rice of any variety – long-grain, short-grain or basmati – is allowed. It will often be used instead of potatoes. Rice cakes (a rice crisp-bread) can be used in place of bread. Additionally, buckwheat, millet, sago and tapioca can be used from time to time, but these are not usually very popular.

Breakfast cereals

Only cornflakes and rice cereals are included in Stage I. They contain a good amount of protein and are fortified with extra vitamin B and iron. Other breakfast cereals are not allowed.

Eggs

Up to seven eggs per week are allowed, unless you are known to have a very high cholesterol level or allergy to egg. Free-range eggs are highly nutritious and very good value for money.

Stage I: Foods to be avoided or severely limited

Wheat, oats, barley and rye

All foods made with these, apart from the exceptions given below, are to be avoided. This means no ordinary cakes, biscuits, puddings, pasta, pastry, pies, porridge or breakfast cereals (apart from cornflakes or rice cereals). Bread is severely limited to two slices of white French bread, made with French flour.

Diary products

Cream and cheese are forbidden – even low-fat cottage cheese is out. Your milk allowance is very low, only 75 ml (3 fl ozs) per day of skimmed milk, 600 ml (1 pint) per week. You can use dried skimmed milk instead, or low-fat plain yoghurt.

Butter or a polyunsaturated low-fat spread is allowed: 2–3 teaspoonfuls per day. However, if you have premenstrual tension, painful breasts, or an elevated blood cholesterol level, you should have a low-fat polyunsaturated spread instead of butter.

Foods containing milk, cream, cheese, milk solids, non-fat milk solids, lactalbumin, whey, caseinates, and should be avoided. The only exception to this is polyunsaturated margarine which often contains a very small amount of milk protein, lactalbumin or whey.

Vegetarians i.e. non-meat or fish eaters can have up to 250ml (8 fl oz) cows' milk per day and probably they should have either one egg per day or good portions of beans, peas, lentils and some nuts or seeds on most days. If you are known to have problems with cows' milk you can use soya milk instead; most supermarkets and health-food shops stock it.

Animal fats and some vegetable fats

Animal fats, some vegetable fats, hard margarines, lard, dripping and suet are out, as are palm oil and coconut oil, and foods containing them. Chemically, these vegetable oils are much more like saturated animal fats than good quality sunflower or corn oil which are high in the healthier polyunsaturates. Hard margarines which are made from hydrogenated vegetable oils, are also off the menu.

Sugar, honey, glucose and fructose (fruit sugar)

Any food made with these should be avoided in the main. This means cakes, biscuits, most ice cream, sweets of all kinds, chocolate, and puddings. This is not as depressing as it sounds. There are plenty of fresh fruit desserts, as you will see on the suggested menus. Leave the large helpings of honey for the bees!

Alcoholic beverages

You name it – alcohol is out. Sorry! Don't do this diet over Christmas. Even low-calorie alcoholic drinks, though they are a great improvement, present too many complications for Stage I. You will, however, get the chance to try out alcohol in the third week of Stage II of the diet.

Yeast-rich foods

This includes any foods containing yeast extract: Bovril, Marmite, Oxo, Knorr and other stock cubes, vinegar, any pickled food, chutneys, piccalilli, sauces, or condiments containing yeast extract or vinegar.

Salt

Salt should not be used in cooking or at the table. This is particularly true if you experience fluid retention or high blood pressure. Salty food such as ham, bacon, and any other salted meats should be eaten sparingly. Crisps, peanuts and many convenience dinners are not on the menu at all. If you really cannot do without salt, then use a very small amount only. Put it on the side of your plate. Try flavouring any salads, vegetables, or cooked main dishes with pepper or herbs instead of salt. You should find that your taste for salt becomes less as you progress through the diet programme.

Foods with additives

These cannot be avoided completely, but it is best to avoid those with some types of colouring and preservatives which can cause asthma, nettle-rash (urticaria), eczema, and possibly migraine.

Avoid the following additives where possible:

E102	Tartrazine
E104	Quinoline Yellow
E110	Sunset Yellow FCF or Orange Yellow
E122	Carmoisine or Azorubine
E123	Amaranth
E124	Ponceau 4R or Cochineal Red A
E127	Erythrosine BS
E131	Patent Blue V
E132	Indigo Carmine or Indigotine
E142	Green S or Acid Brilliant Green BS or Lissamine Green
E151	Black PN or Brilliant Black PN
E180	Pigment Rubine or Lithol Rubine BK
E220–227	Sulphites – these may worsen asthma in very sensitive individuals

Other colourings are not likely to cause any adverse reactions.

Suspect foods

Avoid any foods that you know or suspect do not suit you. For example, many people find some fruits, such as oranges or pineapples, too acidic. Even though they are not particularly high in calories you should avoid them. A not-infrequent problem is an inability to digest beans, peas and some vegetables properly, resulting in excessive wind. Possible vegetables in this group include cabbage, Brussels sprouts, cauliflower, onions and sweetcorn. At this point, trust your own knowledge and experience. After all, it is this that we want to increase, so let's not go against anything you know already. Accordingly you may have to adapt the day's menu to recipes to suit yourself.

Modifications

Vegetarians/vegans should also allow peas, beans, lentils, soya milk, non-fermented soya produce, and increased amounts of nuts, seeds and brown rice.

Symptoms

You may notice during the beginning of Stage I that you experience some withdrawal symptoms as a direct result of giving up certain foods and drinks that you usually consume. These symptoms may be anything from headaches to fatigue, even depression. This will depend on your existing diet. For example, if you are consuming lots of cups of coffee or tea, cola drinks, or refined sweet foods, you may find the first week of the diet is quite a challenge.

It is probably best to begin the diet when you have a quiet week to spare. A word of advice to women of child-bearing age is to begin the diet just after your period has arrived and not in the week your period is due. The reason for this is to prevent additional symptoms occurring at a time when you might be suffering from PMS.

You will need the time to accustom yourself to your new way of eating and to get plenty of relaxation. This doesn't mean that you should take time off work; quite the opposite, as it is preferable that you remain occupied while on the diet. Just keep social engagements that involve eating to a minimum. Then, if you feel tired or experience any withdrawal symptoms, you can go off to rest without any guilty feelings of having let others down.

After the first week or so of following the diet, with any possible withdrawal symptoms behind you, things should look up. By Week Three, you may notice that a number of minor health problems have begun to improve. By Week Four, you should be feeling quite well, perhaps better than you have felt for some time and, you may notice that you have shed a few pounds without really trying. In fact those underweight will need to work at maintaining their weight by consuming nuts, seeds, oily salad dressing and alternative cakes and biscuits.

Stage II

You start becoming a 'nutritional detective' during the second four-week period: trying out groups of foods to see whether they push your weight up or produce unwanted symptoms or side-effects. See the Food list for reintroduction, page 468.

For each week there are different instructions. You will need to follow these very carefully as this is an important stage of the diet. If you follow the instructions precisely, you will end up with a diet that is really tailored to suit your own body.

You may experience some symptoms or side-effects from the foods under test. These should pass off within two or three days. There are a large number of symptoms that could be experienced, but these should only be those that cleared up in Stage I. They include migraine, headaches, eczema, nettle-rash (urticaria), rhinitis, asthma, abdominal bloating and discomfort, constipation, diarrhoea, wind, anxiety, irritability, insomnia, and possibly premenstrual tension. If and when you do have a reaction to individual food groups, you may feel that you have had a setback. On the contrary, any reaction should be regarded as a positive step. It means that you have discovered some foods that don't really suit your body at the moment. Any reaction, should it occur, is unlikely to be worse than you have already experienced, and probably will not last more than three days. If you do experience a reaction, you will need to stop eating the foods that are causing the problem. Keep a diary each day and score any reaction you get on a scale of 0–3, 0 = none, 1 = mild, 2 = moderate and 3 = severe. Keep an ongoing list of foods you react to and another list of suspect foods.

Stage III

During the final two-week period you will be eating a diet composed of the foods you have selected through trial and error in the preceding four weeks. You should continue to lose weight and to feel more and more healthy as the weeks go by.

You will have gained the knowledge of how to tell when a particular food does not suit your body and how to deal with any bloating or other symptoms that may occur as a result. By that stage, you should feel totally at home with your new diet and confident that you can maintain it as a life-style with ease in the place of your former diet. Every so often you can reintroduce the foods that were on your Suspect List to see whether you can tolerate them in small quantities perhaps. Sometimes, once the body has had a rest from a previously irritating substance it can cope with reintroduction without any problems.

The Strict Exclusion Diet

This diet is based on considerable work done in the USA and this country, especially at the hospital for Sick Children, Great Ormond Street, London and at Addenbrooke's Hospital, Cambridge. We recommend it for adults only.

	Excluded	Included
Meat	Beef, pork, preserved meats, bacon, sausages.	Lamb, turkey, rabbit.
Fish	All fish and shellfish, except	Trout, fresh or frozen.
Vegetables	Potatoes, onions, sweetcorn, and many other vegetables. Only those mentioned are allowed.	Carrots, parsnips, swedes, spinach, celery, leeks, lettuce and sweet potatoes.
Fruit	All fruits, except	Peeled bananas, pears, mangoes, pomegranates, paw-paws.
Cereals	Wheat, oats, barley, rye, corn.	Rice (white only), rice flakes, rice flour, sago, tapioca, millet, buckwheat and rice cakes.
Cooking oils	Corn oils, soya oil, vegetable oil, nuts, especially peanuts.	Sunflower oil, safflower oil and olive oil.
Dairy products	Cow's milk, butter, most margarines, cows' milk yoghurt, cheese, eggs. All goats', sheep's and soya milk products.	Vitaquell margarine. Pure sunflower or soya margarine.
Beverages	Tea, coffee (beans, instant and decaffeinated), fruit squashes, orange juice, grapefruit juice, alcohol, tap water.	Herbal teas, e.g. camomile, etc. without milk. Water – filtered or bottled mineral. Rooibosch/Redbush tea.
Miscellaneous	Chocolate, yeast, preservatives. All food additives (see separate list). Herbs, spices, sugar, honey.	Sea salt, unless fluid retention, asthma or high blood pressure are present.

Note: Follow this diet exactly. If a food is not mentioned, it is not allowed. Only those foods in the Included list are allowed.

This diet needs to be followed for one to three weeks, and must be undertaken with medical supervision.

Your progress on an exclusion diet

If your symptoms are due to a food reaction, then there should have been some improvement or even complete disappearance of your symptoms whilst following the appropriate diet. It is now important to reintroduce foods, and by so doing, determine which foods, if any, are responsible for your symptoms. In so doing it is important to bear in mind the following points:

- On introducing foods, reactions can occur within minutes, hours or several days of consuming a new food. The speed with which symptoms occur depends to some degree upon the types of symptoms. Nettle rash or facial swelling due to food allergy can occur within minutes or hours. With muscle aches and pains, or even arthritis, it can sometimes take three or four days before the symptoms appear.
- If the reaction occurs, stop consuming the food that you have just introduced, and wait for it to settle down before re-introducing a further food. This may take two or three days.
- If your symptoms are severe, particularly if it is a migraine, you may try taking a drink of two teaspoons of bicarbonate of soda dissolved in water. Also breathing into a paper bag may help abort a migraine attack. Such measures can be useful in reducing the severity of a reaction.
- If you only consume a small amount of the test food, a positive reaction may be missed. It is important that you consume a normal large portion, not excessive, of the food in question.
- If you are uncertain whether there has been a reaction or not, it is usually advisable to leave the food off, assuming that a positive reaction has occurred. It can be tested later. If, however, you are on a very restricted diet, it may be unwise to do this.
- If on a very restricted diet, it is usually advisable to reintroduce relatively safe foods, i.e. further vegetables, meat and fruits. It is often better to leave common high-risk foods, such as wheat and dairy produce, until later in the diet.

Remember that an exclusion diet is done to determine whether or not you have a food sensitivity. Only by reintroducing foods can this be determined. It is very often the case that a considerable amount of weight is lost on such a diet. It is important that this amount is not excessive, and that before starting an exclusion diet, you do not have any physical signs or symptoms attributable to nutritional deficiencies. If so, your doctor will advise you to take appropriate supplements for several weeks before commencing an exclusion diet.

In the long run, reactions to various foods might be diminished by avoiding excessive consumption of salt, sugar and alcohol, even if you are not sensitive to these. Factors such as cigarette smoking, that interfere with normal digestive processes, could also be a contributory factor. Long-term avoidance of those foods to which one reacts may sometimes result in a reduction of the sensitivity to various foods. It is not uncommon that, with appropriate management, those who were previously sensitive to a food, can after several months of appropriate dietary management, be able to tolerate small quantities of the foods to which they reacted. This is not, however, always the case.

Food list for reintroduction

This list of foods is for people who have been on one of the exclusion diets, and are now ready to test out some foods. By now you should have experienced a significant improvement, and unfortunately, may well experience a return of your old symptoms on testing some of these foods. It is important that you proceed in a strictly ordered fashion, otherwise the picture may become confused.

ADD THE FOLLOWING FOODS OR FOOD GROUPS AT INTERVALS OF FIVE DAYS

Eat a normal larger portion of the food(s) on each day of the trial. The foods should be fresh if possible, and not contain any additives.

Vegetables

Carrots, parsnips, celeriac, fennel, parsley
Brussels sprouts, cabbage, broccoli, cauliflower, kale, mustard, turnip, watercress
Cucumber, courgettes, melon, marrow, pumpkin
Potato
Tomato, peppers, chilli, aubergine, paprika
Sweet potato
Onion, leeks, shallots, garlic, asparagus, chives
Spinach
Peas, beans (dry and green), lentils
Nuts, walnuts, Brazil nuts, hazelnuts, cob-nuts (not peanuts)
Peanuts, plain, no additives, roasted or unroasted
Soy beans, soy sauce

Fruits

Apples, pears with skins (and juices)
Oranges, lemons, grapefruits, pomelo, ugli fruit, lime, mandarin, tangerine, satsuma, etc. (and juices)
Peach, apricot, nectarine, prune, cherries
Raspberry, loganberry, strawberry, blackberry
Bananas
Bilberry, blueberry, cranberry
Blackcurrant, redcurrant, gooseberry
Pineapple
Dried fruits

Meats

Test plain meats, not meat products, such as pies, sausages, salami, etc.
Beef, plain, e.g. steak, roast joint, hot or cold
Pork, not bacon, ham and gammon or pâtés
Bacon, ham and gammon
Fish
Shellfish
Chicken and eggs

Grains

Wheat as wholemeal pasta and pastry, not wholemeal bread
Oats
Rye, e.g. Ryvita
Wholemeal bread
Corn maize

Dairy

Cows' milk, cream, yoghurt, butter
Cows' cheese
Goats' milk
Goats' cheese
Soya milk

Other

Tap water
Oxo, Marmite, Bovril, stock cubes
Alcohol, vinegar
Mushrooms
Tea
Coffee
Chocolate
Sugar

It may well help to keep a written record of any reactions you experience after testing various foods.

Further reading: The Allergy Diet, by Workman, Hunter, Alun Jones (Vermilion). This has many invaluable lists of foods which contain wheat, cows' milk, corn, eggs, etc.

Exclusion Menus for Specific Ailments

MENU FOR ACNE

Acne sufferers should have a low-fat and low-sugar diet and concentrate on eating foods that are high in B vitamins and the minerals zinc and selenium.

Rich sources of zinc are:

liver	lentils	cheese
wholegrains	pilchards	oysters and cockles
nuts	spinach	
beans	milk	

Selenium-rich foods are:

herring	wheatgerm	lamb
cod	milk	turnips
scallops	brown rice	garlic
shrimps	eggs	orange juice
Brazil nuts	steak	

Many of these foods are also rich sources of B vitamins.
For further details see Nutritional Content of Food list which commence on page 483.

Breakfast

Fresh grapefruit and orange salad with sunflower seeds
Toast and dried fruit conserve
Dandelion coffee

Mid-morning snack

Brazil nuts and raisins
Rooibosch or Redbush herbal tea look-alike

Lunch

Mackerel in spicy tomato sauce
Mixed salad with mung beans
Barley Cup or NoCaf

Snack

Dried apricots and figs
Cranberry and Apple Tea

Dinner

Lamb steak with jacket potato, spring greens and cauliflower
Carrot cake
Decaffeinated coffee

MENU FOR BREAST TENDERNESS

For every one woman with breast cancer there are ten other women who suffer with benign lumps (non-cancerous) or breast tenderness. Any breast problem should be checked out with your doctor. Once you have established that nothing sinister is going on then you would be advised to change your diet.

- Eat leaner cuts of meat, avoid processed meats like pies and sausages which have a high-fat content, and leave the chicken or fish skin on your plate.
- All meat and fish should be grilled and your dairy intake should be limited, replacing full-cream milk with skimmed or semi-skimmed. Eat low-fat cheese, poly-unsaturated spreads instead of butter, and avoid cream altogether.
- Eat plenty of fibre in the form of fruit, vegetables and salads and steer away from alcohol, sugar, tea, coffee and tobacco.
- Efamol evening primrose oil can be helpful – but you need to take 6–8 x 500 ml capsules per day.

Breakfast

Cornflakes with chopped apple, crumbled pecan nuts and skimmed milk
Rooibosch or Redbush herbal tea look-alike

Mid-morning snack

Two carrots and two sticks of celergy with a hummus dip
Dandelion Coffee

Lunch

Selection of mixed vegetables and brown rice stir-fry, with 2 tablespoons of mixed nuts or beans
Raspberry and Ginseng Tea

Mid-afternoon snack

Rye crackers and mashed banana
Rooibosch/Redbush Tea

Dinner

Poached salmon with courgettes, boiled potatoes and green salad
Fresh fruit salad
Mixed Berry Tea

MENU FOR FATIGUE

Diet and nutrition play a very important part in causing – and alleviating – fatigue. Many people need extra iron, magnesium and vitamin B in their diet, especially women of child-bearing age. Eating a more nutritious, high-protein diet should give you more vitality.

Drinking too much tea, coffee and alcohol and eating too much sugar or sweet and processed foods can also contribute to fatigue. So eat good food, with three regular meals per day and nutritious energy-sustaining snacks.

Breakfast

Oat crunch cereal
Scrambled egg on toast
Decaffeinated coffee

Mid-morning snack

Plain yoghurt with grated apple and sunflower seeds
Mixed Berry Tea

Lunch

Jacket potato with grated cheese or tuna filling
Mixed salad
Barley Cup or NoCaf

Mid-afternoon snack

Wholemeal toast and peanut butter
Herb tea or Rooibosch or Redbush tea

Dinner

Chicken curry with rice, mixed vegetables and poppadoms
Apple pie
Jasmine tea

MENU FOR IRRITABLE BOWEL SYNDROME (IBS)

Between ten and 15 per cent of people in Britain have irritable bowel syndrome, and suffer with abdominal pain, constipation or diarrhoea, and sometimes indigestion. The causes are thought to be related to stress, lack of fibre and, for some, food intolerance.

Eat lots of fibre in the form of fruit and vegetables, and not in the form of wholewheat and bran which can aggravate the symptoms.

It is important to isolate the foods that irritate your condition. Many books on diet and allergies suggest using exclusion diets to relieve symptoms.

Breakfast
Rice Krispies with chopped banana and soya milk
Rooibosch or Redbush tea

Snack
Apple and pecan nuts
Cranberry and Apple Tea

Lunch
Sardines in tomato sauce with jacket potato and green salad
Dandelion Coffee

Mid-afternoon snack
Two Rice Cakes with low-sugar jam
Rooibosch or Redbush tea

Dinner
Grilled lamb chop with French beans, carrots and peas
Baked apple
Mixed Berry Tea

MENU FOR MIGRAINE

A variety of factors can trigger a migraine attack, including stress, diet, hormonal changes, missing meals, drinking too much tea or coffee – or cutting back on them too suddenly – high blood pressure and, in rare cases, neurological problems. Key foods are known to cause attacks. Try avoiding:

cheese	alcohol	liver
chocolate	yeast extract	oranges
tea	pickled foods	artificial colourings
coffee	soya sauce	monosodium glutamate

After a few weeks, add these items back to your diet one by one. If you experience a headache discontinue that particular substance, wait a few days until you feel well again before introducing the next type of food or drink. Keep careful records to avoid confusion.

Breakfast
Boiled egg and two slices of Ryvita
Rooibosch or Redbush tea

Mid-morning snack

Apple and walnuts
Dandelion Coffee

Lunch

Stir-fry prawns and vegetables with ginger
Raspberry and Ginseng Tea

Mid-afternoon snack

Almond macaroon
Rooibosch or Redbush tea

Dinner

Lean ham with a portion of hummus and mixed salad
Rhubarb and ginger mousse
Apple and Cinnamon Tea

MENU FOR PMS

Mild to severe

Breakfast

Oat based Muesli with fresh chopped fruit and semi-skimmed milk
Rooibosch/Redbush tea or Barley Cup

Mid-morning snack

Fresh banana and a bio yogurt with pumpkin and sunflower seeds

Lunch

Glass of orange juice
Jacket potato with sardines in tomato sauce, with a mixed salad and
    grated raw carrot

Mid-afternoon snack

Rice cakes with almond nut butter
Pear

Dinner

Grilled trout with cauliflower, carrots and mixed root vegetables
Fresh fruit salad

MENU FOR PMS
Severe

Breakfast

Muesli made with cornflakes, puffed rice, chopped almonds, dried apricots, sunflower seeds and raisins with chopped fresh fruit, bio yogurt and semi-skimmed milk.

Rooibos/Redbush herbal tea lookalike or Barley Cup

Mid-morning snack

Yogurt, apple, almonds and pecan nuts

Lunch

Glass of orange juice
Rice salad with hummus and crudit

Mid-afternoon snack

Rice cakes with pure fruit spread

Dinner

Stir-fry chicken and vegetables with chilli and ginger
Berry mousse and Raspberry and Ginseng Tea

Variations

Premenstrual cravings for sweet food

- Concentrate on eating foods rich in the minerals Chromium and Magnesium and B vitamins (see page 483).
- Your calorie requirements in your premenstrual week increase by up to 500 calories per day so you will need to eat little and often.
- In your premenstrual week have a wholesome mid-morning and mid-afternoon snack.

Premenstrual breast tenderness

- Cut down on animal fat and increase your consumption of fruit and vegetable fibre.
- Eat a low-salt diet.
- Cut out caffeine in the form of tea, coffee, chocolate and cola-based drinks.
- Keep alcohol consumption to a minimum.
- Cut down or better still, cut out, cigarettes.
- Restrict your intake of dairy products.
- Take daily supplements of Efamol Evening Primrose Oil (6–8 500 IU capsules per day).

Premenstrual constipation

- Avoid all foods containing wheat and modified starch.
- Eat plenty of fruit and vegetables.
- Take regular exercise.
- Massage your tummy and lower back with sweet almond oil with a few drops of lavender or geranium essential oil.
- Take 2 tablespoons of organic golden linseeds every day with your cereal.
- Spend 15–20 minutes relaxing each day (see page 000).

Period Pains

- Concentrate on foods rich in magnesium and B vitamins (see page 000).
- Take regular exercise.
- Massage the tummy and lower back with sweet almond oil or a few drops of lavender or geranium essential oil.
- Take extra supplements of magnesium (preferably amino acid chelate.
- Apply a heat pad to help relax the muscles.

MENU FOR SUGAR CRAVING

In order to overcome sugar cravings, you need to stabilise your blood sugar levels, doing so by eating three nutritious meals per day and two or three wholesome snacks in between meals. Blood sugar levels can be controlled by eating low glycaemic index (GI) foods. These are foods which are converted into glucose at a slow rate, therefore keeping blood sugar levels stable for longer, and reducing sugar cravings.

B vitamins, and the minerals magnesium and chromium are all important for maintaining normal blood sugar levels. Eat plenty of:

wholegrains	liver	bananas
green leafy vegetables	potatoes	unsalted nuts
salad	green peppers	black pepper
chicken	chilli	

Breakfast

Poached eggs on toast with grilled tomatoes
Decaffeinated coffee

Mid-morning snack

Small bag of nuts and raisins

Lunch

Tuna fish with coleslaw salad and potato salad
Barley Cup or NoCaf

Mid-afternoon snack
Rye crackers with peanut butter
Decaffeinated tea

Dinner
Stir-fry chicken with mixed vegetables
Dried fruit compôte
Mango and peach tea

The GI is set at 100 and every other food is ranked on a scale from 0 to 100 according to its actual effect on blood sugar levels.

Low		Intermediate		High	
Apple	38	Apricots	57	Bagel	74
Buckwheat	54	Wholemeal bread	69	Cornflakes	84
Butter beans	31	Couscous	65	Puffed wheat	80
Lentils	30	Sweetcorn	55	Corn chips	72
Orange	44	Pineapple	66	Potatoes	75
Pasta	55	Sweet potato	54	Watermelon	72
Pear	38	Raisins	64	Pumpernickel	80
Porridge	46	White bread	70	French bread	96
Rice bran	46	Oat bran	55	Rye bread	76
Skimmed milk	32	Digestive biscuit	59	White rice	87
Yogurt	33	Banana	55	Brown rice	76
Soya beans	14	Basmati rice	58	Parsnips	97

Sample WNAS Programmes

NORMAL MENOPAUSE
(late 40s/early 50s)

If you are not particularly planning to take HRT, and have no real family history of osteoporosis you should concentrate on:

- dietary changes and including phytoestrogens, foods rich in naturally occurring oestrogen, in your diet
- a supplement programme (see page 478)
- relaxation
- weight-bearing exercise.

Sample menu

Breakfast

Cornflakes with chopped fresh fruit, pecan nuts, sunflower seeds, organic
golden linseeds and soya milk
Rooibos or Redbush herbal tea look-alike

Mid-morning snack

Bio yoghurt, apple and raisins

Lunch

Sardines with a celery, fennel and pumpkin seed salad and jacket potato
Stewed rhubarb and a glass of soya milk

Mid-afternoon snack

Carrot cake or rice cakes with sugar-free spread
Or phyto-rich Wallaby bar

Dinner

Stir-fry vegetables with almonds and prawns
Lemon mousse or tofu fruit whip or soya dessert
Raspberry & Ginseng Tea

NB This menu provides approximately 1600 mg of calcium.

Supplement programme

- Multi-vitamins and minerals to correct nutrient balance.
- Novogen red clover to help control the hot flushes and night sweats.
- Evening primrose oil, marine fish oil and calcium reduce your chances
  of osteoporosis.

Relaxation/creative visualisation

15–20 minutes per day to help control the hot flushes.

Exercise

At least three 30 minute sessions of low-impact aerobic and weight-
bearing exercise per week, to help keep the heart healthy and prevent
osteoporosis.

EARLY MENOPAUSE (NATURAL, CHEMICAL OR SURGICAL)

If you have a family history of osteoporosis or history of fractures
we suggest:

- a bone density scan
- a blood test to determine if you are a 'fast-loser'
- you consider taking HRT if you have severe symptoms or low bone mineral density
- you follow the WNAS recommendations.

You should also concentrate on:

- dietary changes and including phytoestrogens, foods containing naturally occurring oestrogen in your diet
- consuming extra calcium
- five sessions of exercise per week.

Sample menu

Breakfast

Orange juice

Oat-based muesli with 1–2 tablespoons of organic golden linseeds and soya milk

Rye toast and sugar free spread

Mid-morning snack

Dried apricots, sunflower and pumpkin seeds

Lunch

Cheese omelette and a salad of sprouted soya beans, alfalfa, fennel and celery

Fresh banana with a glass of soya milk

Mid-afternoon snack

Almond macaroon or almonds and raisins

Dinner

Grilled salmon with broccoli, courgettes, carrots and new potatoes

Crème caramel made with soya milk with fresh berries

NB This menu provides approximately 1700 mg of calcium.

Supplement programme

- Multi-vitamins and minerals to correct nutrient balance.
- Novogen red clover to help control the hot flushes and night sweats.
- Evening primrose oil, marine fish oil and calcium reduce your chances of osteoporosis.

Relaxation

15–20 minutes per day to help control the hot flushes.

Exercise

At least three 30 minute sessions of low impact aerobic and weight-bearing exercise per week, to help keep the heart healthy and prevent osteoporosis.

Sample phytoestrogen-rich menu

Breakfast

Phyto Muesli with a piece of chopped fresh fruit and soya milk

Bio yogurt with a piece of chopped fresh fruit, pumpkin seeds, sunflower seeds and golden linseeds

Banana or fruit soya smoothie followed by toasted wheat-free soya and linseed loaf with Meridian pure fruit spread

Toasted wheat-free soya and linseed loaf with scrambled egg and grilled mushrooms

Porridge oats soaked in soya milk, with chopped organic dried apricots, sunflower seeds, pumpkin seeds and golden linseeds

Fruit and nut compôte with soya yogurt

Lunch

A salad with

A jacket potato with a filling of you choice
Salmon and chives
Tuna and sweetcorn
Baked beans
Hummus
Avocado and cottage cheese with sesame seeds

'Home made' lentil or bean soup made with soya 'milk' soup – soup is a wholesome snack, and very easy to make. Incorporate a combination of vegetables and enhance with herbs and mild spices. Alternatively you can buy some very good organic (and wheat free) ready made soups from the supermarket.

Any form of protein, preferably oily fish, poultry or phytoestrogen-rich vegetarian alternatives like nuts, seeds, pulses, tofu and hoummus

Cheese, spinach and mushroom omlette made with soya milk

Fresh fruit or a whipped tofu dessert or fruit shake made with soya 'milk'

NB Fruit may be served as a snack at tea time and/or mid morning.

Dinner

A good serving of protein – again oily fish, poultry, game or vegetarian protein, plus three servings of vegetables, including one green variety like cabbage, spinach or broccoli

Dessert

Fresh fruit salad with soya yogurt
Prune and tofu whip
Apple and oat crumble and custard made with soya milk

Beverages

Rooibosch/Redbush herbal tea 'look-alike'
Fruit herbal teas
Ground dandelion coffee or any caffeine-free alternatives (Whole Earth No Caf is particularly good)
Soya milk
Fresh fruit juice
Carbonated water mixed with fruit juice
Organic fruit cordials

Other 'phyto fixes'

One or two slices of wheat free soya and linseed loaf with Meridian pure fruit spread or honey
Soya yogurt with a handful of sunflower and pumpkin seeds
A glass of soya milk
Phyto rich Wallaby bar
A soya fruit shake or smoothie
A slice of any of the wholesome, phyto-rich, wheat free cakes in *The Phyto Factor*
Soya dessert

PREVENT OSTEOPOROSIS
(Heavy exerciser/athlete)

If you are menstruating regularly we suggest you follow the plan below. If you have no periods or irregular ovulation, we suggest:

- a bone density scan.
- you consider taking one of the bisphosphates if established osteoporosis exists.
- you follow the WNAS recommendations.

You should also concentrate on:

- consuming extra calories to meet your energy output.
- consuming a diet rich in calcium.
- reducing your exercise to five sessions per week if it is a hobby.
- taking regular supplements of multi-vitamins and minerals and Efacal to increase the uptake of calcium and help to prevent osteoporosis.

Sample menu

Breakfast

Oat-based muesli, with fresh fruit and soya milk fortified with calcium
Cheese omelette and toast

Mid-morning snack

Rye crackers and nut butter spread

Lunch

Jacket potato with cheese and bean filling
Salad of sprouted soya beans, fennel, celery and walnuts
Glass of soya milk fortified with calcium

Mid-afternoon snack

Bio yoghurt, almonds and fresh fruit or cheese and biscuits with grapes

Dinner

Raw vegetable crudités with hummus
Grilled fish with broccoli, carrots, courgettes and new potatoes
Berry mousse made with silken tofu or fresh fruit salad with soya yoghurt

NB This menu provides approximately 2300 mg of calcium.

Sample high calcium menu

Breakfast

Cornflakes with chopped fresh fruit, a tablespoon of organic golden
    linseeds, and soya milk fortified with calcium
Hovis toast with almond butter spread
A mug of either decaffeinated tea or coffee, or herbal tea or coffee
    substitute

Lunch

Baked beans on toast
Low-fat bio yoghurt with chopped almonds and grapes
Glass of milk

Dinner

Sardines, with baked potato, and fennel and mixed pepper salad
Cheddar cheese and biscuits with fresh grapes
Herb tea or decaffeinated coffee

This menu will provide over 1800 mg of calcium, as well as a good quantity of naturally occurring oestrogen. Bear in mind that up to two-thirds
of dietary calcium fails to be absorbed by the body, so it may be that you
will benefit from approximately 600 mg.

Appendix I
Nutritional Content of Food

Unless stated otherwise, foods listed are raw.

Vitamin A – Retinol
Micrograms per 100 g (3.5 oz)

Skimmed milk	1
Semi-skimmed milk	21
Grilled herring	49
Whole milk	52
Porridge made with milk	56
Cheddar cheese	325
Margarine	800
Butter	815
Lamb's liver	15,000

Vitamin B1 – Thiamin
Milligrams per 100 g (3.5 oz)

Peaches	0.02
Cottage cheese	0.02
Cox's apple	0.03
Full-fat milk	0.04
Skimmed milk	0.04
Semi-skimmed milk	0.04
Cheddar cheese	0.04
Bananas	0.04
White grapes	0.04
French beans	0.04
Low-fat yoghurt	0.05
Cantaloupe melon	0.05
Tomato	0.06
Green peppers, raw	0.07
Boiled egg	0.08
Roast chicken	0.08
Grilled cod	0.08
Haddock, steamed	0.08
Roast turkey	0.09
Mackerel, cooked	0.09
Savoy cabbage, boiled	0.10
Oranges	0.10
Brussels sprouts	0.10
Potatoes, new, boiled	0.11
Soya beans, boiled	0.12
Red peppers, raw	0.12
Lentils, boiled	0.14
Steamed salmon	0.20
Corn	0.20
White spaghetti, boiled	0.21
Almonds	0.24
White self-raising flour	0.30
Plaice, steamed	0.30
Bacon, cooked	0.35
Walnuts	0.40
Wholemeal flour	0.47
Lamb's kidney	0.49
Brazil nuts	1.00
Cornflakes	1.00
Rice Krispies	1.00
Wheatgerm	2.01

Vitamin B2 – Riboflavin
Milligrams per 100 g (3.5 oz)

Cabbage, boiled	0.01
Potatoes, boiled	0.01
Brown rice, boiled	0.02
Pear	0.03
Wholemeal spaghetti, boiled	0.03
White self-raising flour	0.03
Orange	0.04
Spinach, boiled in salted water	0.05
Baked beans	0.06
Banana	0.06
White bread	0.06
Green peppers, raw	0.08
Lentils, boiled	0.08

Hovis	0.09
Soya beans, boiled	0.09
Wholemeal bread	0.09
Wholemeal flour	0.09
Peanuts	0.10
Baked salmon	0.11
Red peppers, raw	0.15
Full-fat milk	0.17
Avocado	0.18
Grilled herring	0.18
Semi-skimmed milk	0.18
Roast chicken	0.19
Roast turkey	0.21
Cottage cheese	0.26
Soya flour	0.31
Boiled prawns	0.34
Boiled egg	0.35
Topside of beef, cooked	0.35
Leg of lamb, cooked	0.38
Cheddar cheese	0.40
Muesli	0.70
Almonds	0.75
Cornflakes	1.50
Rice Krispies	1.50

Vitamin B3 – Niacin
Milligrams per 100 g (3.5 oz)

Boiled egg	0.07
Cheddar cheese	0.07
Full-fat milk	0.08
Skimmed milk	0.09
Semi-skimmed milk	0.09
Cottage cheese	0.13
Cox's apple	0.20
Cabbage, boiled	0.30
Orange	0.40
Baked beans	0.50
Potatoes, boiled	0.50
Soya beans, boiled	0.50
Lentils, boiled	0.60
Banana	0.70
Tomato	1.00
Avocado	1.10
Green peppers, raw	1.10
Brown rice	1.30
Wholemeal spaghetti, boiled	1.30
White self-raising flour	1.50
Grilled cod	1.70
White bread	1.70
Soya flour	2.00
Red peppers, raw	2.20

Almonds	3.10
Grilled herring	4.00
Wholemeal bread	4.10
Hovis	4.20
Wholemeal flour	5.70
Muesli	6.50
Topside of beef, cooked	6.50
Leg of lamb, cooked	6.60
Baked salmon	7.00
Roast chicken	8.20
Roast turkey	8.50
Boiled prawns	9.50
Peanuts	13.80
Cornflakes	16.00
Rice Krispies	16.00

Vitamin B6 – Pyridoxine
Milligrams per 100 g (3.5 oz)

Carrots	0.05
Full-fat milk	0.06
Skimmed milk	0.06
Semi-skimmed milk	0.06
Satsuma	0.07
White bread	0.07
White rice	0.07
Cabbage, boiled	0.08
Cottage cheese	0.08
Cox's apple	0.08
Wholemeal pasta	0.08
Frozen peas	0.09
Spinach, boiled	0.09
Cheddar cheese	0.10
Orange	0.10
Broccoli	0.11
Hovis	0.11
Baked beans	0.12
Boiled egg	0.12
Red kidney beans, cooked	0.12
Wholemeal bread	0.12
Tomatoes	0.14
Almonds	0.15
Cauliflower	0.15
Brussels sprouts	0.19
Sweetcorn, boiled	0.21
Leg of lamb, cooked	0.22
Grapefruit juice	0.23
Roast chicken	0.26
Lentils, boiled	0.28
Banana	0.29
Brazil nuts	0.31
Potatoes, boiled	0.32

Roast turkey	0.33
Grilled herring	0.33
Topside of beef, cooked	0.33
Avocado	0.36
Grilled cod	0.38
Baked salmon	0.57
Soya flour	0.57
Hazelnuts	0.59
Peanuts	0.59
Walnuts	0.67
Muesli	1.60
Cornflakes	1.80
Rice Crispies	1.80
Special K	2.20

Vitamin B12 – Cyanocobalamine

Micrograms per 100 g (3.5 oz)

Tempeh	0.10
Miso	0.20
Quorn	0.30
Full-fat mik	0.40
Skimmed milk	0.40
Semi-skimmed milk	0.40
Marmite	0.50
Cottage cheese	0.70
Choux buns	1.00
Eggs, boiled	1.00
Eggs, poached	1.00
Halibut, steamed	1.00
Lobster, boiled	1.00
Sponge cake	1.00
Turkey, white meat	1.00
Waffles	1.00
Cheddar cheese	1.20
Eggs, scrambled	1.20
Squid	1.30
Eggs, fried	1.60
Shrimps, boiled	1.80
Parmesan cheese	1.90
Beef, lean	2.00
Cod, baked	2.00
Cornflakes	2.00
Pork, cooked	2.00
Raw beef mince	2.00
Rice Krispies	2.00
Steak, lean, grilled	2.00
Edam cheese	2.10
Eggs, whole, battery	2.40
Milk, dried, whole	2.40
Milk, dried, skimmed	2.60

Eggs, whole, free-range	2.70
Kambu seaweed	2.80
Squid, frozen	2.90
Taramasalata	2.90
Duck, cooked	3.00
Turkey, dark meat	3.00
Grapenuts	5.00
Tuna in oil	5.00
Herring, cooked	6.00
Herring roe, fried	6.00
Steamed salmon	6.00
Bovril	8.30
Mackerel, fried	10.00
Rabbit, stewed	10.00
Cod's roe, fried	11.00
Pilchards canned in tomato juice	12.00
Oysters, raw	15.00
Nori seaweed	27.50
Sardines in oil	28.00
Lamb's kidney, fried	79.00

Folate/Folic Acid

Micrograms per 100 g (3.5 oz)

Cox's apple	4.00
Leg of lamb, cooked	4.00
Full-fat milk	6.00
Skimmed milk	6.00
Semi-skimmed milk	6.00
Porridge with semi-skimmed milk	7.00
Turnip, baked	8.00
Sweet potato, boiled	8.00
Cucumber	9.00
Grilled herring	10.00
Roast chicken	10.00
Avocado	11.00
Grilled cod	12.00
Banana	14.00
Roast turkey	15.00
Carrots	17.00
Sweet potato	17.00
Tomatoes	17.00
Topside of beef, cooked	17.00
Swede, boiled	18.00
Strawberries	20.00
Brazil nuts	21.00
Red peppers, raw	21.00
Green peppers, raw	23.00
Rye bread	24.00

Dates, fresh	25.00	Red kidney beans	1.00
New potatoes, boiled	25.00	Carrots	2.00
Grapefruit	26.00	Cucumber	2.00
Oatcakes	26.00	Muesli with dried fruit	2.00
Cottage cheese	27.00	Apricots, raw	6.00
Baked salmon	29.00	Avocado	6.00
Cabbage, boiled	29.00	Pear	6.00
Onions, boiled	29.00	Potato, boiled	6.00
White bread	29.00	Spinach, boiled	8.00
Orange	31.00	Cox's apple	9.00
Baked beans	33.00	Turnip	10.00
Cheddar cheese	33.00	Banana	11.00
Clementines	33.00	Frozen peas	12.00
Raspberries	33.00	Lamb's liver, fried	12.00
Satsuma	33.00	Pineapple	12.00
Blackberries	34.00	Dried skimmed milk	13.00
Rye crispbread	35.00	Gooseberries	14.00
Potato, baked in skin	36.00	Raw dates	14.00
Radish	38.00	Melon	17.00
Boiled egg	39.00	Tomatoes	17.00
Hovis	39.00	Cabbage, boiled	20.00
Wholemeal bread	39.00	Canteloupe melon	26.00
Red kidney beans, boiled	42.00	Cauliflower	27.00
Potato, baked	44.00	Satsuma	27.00
Frozen peas	47.00	Peach	31.00
Almonds	48.00	Raspberries	32.00
Parsnips, boiled	48.00	Bran flakes	35.00
Cauliflower	51.00	Grapefruit	36.00
Green beans, boiled	57.00	Mangoes	37.00
Broccoli	64.00	Nectarine	37.00
Walnuts	66.00	Kumquats	39.00
Artichoke	68.00	Broccoli	44.00
Hazelnuts	72.00	Lychees	45.00
Spinach, boiled	90.00	Unsweetened apple juice	49.00
Brussels sprouts	110.00	Orange	54.00
Peanuts	110.00	Kiwi fruit	59.00
Muesli	140.00	Brussels sprouts	60.00
Sweetcorn, boiled	150.00	Strawberries	77.00
Asparagus	155.00	Blackcurrants	115.00
Chickpeas	180.00		
Lamb's liver, fried	240.00		
Cornflakes	250.00		

Vitamin D
Micrograms per 100 g (3.5 oz)

Rice Krispies	250.00
Calf's liver, fried	320.00

Vitamin C
Milligrams per 100 g (3.5 oz)

Full-fat milk	1.00
Skimmed milk	1.00
Semi-skimmed milk	1.00

Vitamin D
Micrograms per 100 g (3.5 oz)

Skimmed milk	0.01
Whole milk	0.03
Fromage frais	0.05
Cheddar cheese	0.26
Cornflakes	2.80
Rice Krispies	2.80
Kellogg's Start	4.20
Margarine	8.00

Vitamin E
Milligrams per 100 g (3.5 oz)

Semi-skimmed milk	0.03
Boiled potatoes	0.06
Cucumber	0.07
Cottage cheese	0.08
Full-fat milk	0.09
Cabbage, boiled	0.10
Leg of lamb, cooked	0.10
Cauliflower	0.11
Roast chicken	0.11
Frozen peas	0.18
Red kidney beans, cooked	0.20
Wholemeal bread	0.20
Orange	0.24
Topside of beef, cooked	0.26
Banana	0.27
Brown rice, boiled	0.30
Grilled herring	0.30
Lamb's liver, fried	0.32
Baked beans	0.36
Cornflakes	0.40
Pear	0.50
Cheddar cheese	0.53
Carrots	0.56
Lettuce	0.57
Cox's apple	0.59
Grilled cod	0.59
Rice Krispies	0.60
Plums	0.61
Unsweetened orange juice	0.68
Leeks	0.78
Sweetcorn, boiled	0.88
Brussels sprouts	0.90
Broccoli	1.10
Boiled egg	1.11
Tomato	1.22
Watercress	1.46
Parsley	1.70
Spinach, boiled	1.71
Olives	1.99
Butter	2.00
Onions, dried raw	2.69
Mushrooms, fried in corn oil	2.84
Avocado	3.20
Muesli	3.20
Walnuts	3.85
Peanut butter	4.99
Olive oil	5.10
Sweet potato, baked	5.96
Brazil nuts	7.18
Peanuts	10.09
Pine nuts	13.65
Rapeseed oil	18.40
Almonds	23.96
Hazelnuts	24.98
Sunflower oil	48.70

Calcium
Milligrams per 100 g (3.5 oz)

Cox's apple	4.00
Brown rice, boiled	4.00
Potatoes, boiled	5.00
Banana	6.00
Topside of beef, cooked	6.00
White pasta, boiled	7.00
Tomato	7.00
White spaghetti, boiled	7.00
Leg of lamb, cooked	8.00
Red peppers, raw	8.00
Roast chicken	9.00
Roast turkey	9.00
Avocado	11.00
Pear	11.00
Butter	15.00
Cornflakes	15.00
White rice, boiled	18.00
Grilled cod	22.00
Lentils, boiled	22.00
Baked salmon	29.00
Green peppers, raw	30.00
Young carrots	30.00
Grilled herring	33.00
Wholemeal flour	38.00
Turnips, baked	45.00
Orange	47.00
Baked beans	48.00
Wholemeal bread	54.00
Boiled egg	57.00
Peanuts	60.00
Cottage cheese	73.00
Soya beans, boiled	83.00
White bread	100.00
Full-fat milk	115.00
Hovis	120.00
Muesli	120.00
Skimmed milk	120.00
Semi-skimmed milk	120.00
Prawns, boiled	150.00
Spinach, boiled	150.00
Brazil nuts	170.00
Yoghurt, low-fat, plain	190.00
Soya flour	210.00
Almonds	240.00

White self-raising flour	450.00
Sardines	550.00
Sprats, fried	710.00
Cheddar cheese	720.00
Whitebait, fried	860.00

Chromium
Micrograms per 100 g (3.5 oz)

Egg yolk	183.00
Molasses	121.00
Brewer's yeast	117.00
Beef	57.00
Hard cheese	56.00
Liver	55.00
Fruit juices	47.00
Wholemeal bread	42.00

Iron
Milligrams per 100 g (3.5 oz)

Semi-skimmed milk	0.05
Skimmed milk	0.06
Full-fat milk	0.06
Cottage cheese	0.10
Orange	0.10
Cox's apple	0.20
Pear	0.20
White rice	0.20
Banana	0.30
Cabbage, boiled	0.30
Cheddar cheese	0.30
Avocado	0.40
Grilled cod	0.40
Potatoes, boiled	0.40
Young carrots, boiled	0.40
Brown rice, boiled	0.50
Tomato	0.50
White pasta, boiled	0.50
Baked salmon	0.80
Roast chicken	0.80
Roast turkey	0.90
Grilled herring	1.00
Red peppers, raw	1.00
Boiled prawns	1.10
Green peppers, raw	1.20
Baked beans	1.40
Wholemeal spaghetti, boiled	1.40
White bread	1.60
Spinach, boiled	1.70
Boiled egg	1.90
White self-raising four	2.00
Brazil nuts	2.50
Peanuts	2.50

Leg of lamb, cooked	2.70
Wholemeal bread	2.70
Topside of beef, cooked	2.80
Almonds	3.00
Soya beans, boiled	3.00
Lentils, boiled	3.50
Hovis	3.70
Wholemeal flour	3.90
Muesli	5.60
Cornflakes	6.70
Rice Krispies	6.70
Soya flour	6.90

Magnesium
Milligrams per 100 g (3.5 oz)

Butter	2.00
Cox's apple	6.00
Turnip, baked	6.00
Young carrots	6.00
Tomato	7.00
Cottage cheese	9.00
Orange	10.00
Full-fat milk	11.00
White rice, boiled	11.00
Semi-skimmed milk	11.00
Skimmed milk	12.00
Boiled egg	12.00
Cornflakes	14.00
Potatoes, boiled	14.00
Red peppers, raw	14.00
White pasta, boiled	15.00
Wholemeal spaghetti, boiled	15.00
White self-raising flour	20.00
Green peppers, raw	24.00
Roast chicken	24.00
Topside of beef, cooked	24.00
White bread	24.00
Avocado	25.00
Cheddar cheese	25.00
Grilled cod	26.00
Roast turkey	27.00
Leg of lamb, cooked	28.00
Baked salmon	29.00
Baked beans	31.00
Spinach, boiled	31.00
Grilled herring	32.00
Banana	34.00
Lentils, boiled	34.00
Boiled prawns	42.00
Wholemeal spaghetti, boiled	42.00
Brown rice, boiled	43.00
Hovis	56.00

Soya beans, boiled	63.00
Wholemeal bread	76.00
Muesli	85.00
Wholemeal flour	120.00
Peanuts	210.00
Soya flour	240.00
Almonds	270.00
Brazil nuts	410.00

Selenium
Micrograms per 100 g (3.5 oz)

Full-fat milk	1.00
Semi-skimmed milk	1.00
Skimmed milk	1.00
Baked beans	2.00
Cornflakes	2.00
Orange	2.00
Peanuts	3.00
Almonds	4.00
Cottage cheese	4.00
White rice	4.00
White self-raising flour	4.00
Soya beans, boiled	5.00
Boiled egg	11.00
Cheddar cheese	12.00
White bread	28.00
Wholemeal bread	35.00
Lentils, boiled	40.00
Wholemeal flour	53.00

Zinc
Milligrams per 100 g (3.5 oz)

Butter	0.10
Pear	0.10
Orange	0.10
Red peppers, raw	0.10
Banana	0.20
Young carrots	0.20
Cornflakes	0.30
Potatoes, boiled	0.30
Avocado	0.40
Full-fat milk	0.40
Skimmed milk	0.40
Green peppers, raw	0.40
Semi-skimmed milk	0.40
Baked beans	0.50
Grilled cod	0.50
Grilled herring	0.50
White pasta	0.50
Tomatoes	0.50

Cottage cheese	0.60
Spinach, boiled	0.60
White bread	0.60
White self-raising flour	0.60
Brown rice	0.70
White rice	0.70
Soya beans, boiled	0.90
Wholemeal spaghetti, boiled	1.10
Boiled egg	1.30
Lentils, boiled	1.40
Roast chicken	1.50
Boiled prawns	1.60
Wholemeal bread	1.80
Hovis	2.10
Cheddar cheese	2.30
Roast turkey	2.40
Muesli	2.50
Wholemeal flour	2.90
Almonds	3.20
Peanuts	3.50
Brazil nuts	4.20
Leg of lamb, cooked	5.30
Topside of beef, cooked	5.50

Essential Fatty Acids

Exact amounts of these fats are hard to quantify. Good sources for the two families of essential fatty acids are given.

Omega-6 Series Essential Fatty Acids

Sunflower oil
Rapeseed oil
Corn oil
Almonds
Walnuts
Brazil nuts
Sunflower seeds
Soya products including tofu

Omega-3 Series Essential Fatty Acids

Mackerel ⎱ fresh cooked or
Herring ⎰ smoked/pickled
Salmon
Walnuts and walnut oil
Rapeseed oil
Soya products and soy bean oil

Appendix II
Recommended Reading

Note
UK, USA and **A** denotes the following books are available in Great Britain, the United States and Australia.

General Health
Acupuncture, Dr Michael Nightingale (Vermilion). **UK USA A**
Alexander Technique, Chris Stevens (Vermilion).
Alternative Health Care for Women, Patsy Westcott (Thorsons).
Alternative Health Osteopathy, Stephen Sandler (Optima). **UK USA A**
Aromatherapy, Gill Martin (Vermilion). **UK USA A**
Aromatherapy for Women and Children, Jane Dye (C.W. Daniel). **UK USA**
Beauty Bible, The, J. Fairley and S. Stacey (Kyle Cathie).
Better Health Through Natural Healing, R. Trattler (Thorsons).
Bone Boosters – Natural Ways to Beat Osteoporosis, Diana Moran and Helen Franks (Boxtree). **UK**
Book of Massage, The (Ebury Press). **UK**
Candida Albicans, Gill Jacobs (Optima). **UK USA A**
Candida Albicans: Could Yeast Be Your Problem?, Leon Chaitow (Thorsons). **UK USA A** (Lothian Publishing Co.)
Candida – Diet Against It, Luc de Schepper (Foulsham).
Coming Off Tranqullizers, Shirley Trickett (Thorsons). **UK USA A** (Lothian Publishing Co.)
Conquering Cystitis, Dr Patrick Kingsley (Ebury Press). **UK**
Contraception – Your Questions Answered, 3rd edn, John Guillebaud (Churchill Livingstone).
Creating Kids Who Can, Jean Robb and Hilary Letts (Hodder & Stoughton).
Creating Kids Who Can Concentrate, Jean Robb and Hilary Letts (Hodder & Stoughton).
Creative Journal for Parents, The, Lucia Capacchione (Shambhala).
Diet and Arthritis, G. Darlington and Linda Gamlin (Vermilion).
Do-It-Yourself Shiatsu, W. Ohashi (Unwin Hyman). **UK**
Escape from Tranquillisers and Sleeping Pills, Larry Neild (Bloomsbury). **UK A**
Evening Primrose Oil, Judy Graham (Thorsons).
Fats that Heal, Fats that Kill, Udo Erasmus (Alive Books).
Feel Fabulous Forever, J. Fairley and S. Stacey (Kyle Cathie).
Fibromyalgia and Muscle Pain, Leon Chaitow (Thorsons).
Food Allergy and Intolerance, Jonathan Brostoff and Linda Gamlin (Bloomsbury). **UK A**
Food for Fitness, Amanda Bean (A&C Black).

Food Irradiation: The Facts, Tony Webb and Dr Tim Lang (Thorsons).
Food Scandal, The, Caroline Walker and Geoffrey Cannon (Century). **UK A**
Getting Sober and Loving It, Joan and Derek Taylor (Vermilion). **UK A**
Guide to Herbal Remedies, A, Mark Evans (C.W. Daniel). **UK USA**
Holistic Approach to Cancer, The, Ian C.B. Pearce (C.W. Daniel). **UK USA**
Homoeopathy for the First Aider, Dr Dorothy Shepherd (C.W. Daniel). **UK USA**
Hyperactivity: What's the Alternative?, Maggie Jones (Element Books).
Hysterectomy – New Options and Advances, Lorraine Dennerstein, Carl Wood
    and Ann Westmore, 2nd edition (Oxford University Press, Melbourne).
Memory Power, Ursula Markham (Vermilion). **UK A**
Mental Health: the Nutrition Connection, Patrick Holford (Piatkus).
Migraine Handbook, The, Jenny Lewis (Vermilion). **UK**
Migraine Revolution, The – The New Drug-free Solution, Dr John Mansfield
    (Thorsons). **UK USA A** (Lothian Publishing Co.)
MSM The Natural Pain Relief, Deborah Mitchell (Wholecare).
Natural Hormone Health, Arabella Melville (Thorsons). **UK USA A**
Nutritional Health Bible, The, Linda Lazarides (Thorsons).
Nutritional Medicine, Dr Stephen Davies and Dr Alan Stewart (Pan Books). **UK A**
Optimal Wellness, Ralph Golan (Ballantine Books).
Osteoporosis, Kathleen Mayes (Thorsons). **UK**
Pain-free Periods, Stella Weller (Thorsons). **UK**
Pure, White and Deadly, Professor John Yudkin (a book about sugar) (Viking).
    UK A
Seed Handbook, The, Lynne Franks (Thorsons).
Simple Soybean and Your Health, The, M. Messina, V. Messina and K. Setchell
    (Avery).
Success in Exams, Triumph in Tests, Jean Robb and Hilary Letts (Hodder &
    Stoughton).
Tired All the Time, Dr Alan Stewart (Vermilion). **UK USA A**
Understanding Cystitis, Angela Kilmartin (Arrow Books). **UK A**
Well Woman's Self-help Book, The, Nikki Bradford (Sidgwick and Jackson).
Why I Can't Remember, Pavel Yutsis and Lynda Toth (Avery).
Women's Guide to Homeopathy, The, Dr Andrew Lockie and Dr Nicola Geddes
    (Hamish Hamilton). **UK**

Food

Allergy Diet, The, Elizabeth Workman SRD, Dr John Hunter and Dr Virginia
    Alun Jones (Vermilion). **UK USA**
Beat Sugar Craving, Maryon Stewart (Vermilion). **UK A**
Food Allergy and Intolerance, Jonathan Brostoff and Linda Gamlin
    (Bloomsbury). **UK A**
Food Intolerance Diet, The, Elizabeth Workman SRD, Dr John Hunter and Dr
    Virginia Alun Jones (Martin Dunitz). **UK USA**
Food Bible, The, Judith Wills (Quadrille).
Foods that Harm, Foods that Heal (Reader's Digest).
Foresight Index Number Decoder (Packet Additive Dictionary) available from
    Foresight (address in Useful Addresses). **UK**
New Foods Guide, The, John Elkington and Julia Hailes (Gollancz).

New Raw Energy, The, Leslie and Susannah Kenton (Vermilion). **UK A** (Doubleday Publishing Co.)

New Why You Don't Need Meat, The, Peter Cox (Bloomsbury). **UK A**

Organic Consumer Guide/Food You Can Trust, edited by David Mabey and Alan and Jackie Gear (Thorsons).

Potatoes Not Prozac, Kathleen Desmaisons (Simon & Schuster).

Real Food Shop and Restaurant Guide, The, Clive Johnstone (Ebury Press).

Salt-free Diet Book, The, Dr Graham McGregor (Martin Dunitz). **UK USA**

Vitality Diet, The, Maryon Stewart and Dr Alan Stewart (Optima) (WNAS Mail Order Service).

Stress

Book of Massage, The, Lucy Lidell (Ebury Press). **UK**

Book of Yoga, The, Sivananda Yoga Centre (Ebury Press). **UK A**

Do-It-Yourself Shiatsu, W. Ohashi (Unwin Hyman). **UK**

Lyn Marshall's Instant Stress Cure, Lyn Marshall (Vermilion). **UK A**

Self-Help for Your Nerves, Dr Clair Weekes (Angus and Robertson). **UK USA** (Hawthorn Publishing Co.)

Stress and Relaxation Self-help Techniques for Everyone, Jane Madden (Vermilion). **UK USA A**

Stress Wise, Dr Terry Looker and Dr Olga Gregson (Headway). **UK**

Tranquillisation: The Non-addictive Way, Phyllis Speight (C.W. Daniel). **UK USA**

Recipe Books

Candida Albicans Yeast-free Cook Book, The, Pat Connolly and Associates of the Price Pottenger Nutrition Foundation (Keats). **UK USA**

Cook Organic, Gill Davies (Metro Books).

Cooking Without, Barbara Cousins (Thorsons).

Dairy-free Cookbook, Jane Zukin (Prima).

Estrogen the Natural Way – Over 250 Easy and Delicious Recipes for Menopause, Nina Shandler (Villard Books).

Everyday Wheat Free and Gluten Free Cookbook, The, Michelle Berriedale-Johnson (Grub Street).

Gluten-free and Wheat-free Bumper Bake Book, The, Rita Greer (Bunterbird Ltd). **UK**

Gourmet Vegetarian Cooking, Rose Elliot (Fontana). **UK A**

Healthy Cooking, from Tesco Stores. **UK**

Raw Energy Recipes, Leslie and Susannah Kenton (Vermilion).

Reluctant Vegetarian Cook, The, Simon Hope (Heinemann). **UK**

Sensitive Gourmet, The, Antoinette Savill (Thorsons).

Single Vegan, The, Leah Leneman (Thorsons).

SuperJuice, M. Van Straten (Mitchell Beazley).

Wheat and Gluten Free Cookbook, The, Joan Noble (Vermilion). **UK A**

Whole Earth Cookbook, Hilary Meth (Vermilion). **UK**

Drugs

Forbidden Drugs – Understanding Drugs and How People Take Them, Robson (Oxford University Press).

What Do You Know About Drugs?, Sanders and Myers (Gloucester Press).

Smoking
Easy Way to Stop Smoking, Allen Carr (Penguin).
How to Stop Smoking and Stay Stopped for Good, Gillian Riley (Vermilion). **UK A**

IBS
No More IBS!, Maryon Stewart and Dr Alan Stewart (Vermilion). **UK A**

Exercise and Relaxation
Alexander Technique, The, Wilfred Barlow (Inner Tradition).
Art of Swimming, The, Steven Shaw and A. D'Angour (Ashgrove).
Body Control the Pilates Way, Lynne Robinson and G. Thomas (Pan).
Diana Moran's 3 in 1 Workout video, Diana Moran.
Dynamic Yoga, Godfrey Devereux (Thorsons).
Pure Pilates, Michael King (Mitchell Beazley).
YMCA *Guide to Exercise to Music*, Rodney Cullum and Lesley Mowbray (available from YMCA, see Useful Addresses).
The Y's Way to Physical Fitness, Clayton R. Myers and Lawrence A. Golding (available from YMCA, see Useful Addresses).

PMS
Beat PMS Cookbook, Maryon Stewart and Sarah Tooley (Vermilion). **UK A**
No More PMS!, Maryon Stewart (Vermilion). **UK A**

Menopause
Cruising Through the Menopause, Maryon Stewart (Vermilion). **UK A**

Pregnancy and Baby Books
Breast Book, The, Miriam Stoppard (Dorling Kindersley).
Breast Is Best, Drs Penny and Andrew Stanway (Pan Books).
Breastfeeding Your Baby, Sheila Kitzinger (Dorling Kindersley).
Child Is Born, Lennart Nilsson (Doubleday). **UK USA A**
Complete Book of Massage, The, Clare Maxwell-Hudson (Dorling Kindersley). **UK**
Complete Book of Relaxation Techniques, The, Jenny Sutcliffe (Headline). **UK**
Easy Exercises for Pregnancy, Janet Balaskas (Frances Lincoln).
Green Babies, Penny Stanway (Century). **UK USA**
Healthy Parents, Healthy Baby, Maryon Stewart (Headline). **UK A**
National Childbirth Trust Book of Breast-feeding, The, Mary Smale (Vermilion). **UK USA A**
National Childbirth Trust Book of Pregnancy, Birth and Parenthood, The, Sheila Kitzinger (Oxford University Press). **UK USA**
Natural Fertility Awareness, John and Lucie Davidson (C.W. Daniel). **UK USA**
New Pregnancy and Childbirth, Sheila Kitzinger (Penguin Books).
Planning for a Healthy Baby, Belinda Barnes and Suzanne Gail Bradley (Foresight) (Vermilion). **UK**
Preparation for Pregnancy, S. Bradley and N. Bennet (Argyll Publishing).
Preparing for Birth with Yoga, Janet Balaskas (Element Books).
Your Choices for Pregnancy and Childbirth, Helen Lewison (Ebury Press). **UK USA**

Women's Health
Breast Cancer Prevention and Recovery Diet, The, Suzannah Olivier (Michael Joseph).

Cruising Through the Menopause, Maryon Stewart (Vermilion).

Endometriosis – A Key to Healing Through Nutrition, Dian Shepperson Mills and Michael Vernon (Element Books).

Natural Treatment of Fibroid Tumours and Endometriosis – Effective Natural Solutions for Relieving Heavy Bleeding, Cramps and Infertility that Accompany these Common Female Problems, Susan M. Lark MDE (Keats).

Natural Way, The – Infertility, Belinda Whitworth (Element Books).

No More PMS!, Maryon Stewart (Vermilion).

The Phyto Factor, Maryon Stewart (Vermilion).

Preventing and Reversing Osteoporosis, Alan Gaby (Prima).

Woman's Guide to Dealing with Polycistic Ovary Syndrome, A, Collette Harris with Dr Adam Carey (Thorsons).

Women, Hormones and the Menstrual Cycle, Ruth Trickey (Allen & Unwin).

Allergies

Asthma – The Complete Guide, Johnathon Brostoff and Linda Gamlin (Bloomsbury).

Complete Guide to Food Allergy and Intolerance, The, Prof Johnathon Brostoff and Linda Gamlin (Bloomsbury).

Digestive Health

Candida Albicans, Leon Chaitow (Inner Traditions).

Digestive Wellness, Elizabeth Lipski (Keats).

No More IBS!, Maryon Stewart and Dr Alan Stewart (Vermilion).

Overcoming Candida, Xandria Williams (Element Books).

Superbug, Geoffrey Cannon (Virgin).

Complementary Therapies

Creative Journal, The – The Art of Finding Yourself, Lucia Capacchione (Newcastle Publishing).

Family Guide to Homeopathy, The, Andrew Lockie (Hamish Hamilton).

Mind Magic, Betty Shine (Corgi).

Mind Power into the 21st Century, John Kehoe (Zoetic Inc. Publishing).

Qi Gong for Beginners, Stanley Wilson (Rudra Press).

Power of Your Other Hand, The, Lucia Capacchione (Newcastle Publishing).

Power of Your Subconscious Mind, The, Dr Joseph Murphy (Pocket Books).

Practical Reiki, Mari Hall (Thorsons).

Recovery of Your Inner Child, Lucia Capacchione (Fireside).

Visioning – Ten Steps to Designing the Life of Your Dreams, Lucia Capacchione (Putnam Publishing).

You Can Heal Your Life, Louise L. Hay (Eden Grove Editions).

Herbs

Complete Woman's Herbal, Anne McIntyre (Gaia Books).

Kava, Chris Kilham (Park Street Press).

Kitchen Pharmacy, Rose Elliot and C. Paoli (Orion).

New Green Pharmacy, Barbara Griggs (Vermilion).

New Herb Relief, The, Earl Mindell (Fireside Books).

St John's Wort, Norman Rosenthal (Thorsons).

Appendix III
References

Standard References:

Encyclopedia of Complementary Medicine – The definitive guide to the best treatment options for 200 health problems, Woodham, A. and Peters, Dr D., Dorling Kindersley, 1997.

Environmental Medicine in Clinical Practice, Anthony, H. *et al*, BSAENM Publications, 1997.

Human Nutrition and Dietetics, Passmore, R., Eastwood, M.A., 8th edition, Churchill Livingstone, 1986.

Hysterectomy – New Options and Advances, Dennerstein, L., Wood, C., Westmore, A., 2nd edition, Oxford University Press.

Nutritional Influences on Illness, Werbach, M.R., MD, Thorsons, 1989.

Nutritional Influences on Mental Illness, Werbach, M.R., MD, Third Line Press Inc. (California), 1991.

Nutritional Medicine, Davies, Dr Stephen, Stewart, Dr Alan, Pan Books, 1987.

Oxford Textboook of Medicine, 3rd edition, ed. Weatherall, D.J., Ledingham, J.G.G., Warrell, D.A., Oxford Medical Publications, 1996.

Prescription for Nutritional Healing, 2nd edition, Balch, J., Balch, P., Avery, 1997.

Textbook of Natural Medicine – Volume 1 & 2, Pizzorno, J., Murray, M., Churchill Livingstone, 1999.

Textbook of Nutritional Medicine, Werbach, M., Moss, J., Third Line Press, 1999.

Abdominal Wind and Bloating

Calloway, S.P., Fonagy, P., 'Aerophagia and irritable bowel syndrome', *The Lancet*, 1985; 2: 1368.

Cannon, Geoffrey, *Superbug*, Virgin.

Chaitow, Leon, *Candida Albicans*, Inner Tradition International, 1999.

Christi, S.U., Gibson, G.R., Cummings, J.H., 'Role of dietary sulphate in the regulation of methanogenesis in the human large intestine', *Gut*, 1992; 33: 1234–8.

Cummings, J.H., 'Fermentation in the human large intestine: evidence and implications for health', *The Lancet*, 1983; 1: 1206–9.

Editorial, 'The colon, the rumen, and d-lactic acidosis', *The Lancet*, 1990; 336: 599–600.

Hunter, J.O., 'Food allergy – or enterometabolic disorder?', *The Lancet*, 1991; 2: 495–6.

Lipski, Elizabeth, *Digestive Wellness*, Keats, 1996.

Levitt, M.D., Lasser, R.N., Schwartz, J.S., Bond, J.H., 'Studies of a flatulent patient', *The New England Journal of Medicine*, 1976; 295: 260–2.

Maxton, D.G., Martin, D.F., Whorwell, P.J., Godfrey, M., 'Abdominal distension in female patients with irritable bowel syndrome; exploration of possible mechanisms', *Gut*, 1991; 32: 62–4.

Stewart, Maryon, Stweart, Dr Alan, *No More IBS!*, Vermilion, 1999.

Trotman, I.F., Price, C.C., 'Bloated irritable bowel syndrome defined by dynamic 99m Tc Bran Scan', *The Lancet*, 1986; 2: 364–6.

Williams, Xandria, *Overcoming Candida*, Element Books, 1998.

Acne
Standard References

Acne Rosacea
Standard References

Ageing
Standard References

Agoraphobia (see **Anxiety**)
Standard References
Burns, L.E., Thorpe, G.L., 'Fears and clinical phobias: epidemiological aspects and the national survey of agoraphobics', *Journal of International Medical Research*, Vol. 5(1), 1977.

Alcoholism
Standard References

Allergy and Intolerance
Standard References
Brostoff, Prof Johnathon, Gamlin, Linda, *The Complete Guide to Food Allergy and Intolerance*, Bloomsbury, 1989.
'Food Intolerance and Food Aversion', Royal College of Physicians and the British Nutrition Foundation, 1984.

Anaemia
Standard References
Lucas, C.A., Logan, E.C.N., Logan, R.A., 'Audit of the investigation and outcome of iron deficiency anaemia in one health district', *Journal of the Royal College of Physicians of London, 1996*; 33–5.

Anxiety
Standared References
Durham, R.C., Allan, T., 'Psychological treatment of generalised anxiety disorder: a review of the clinical significance of results in outcome studies since 1980', *British Journal of Psychology*, 1993; 163: 19–26.

Arthritis and Musculo-skeletal Problems
Standard References
Darlington, G., Gamlin, Linda, *Diet and Arthritis*, Vermilion, 1996.

Asthma, Allergic Rhinitis and Viral Chest Infections
Britton, J. *et al*, 'Dietary magnesium, lung function, wheezing and airway hyper-

reactivity in a random adult population sample', *The Lancet*, 1994; 344: 357–62.

Fantidis, P. *et al*, 'Intercellular (polymorphonuclear) magnesium content in patients with bronchial asthma between attacks', *Journal of the Royal Society of Medicine*, 1995: 441–5.

Kaliner, M., Lemanske, R., 'Rhinitis and asthma', *Journal of the American Medical Association*, 1992; 286: 2807–29.

Peacock, S., Murray, V., Turton, C., 'Respiratory distress and royal jelly', *British Medical Journal*, 1995; 311: 1472.

Platts-Mills, T.A.E., Rakes, G.P., Heymann, P.W., 'Role of viral infections in exacerbations of asthma: allergy must also be a factor', *British Medical Journal* 1995; 311: 629–30.

Royal College of General Practitioners, *Guidelines for the care of patients with asthma*, RCGP Publication, 1993.

Back Pain
Standard References

Breast Pain
Boyd, E.M.F. *et al*, 'The effect of a low-fat, high complex-carbohydrate diet on symptoms of cyclical mastopathy', *The Lancet* 1988; 2: 128–32.

Boyle, C.A. *et al*, 'Caffeine consumption and fibrocystic breast disease: a case control epidemiologic study', *JNCI*, 1984; 72:1015–19.

Gateley, G.A. *et al*, 'Drug treatments for mastalgia: 17 years' experience in the Cardiff mastalgia clinic', *Journal of the Royal Society of Medicine*, 1992; 85: 12–15.

Hughes, L.E. *et al*, *Benign Disorders and Diseases of the Breast*, Baillière Tindal, 1989.

London, R.S. *et al*, 'The effect of alpha-tocopherol on premenstrual symptomatology: a double-blind study 2. Endocrine correlates', *Journal of American College of Nutrition*, 1984; 3: 351–6.

Mansel, R.E., 'Breast Pain, "ABC of Breast Diseases" ', *British Medical Journal*, 1994; 309: 866–8.

Cancer
Stewart, Maryon, *The Phyto Factor*, Vermilion, 2000.

Williams, M.C., Dickerson, J.W.D., 'Nutrition in cancer – some biochemical mechanisms', *Nutrition Research Reviews*, 1990; 3: 75–100.

Candida and Thrush
Standard References

Lipski, Elizabeth, *Digestive Wellness*, Keats, 1996.

Williams, Xandria, *Overcoming Candida*, Element Books, 1998.

Carpal Tunnel Syndrome
Standard References

Cerebrovascular Disease
De Keyser, J., De Kippel, N., Merkx, H., Vervaek, M., Herroelen, L., 'Serum concentrations of vitamins A and E and early outcome after ischaemic stroke', *The Lancet*, 1992; 339: 1562–5.

Coeliac Disease
Standard References

Constipation
Alun Jones, V., McLaughlan, P., Shorthouse, M., Workman, E., Hunter, J.O., 'Food intolerance: a major factor in the pathogenesis of irritable bowel syndrome', *The Lancet*, 1982; 2: 1115–17.

Cann, P.A., Read, N.W., Holdsworth, C.D., 'What is the benefit of wheat bran in patients with irritable bowel syndrome?', *Gut*, 1984; 25: 168–73.

Editorial, 'Constipation in young women', *The Lancet*, 1986; 1: 778–9.

Hojgaard, L., Arffman, S., Jorgensen, M., Kragg, E., 'Tea consumption: a cause of constipation', *British Medical Journal*, 1981; 282: 864.

Letter, 'Food intolerance and irritable bowel syndrome', *The Lancet*, 1983; 2: 633–4.

Preston, D.M., Lennard-Jones, J.E., 'Severe chronic constipation of young women: "idiopathic slow transit constipation" ', *Gut*, 1986; s7: 41–8.

Taylor, R., 'Management of constipation', *British Medical Journal*, 1990; 300: 1065–7.

Turnbull, G.K., Lennard-Jones, J.E., Bartram, C.I., 'Failure of rectal expulsion as a cause of constipation: why fibre and laxatives sometimes fail', *The Lancet*, 1986; 1767–9.

Crohn's Disease
Standard References

Lennard Jones, L.E., 'Nutrition and Crohn's disease', *Annals of the Royal College of Surgeons of England*, 1990; 72: 152–4.

Rampton, S., 'Management of Crohn's disease', *British Medical Journal*, 1999; 319: 1480–5.

Chronic Fatigue Syndrome (see Fatigue
Behan, P., Goldberg, G., Mowbray, J.F., 'Post-viral fatigue syndrome', *British Medical Bulletin*, 47, No. 4, 1991.

Gold, M.S., Pottash, A.L.C., Extein, I., 'Hypothyroidism in depression', *Journal of the American Medical Association*, 1981; 245: 1919–22.

Jenkins, R., Mowbray, W. (eds), *Post-viral Fatigue Syndrome*, John Wiley & Sons, 1990.

Kroenke, K., Wood, D.R., Mangelsdorff, B., Meier, N.J., Powell, J.D., 'Chronic fatigue in primary care', *JAMA*, 1988; 260: 929–34.

Lloyd, A.R., Hickie, Il, Broughton, C.R., Spencer, Ol, Wakefield, D., 'Prevalence of chronic fatigue syndrome in an Australian population', *Medical Journal of Australia*, 1990; 153: 522–8.

Manu, P., Lane, T.J., Matthews, D.A., 'The frequency of chronic fatigue syndrome in patients with persistent fatigue', *Annals of International Medicine*, 1988; 109: 554–6.

Marrie, T.J., Ross, L., Mantague, T.J., Doan, B., 'Post-viral fatigue syndrome', *Clinical Ecology*, 1978; 5: 5–10.

Morrison, J.D., 'Fatigue as a present complaint in family practice', *Journal of Family Practitioners*, 1980; 10: 795–801.

Sharpe, M., Horton, K., Seagrott, B., Pasvol, G., 'Follow up patients presenting with fatigue to an infectious disease clinic', *British Medical Journal*, 1992; 305: 147–52.

Stewart, A., *Tired All the Time*, Vermilion, 1993.

Valdini, A., Steinhardt, S., Feldman, E., 'The usefulness of a standard battery of laboratory tests in investigating chronic fatigue in adults', *Family Practitioner*, 1989; 6: 286–91.

Wood, G.C., Bentall, R.P., Gopfert, N., Edwards, R.H.T., 'The comparative psychiatric assessment of patients with chronic fatigue syndrome and muscle disease', *Psychological Medicine*, 1991; 21: 619–28.

Cystitis
Standard References

Kilmartin, A., *Understanding Cystitis*, Arrow Books, 1989.

Dementia
Standard References

Depression and Mood Swings
Standard References

Dermatitis
Hunter, J.A.A., Herd, R.M., 'Recent advances in atopic dermatitis', *Quarterly Journal of Medicine*, 1994; 87: 323–7.

Diabetes Mellitus
Coelingh Bennink, H.J.T., Schreurs, W.H.P., 'Improvement of oral glucose tolerance in gestational diabetes by pyridoxine', *British Medical Journal*, 1975; 3: 13–15.

McNair, *et al*, 'Hypomagnesemia: a risk factor in diabetic retinopathy', *Diabetes*, 1978; 27: 1075–7.

Moles, K.W., McMullen, J.K., 'Insulin resistance and hypomagnesaemia', case report, *British Medical Journal*, 1982; 285: 262.

Diarrhoea
Arnason, J.A., Gudjonsson, H., Freysodottir, J., Jonsdottir, I., Valdimarsson, H., 'Do adults with high gliadin antibody concentrations have subclinical gluten intolerance?' *Gut*, 1992; 33: 194–7.

Bennett, J.R., Progress report: 'Smoking and the gastrointestinal tract', *Gut*, 1972; 13: 658–65.

Cooper, B.T., Holmes, G.K.T., Ferguson, R.A., Thompson, R.N.A., Cooke, W.T., 'Gluten-sensitve diarrhoea without evidence of coeliac disease', *Gastroenterology*, 1980; 79: 801–6.

Editorial, 'Hastening gut transit', *The Lancet*, 1990; 2: 974.

Editorial, 'Milk fat, diarrhoea and the ileal brake', *The Lancet*, 1986; 2: 658.

Merliss, R.R., Hofman, A., 'Steatorrhoea following the use of antibiotics', *The New England Journal of Medicine*, 1951; 245: 328–30.

Royal College of Physicians, 'Food allergy and intolerance', Report, 1984.

Eating Disorders
Lacey, J.H., 'Bulimia nervosa, binge eating and psychogenic vomiting: a controlled treatment study and long-term outcome', *British Medical Journal*, 1993; 286: 1609–13.

Eczema

Morse, P.F. *et al*, 'Meta-analysis of placebo-controlled studies of the efficacy of Epogam in the treatment of atopic eczema; relationship between essential fatty acid changes and clinical response', *British Journal of Dermatology*, 1989; 121: 75–90.

Sloper, K.S., Wadsworth, J., Brostoff, J., 'Children with atopic eczema. 1: Clinical response to food elimination and subsequent double-blind food challenge', *Quarterly Journal of Medicine*, 1991; 80: 677–93.

Endometriosis (see Pelvic Pain)

Standard References

Dennerstein, L. *et al*, *Hysterectomy, New Options and Advances*, Oxford University Press, 1995.

Lark, Susan, M., M.DE., *Natural Treatment of Fibroid Tumours and Endometriosis – effective natural solutions for relieving heavy bleeding, cramps and infertility that accompany these common female problems*, Keats.

McPherson, Ann, *Women's Problems in General Practice*, Oxford University Press, 1995.

Mills, D., Vernon, M., *Endometriosis – a key to healing through nutrition*, Element Books, 1999.

Eye Problems

Hankinson, S.E. *et al*, 'Nutrient intake in cataract extraction in women: a prospective study', *British Medical Journal*, 1992; 305: 335–9.

Sedden, J.M. et al, 'Dietary carotenoids, vitamin A, vitamin C and E, and advanced age-related macular degeneration', *Journal of the American Medical Association*, 1994; 272: 1413–20.

Fatigue

Behan, P., Goldberg, G., Mowbray, J.F., 'Post-viral fatigue syndrome', *British Medical Bulletin*, 47, No. 4, 1991.

Jenkins, R., Mowbray, W. (eds), *Post-viral Fatigue Syndrome*, John Wiley & Sons, 1990.

Manu, P., Lane, T.J., Matthews, D.A., 'The frequency of chronic fatigue syndrome in patients with persistent fatigue', *Annals of International Medicine*, 1988; 109: 554.

Stewart, A., *Tired All the Time*, Vermilion, 1996.

Fibroids (see Pelvic Pain)

Standard References

Dennerstein, L., Wood, C., Westmore, A., *Hysterectomy – New Options and Advances*, 2nd edition, Oxford University Press, 1995.

Lark, Susan M., M.DE., *Natural Treatment of Fibroid Tumours and Endometriosis – effective natural solutions for relieving heavy bleeding, cramps and infertility that accompany these common femal problems*, Keats.

Fibromyalgia (see Arthritis)

Standard References

Romano, T.J., Stiller, J.W., 'Magnesium deficiency in fibromyalgia', presented at the 7th World Congress of Rheumatology, Paris, Dec. 1993.

Fluid Retention
Standard References

Food Craving
Standard References
Stewart, M., *Beat Sugar Craving*, Vermilion, 1992.

Gallstones
Standard References

Genital Herpes
Standard References
Griffith, R.S., Norrins, R.L., Kagan, C., 'A multi-centred study of lysine therapy in herpes simplex infection', *Dermatologica*, 1978; 156: 257–67.
Oates, J.K., 'Genital herpes', *British Journal of Hospital Medicine*, Jan. 1983; 13–22.

Gout (see Arthritis)
Standard References
Stein, H.B., Hassan, A., Fox, I., 'Ascorbic acid-induced uricosuria', *Annals of International Medicine*, 1976; 84: 385–8.

Haemorrhoids
Standard References

Hair Loss
Standard References

Halitosis
Standard References
Kerr, D.A., Major, M. Ash, Jnr, *Oral Pathology*, Lea & Febiger, 6th edition, Philadelphia, 1992.

Hay Fever (see Asthma)
Standard References

Headaches
Standard References
Verne, S., et al, 'Medical intelligence, current concepts – headache', *The New England Journal of Medicine*, 1980; Vol. 302: 8: 446–50.

Heart Failure
Standard References

High Blood Pressure
Standard References

Hysterectomy
Standard References
Anon, 'Complementary medicine: a popular adjunct', *Montage* (Monash University, Melbourne), 1994; Vol. 4; 5: 15.
Bone, K., 'Vitex agnus castus, scientific studies and clinical applications', Mediherb Newsletter, 1994; 42: 1.

Beecher, H.K., 'The powerful placebo', *Journal of the American Medical Association*, 1995; Vol. 159; 17: 1602–6.

Carlson, K., et al, 'The Maine Women's Health Study. 1: Outcomes of hysterectomy', *Obstetrics and Gynaecology*, 1994; Vol. 83: 556–65.

Dennerstein, L. et al, 'Psychosocial and mental health aspects or women's health', Monograph 1, World Health Organisation, Geneva, 1993.

Dennerstein, L., Wood, C., Westmore, A., *Hysterectomy – New Options and Advances*, Oxford University Press, 1995.

Fraser, I., 'Prostaglandins, prostaglandin inhibitors and menstrual disorders. Part 11: Menorrhagia and premenstrual syndrome', *Health-right*, 1988; 8: 31–5.

Helms, J., 'Acupuncture for the management of primary dysmenorrhea', *Obstetrics and Gynaecology*, Vol. 69; 1: 51–5.

Hirsch, N., 'Technologies for the treatment of menorrhagia and uterine myomas', Australian Institute of Health and Welfare Health Care Technology Series, Canberra, 1993; 10: 1.

Morse, C. *et al*, 'A comparison of hormone therapy, coping skills training, and relaxation for the relief of premenstrual syndrome', *Journal of Behavioural Medicine*, 1991; Vol. 14; 5: 469–89.

Indigestion
Standard References

Infertility

Calloway, D.H., 'Nutrition and reproductive function and men', nutrition abstracts and reviews in *Clinical Nutrition*, Series A, 1983; 53(5): 361–80.

Editorial, 'Declining fertility: egg or uterus?', *The Lancet*, 1991; 338: 285–6.

Hargreave, T.B., 'Non-specific treatment to improve infertility', in *Male Fertility*, ed. Hargreave, T.B., Springer-Verlag, 1983, 227–45.

Healey, D.L., Trounston, A.O., Andersen, A.N., 'Female infertility: causes and treatment', *The Lancet*, 1994; 343: 1539–44.

Rowe, P.J., Comhaire, F.H., Hargreave, T.B., Mellows, H.J., *World Health Organisation Manual for the Standard Investigation and Diagnosis of the Infertile Couple*, Cambridge University Press, 1993.

Skakkebaek, N.E., Giwercman, A., De Krester, D., 'Pathogenesis and management of male infertility', *The Lancet*, 1994; 343: 1473–9.

Influenza, Recurrent Coughs, Colds and Sore Throats
Standard References

Insomnia
Standard References

Coyle, K., Watts, F.N., The factorial structure of sleep dissatisfaction, *Behave Res Ther*, 1991; 29: 315–20.

Ford, D.E., Kamerow, D.B., 'Epidemiological study of sleep disturbances and psychiatric disturbances, *JAMA*, 1989; 262: 1479–84.

Lader, Malcolm (ed), *The Medical Management of Insomnia in General Practice*, Royal Society of Medicine, London, 1992.

Irritable Bowel Syndrome

Connell, A.M., Hilton, C., Irvine, G. et al, 'Variation of bowel habit in two population samples', *British Medical Journal*, 1965; 2: 1095–9.

Danivat, D., Tankeyoon, M., Sritratanaban, A., 'Prevalence of irritable bowel syndrome in a non-Western population', *British Medical Journal*, 1988; 296: 171.

Drossman, D.A., Sandler, R.S., McKee, D.C., Lovitz, A.J., 'Bowel patterns among subjects not seeking health care', *Gastroenterology*, 1982; 83: 529–34.

Heaton, K.W., O'Donnell, L.J.D., Braddon, F.E.M., Mountford, R.A., Hughes, A.O., Cripps, P.J., *Gastroenterology*, 1992, 102: 1962–7.

Isgar, B., Harman, M., Kaye, M.D., Whorwell, P.J., 'Symptoms of irritable bowel syndrome in ulcerative colitis in remission', *Gut*, 1983; 24: 190–2.

Jones, R., Lydeard, S., 'Irritable bowel syndrome in the general population', *British Medical Journal*, 1992; 304: 87–90.

Lipski, E., *Digestive Wellness*, Keats, 1996.

Stewart M., Stewart, Dr Alan, *No More IBS!*, Vermilion, 1997.

Thompson, W.G., 'Irritable bowel syndrome: pathogenesis and management', *The Lancet*, 1993; 341: 1569–72.

Whitehead, W.E. et al, 'Effects of stressful life events on bowel symptoms: subjects with irritable bowel syndrome compared with subjects without bowel dysfunction', *Gut*, 1992; 33: 825–30.

Ischaemic Heart Disease

Haq, I.U., Jackson, P.R., Yeo, W.W., Ramsay, L.E., 'Sheffield risk and treatment table for cholesterol lowering for primary prevention of coronary heart disease', *The Lancet*, 1995; 346: 1467–71.

Stampfer, M.J., Rimm, E.B., 'Epidemiological evidence for vitamin E in the prevention of cardiovascular disease', *American Journal of Nutrition*, 1995; 62 (suppl) 1365S–9S.

Kidney Stones

Standard References

Buck, A.C., Smellie, W.S., Jenkins, A., Meddings, R., James, A., Horrobin, D., 'The treatment of idiopathic recurrent urolithiasis with fish oil and evening primrose oil – a double blind story', 1996, in press.

Libido, Loss of

Standard References

Mastitis

Standard References

Menopause

Adlercreutz, H., Mazur, W. 'Phyto-oestrogens and Western diseases', The Finnish Medical Society DUODECIM, *Annals of Medicine*, 1997, 29: 95–120.

Cowan, M.M., Gregory, L.W., 'Responses of pre- and postmenopausal females to aerobic conditioning', *Medical Science, Sports and Exercise*, 1985; 17: 138–43.

Davies, S, Stewart, A., *Nutritional Medicine*, Pan Books, 1987.

Eden, J. 'Phytoestrogens and the menopause', *Baillière's Clinical Endocrinology and Metabolism*, 1998; 12 (4): 581–7.

France, K., Schofield, M.J., Lee, C., 'Patterns and correlates of hormone replacement therapy use among middle-aged Australian women', *Women's Health*, 1997, Summer: 3 (2): 121–38.

Greist, J.H. *et al*, 'Running as treatment for depression', *Comprehensive Psychiatry*, 1979; 20: 41–3.

Haas, S., Schiff, I., 'Symptoms of oestrogen deficiency', in *The Menopause*, eds Studd, J.W.W., Whitehead, M.I., Blackwell Scientific Publications, 1988; 1–14.

Hunt, K., Vessey, M., McPherson, K., 'Mortality in a cohort of long-term users of hormone replacement therapy: an updated analysis', *British Journal of Obstetrics and Gynaecology*, 1990; 97: 1080–6.

Jacobs, H.S., Loeffler, F.E., 'Postmenopausal hormone replacement therapy', *British Medical Journal*, 1992; 305: 1403–8.

McLaren, H.C., 'Vitamin E and the menopause', *British Medical Journal*, 1949; Dec 17: 1378–81.

MacLennan, A.H., Wilson, D.H., Taylor, A.W., 'Hormone replacement therapies in women at risk of cardiovascular disease and osteoporosis in South Australia in 1997', *Med J Aust*, 1999, Jun 7; 170 (11): 524–7.

Martin, K.A., Freeman, M.W., 'Postmenopausal hormone-replacement therapy', *The New England Journal of Medicine*, 1993; 328: 1115–17.

Mazur, W., 'Phytoestrogen content in foodss', *Baillière's Clinical Endocrinology and Metabolism*, 1998, Dec; 12 (4): 729–42.

Nachtigall, L.B., Nachtigall, M.J., Nachtigall, L.E., 'Nonprescription alternatives to hormone replacement therapy', *The Female Patient*, June 1999, Vol. 24: 45–50.

Notelovitz, M., 'The non-hormonal management of the menopause', in *The Modern Management of the Menopause*, eds Berg, G., Hammer, M., Parthenon Publishing, 1994.

Novogen Ltd, 'Clinical evidence that Novogen product protects against bone and heart disease', Press Release, 24/9/99.

Punnonen, R., Lukola, A., 'Oestrogen-like effect of ginseng', *British Medical Journal*, 1980; 281: 110.

St Clair, R.W., 'Estrogens and Atherosclerosis: phytoestrogens and selective estrogen receptor modulators', *Curr Opin Lipidol*, 1998; 9 (5): 457–63.

Stewart, M. *Cruising Through the Menopause*, Vermilion, 2000.

Stewart, M., Stewart, Dr Alan, *The Phyto Factor*, Vermilion, 2000.

Tham, D. *et al*, 'Potential health benefits of dietary phytoestrogens: a review of the clinical, epidemiological, and mechanistic evidence', *Journal of Clinical Endocrinology and Metabolism*, 1998, 83 (7): 2223–35.

Wilbush, J., 'Climacteric disorders – historical perspectives', in *The Menopause*, eds Studd, J.W.W., Whitehead, M.I., Blackwell Scientific Publications, 1988; 1–14.

Wilcox, G., Wahlqvist, M.L., Burger, H.G., Medley, G., 'Oestrogenic effect of plant foods in postmenopausal women', *British Medical Journal*, 1990; 301: 905.

Wilson, R.C.D., *Understanding HRT and the Menopause*, Consumers' Association, 1992.

Migraine
Buring, J.E., Peto, R., Hennekens, C.H., 'Low-dose aspirin for migraine prophylaxis', *JAMA*, 1990; 264: 1711–13.

Egger, J., Carter, C.M., *et al*, 'Is migraine a food allergy? A double-lind controlled trial of oligoantigenic diet treatment', *The Lancet*, ii, 1983, 865–9.

Egger, J., 'Psychoneurological aspects of food allergy', *European Journal of Clinical Nutrition*, 1991; 45 (Suppl. 1); 35–45.

Epstein, M.T., Hockaday, J.M., Hockaday, T.D.R., 'Migraine and reproductive hormones throughout the menstrual cycle', *The Lancet*, 1975; 543–8.

Grant, E., 'Food allergies in migraine', *The Lancet*, I, 1979: 966–9.

Hannington, E., Jones, R.J. et al, 'Migraine: a platelet disorder', *The Lancet*, ii, 1981: 720–3.

Iversen, H.K., Nielsen, T.H., Olesen, J., Tfelt-Hansen, P., 'Arterial responses during migraine headaches', *The Lancet*, 1990; 336: 837–9.

Kaiser, H.J., Meienberg, O., 'Deterioration or onset of migraine under oestrogen replacement therapy in the menopause', *Journal of Neurology*, 1993; 240: 195–7.

Kew, J., McKeran, R., 'Prophylactic treatment of migraine', *Maternal and Child Health*, 1991: 46–51.

Lance, J.W., 'Treatment of migraine', *The Lancet*, I, 1979: 966–9.

Lockett, D-MC., Campbell, J.F., 'The effects of aerobic exercise on migraine', *Headache*, 1992; 32: 50–4.

Monro, J., Carini, C., Brostoff, J., 'Migraine is a food-allergic disease', *The Lancet*, ii, 1984: 719–21.

Murphy, J.J., Heptinstall, S., Mitchell, J.R.A., 'Randomised double-blind placebo-controlled trial of feverfew in migraine prevention', *The Lancet*, 1988; 189.

Miscarriage

Chard, T., 'Frequency of implantation and early pregnancy loss in natural cycles', *Baillière's Clin Obstet Gynaecol*, 1991; 5: 179–89.

Hay, T.E., Lamont, R.P., Taylor-Robinson, D. *et al*, 'Abnormal bacterial colonization of the genital tract and subsequent pre-term delivery and late miscarriage', *British Medical Journal*, 1994; 308: 295–8.

Katesmark, M., 'Early pregnancy loss', *Maternal & Child Health*, 1996; 21: 4: 84–90.

Kline, J., Shrout, P., Stein, Z.A., 'Drinking during pregnancy and spontaneous abortions', *The Lancet*, 1990; 11: 176–88.

Knudsen, U.B., Hansen, V., Juul, S., Secher, N.J., 'Prognosis of a new pregnancy and spontaneous abortions', *European Journal of Gynaecological Reproductive Biology*, 1991; 29: 31–6.

Regan, L., 'Recurrent miscarriage', *British Medical Journal*, 1991; 302: 543–4.

Tulppala, N. *et al*, 'Thromboxane dominance and prosta-cyclin deficiency in habitual abortion', *The Lancet*, 1991; 337: 879–81.

Warburton, D., fraser, F.C., 'Spontaneous abortion risks in man: data from reproductive histories collected in a medical genetics unit', *Hum Genet*, 1964; 16: 1–25.

Mouth Disorders

Editorial, 'Apthous ulceration', *Journal of the Royal Society of Medicine*, 1994; 77: 1–3.

Ferguson, M.M., 'Disorders of the mouth in clinical practice', *Medicine in Practice*, 1982; Vol. 1: No. 9: 243–7.

Lamey, P.J., Hammond, A., Allam, B.F., McIntosh, W.B., 'Vitamin status of patients with burning mouth syndome and ehe response to replacement therapy', *British Dental Journal*, 1986; 160: 81.

Strean, L.P., Bell, F.T., Gilfillan, E.W., Emerson, G.A., Howe, E.E., 'The importance of pyridoxine in the suppression of dental caries in school children and hamsters', *New York State Dental Journal*, 1958; 24: 133.

Multiple Sclerosis
Standard References

Nail Problems
Standard References

Obesity
Standard References
Garrow, J.S., *Treat Obesity Seriously, A Clinical Manual*, Churchill Livingstone, 1981.

Stewart, M., Stewart, A., *The Vitality Diet*, Optima, 1992.

Osteoarthritis (see Arthritis)
Standard References

Osteoporosis
Berg, G., Hammer, M., eds, *The Modern Management of the Menopause*, Parthenon Publishing, 1994.

Blumsohn, A. et al, 'The effect of calcium supplementation on the circadian rhythm of bone resoption', *Journal of Clinical Endocrinology and Metabolism*, Vol. 79: 730–5.

Buck, A.C., Smellie, W.S., Jenkins, A., Meddings, R., James, A., Horrobin, D., Department of Urology, Glasgow Royal Infirmary, Glasgow, 'The treatment of idiopathic recurrent urolithiasis with fish oil and evening primrose oil – a double blind study', in press

Dixon, A. St J., 'The non-hormonal treatment of osteoporosis', *British Medical Journal*, 1983; 286: 999–1000.

Ettinger, B., Grady, D., 'The waning effect of postmenopausal women', *British Medical Journal*, 1990; 301: 905.

Kanis, J.A. et al, 'Evidence of efficacy of drugs affecting bone metabolism in preventing hip fracture', *British Medical Journal*, 1992; 305: 1124–8.

Liberman, U.A., MD PhD *et al*, 'Effect of oral alendronate on bone mineral density and the incidence of fractures in post meopausal osteoporosis', *The New England Journal of Medicine*, 1995; 333: 1437–43.

Martin, D., Notelovitz, M., 'Effects of aerobic training on bone mineral density of postmenopausal women', *Journal of Bone and Mineral Research*, 1993; 8: 931–6.

Notelovitz, M., 'The non-hormonal management of the menopause', in *The Modern Management of the Menopause*, Berg, G., Hammer, M., eds, Parthenon Publishing, 1994.

Peel, N., Eastell, R., 'Osteoporosis', *British Medical Journal*, 1995; 310: 989–92.

Stewart, M., *Cruising Through the Menopause*, Vermilion, 2000.

Stewart, M., Stewart, Dr Alan, *The Phyto Factor*, Vermilion, 2000.

Studd, John W., Whitehead, Malcolm I., eds, *The Menopause*, Blackwell Scientific Publications, 1988.

Van Papendorp, D.H., Coetzer, H., Kruger, M.C., 'Biochemical profile of osteoporotic patients on essential fatty acid supplementation', Nutrition Research, Vol. 15; No. 3: 325–34.

Wilcox, G. et al, 'Osteogenic effects of plant foods in postmenopausal women', *British Medical Journal*, 1990; 301: 905.

Ovarian Cysts (see Pelvic Pain)
Standard References

Painful Ovulation
Standard References

Palpitations
Standard References

Pancreatic Disease
Standard References

Pelvic Inflammatory Disease (see Pelvic Pain)
Standard References

Peptic Ulcers
Standard References

Period Problems
Standard References

Peripheral Vascular Disease
Standard References

Polycystic Ovaries (see Pelvic Pain)
Standard References

Kiddy, D.S., Hamilton-Fairley, D., Bush, A., Short, F., Anyaoku, V., Reed, M.J., Franks, S., 'Improvements in endocrine and ovarian function during dietary treatment of obese women with polycystic ovary syndrome', *Clinical Endocrinology*, 1992: 36; 105–11.

McCluskey, S.E., Lacey, J.H., Pearce, J.M., 'Binge-eating and polycystic ovaries', *The Lancet*, 1992; 340: 723.

Polson, D.W., Adams, J., Wadsworth, J., Franks, S., 'Polycystic ovaries – a common finding in normal women', *The Lancet*, 1988: 870.

Postnatal Depression (see Anxiety)
Standard References

Dostalova, L., 'Vitamin status during puerperium and lactation', *Annals of Nutrition and Metabolism*, 1984; 28 (6) 385–408.

Riley, D.M., Watt, D.C., 'Hypercalcemia in the etiology of puerperal psychosis', *Society of Biological Psychiatry*, 1985; 20: 479–88.

Preconception

Barker, D.J.P., *Mothers, Babies and Disease in Later Life*, British Medical Journal Publishing Group, 1994.

Barker, D.J.P. et al, 'Foetal nutrition and cardiovascular disease in adult life', *The Lancet*, 1993; 341: 938–41.

Barker, D.J.P. *et al*, 'Weight in infancy and death from ischaemic heart disease', *The Lancet*, 1989; ii: 577–80.

Barker, D.J.P. *et al*, 'The relation of foetal length, ponderal index and head circumference to blood pressure and the risk of hypertension in adult life', *Paediatric and Perinatal Epidemiology*, 1992; 6: 35–44.

Godfrey, K.M. et al, 'Relation of fingerprints and shape of the palm to foetal growth and adult blood pressure', *British Medical Journal*, 1993; 307; 405–9.

Law, C.M. *et al* 'Initiation of hypertension in utero and its amplification throughout life', *British Medical Journal*, 1993; 306: 24–7.

Lucas, A., 'Programming by early nutrition in man', in Bock, G.R., Whelan, J., eds, *The Childhood Environment and Adult Disease*, John Wiley & Sons, 1991; 38–55.

McCance, D.R. *et al*, 'Birthweight and non-insulin dependent diabetes: "thrifty geotype", "thrifty phenotype", or "surviving small baby genotype" ', *British Medical Journal*, 1994; 308: 942–5.

Osmond, C., Barker, D.J.P. *et al*, 'Early growth and death from cardiovascular disease in women', *British Medical Journal*, 1993; 307: 1519–24.

Widdowson, E.M., McCance, R.A., 'A review: new thoughts on growth', *Pediatric Research*, 1975; 9: 154–6.

Wynn, M., Wynn, A., 'New thoughts on maternal nutrition', The Caroline Walker Lecture 1993, Caroline Walker Trust.

Pregnancy

Barker, D.J.P., *Mothers, Babies and Disease in Later Life*, British Medical Journal Publishing Group, 1994.

Chief Medical Officer, *Vitamin A and pregnancy*, Department of Health letters to all doctors, October 1990 and November 1993.

Claoo, J.F., 'The effects of maternal exercise on early pregnancy outcome', *American Journal of Obstetrics and Gynaecology*, 1989; 161: 1453–7.

Czeizel, A.E., 'Periconceptional multivitamin supplementation in prevention of congenital abnormalities', *Maternal and Child Health*, December 1994; 381–4.

Czeizel, A.E. *et al*, 'Smoking during pregnancy and congenital limb deficiency', *British Medical Journal*, 1994; 308: 1473–6.

Dietary Reference Values of Food Energy and Nutrients for the United Kingdom, Department of Health Report of the Panel on Dietary Reference Values of the Committee on Medical Aspects of Food Policy, HMSO, 1991.

Dolan-Mullen, P. et al, 'A meta-analysis of randomized trials of prenatal smoking cessation interventions', *American Journal of Obstetrics and Gynaecology*, 1994; 1328–34.

Editorial, 'Maternal smoking affects blood pressure in offstpring', *Archives of Diseases in Childhood*, 1995; 72: 120–4.

Kirke, P.N., Molloy, A.M., Daly, L.E. *et al*, 'Maternal plasma folate and vitamin

B12 are independent risk factors for neural tube defects', *Quarterly Journal of Medicine*, 1993; 86: 703–8.

Laroque, B. *et al*, 'Effects on birth weight of alcohol and caffeine consumption during pregnancy', *American Journal of Epidemiology*, 1993; 197 (9): 941–50.

McCance, R.A., Widdowson, E.H., *The Composition of Foods*, HMSO, 1976, supplements 1985, 1988, 1989, 1990, 1991 and 1992.

'Routine iron supplements in pregnancy are unnecessary', *British National Formulary*, April 1994.

Spohr, H.L. *et al*, 'Prenatal alcohol exposure and long-term development consequences', *The Lancet*, 1993; 341: 907–10.

Wei, Dr M., 'Foetal loss and caffeine intake', letter to editor, *Journal of the American Medical Association*, 6 July 1994; 272, No. 1.

Premenstrual Syndrome

Ashton, C.H., 'Caffeine and health', *The British Medical Journal*, 1987; 295: 1293–4.

Chakmakjian, Z.H., Higgins, C.E., Abraham, G.E., 'The effect of a nutritional supplement, Optivite, for women with pre-menstrual tension syndromes: 2. The effect of symptomatology, using a double-blind cross-over design', *Journal of Applied Nutrition*, 1986; 37: 1–11.

Green, R., Dalton, K., 'The premenstrual syndrome', *British Medical Journal*, 1953; 1007–14.

Hargrove, J.T., Abraham, G.E., 'The incidence of premenstrual tension in a gynaecologic clinic', *The Journal of Reproductive Medicine*, 1982; 27: 721–4.

Mansel, R.E., Pye, J.K., Hughes, L.E., 'Effects of essential fatty acids on cyclical mastalgia and non-cyclical breast disorders', in Horrobin, D.F. (ed), *Omega-6 Essential Fatty Acids*, Wiley-Liss, 1990; 557–66.

Morton, J.H., Additon, H., Addison, R.G., Hunt, L., Sullivan, J.J., 'A clinical study or premenstrual tension', *American Journal of Obstetrics and Gynaecology*, 1953; 55: 1182–91.

Sherwood, R.A., Rocks, B.F., Stewart, A., Saxton, R.S., 'Magnesium in the premenstrual syndrome', *Annals of Clinical Biochemistry*, 1986; 23: 667–70.

Stewart, M., *Beat PMS Through Diet*, Vermilion, 3rd edition, 1994.

Stewart, M., Stewart, Dr Alan, *No More PMS!*, Vermilion, 1997.

Yudkin, J., *Pure, White and Deadly*, Viking Press, 1986.

Psoriasis

Maurice, P.D.L., Allen, B.R., Barkley, A.S.J., Cockbill, S.R., Stammers, J., Bather, P.C., 'The effects of dietary supplementation with fish oil in patients with psoriasis', *British Journal of Dermatology*, 1987; 117: 599–606.

Menter, A., Barker, J.N.W.N., 'Psoriasis in practice', The Lancet, 1991; 338: 231–4.

Michaelsson, G., Gerden, B., Ottosson, M. et al, 'Patients with psoriasis often have increased serum levels of IgA antibodies to gliadin', *British Journal of Dermatology*, 1993; 129: 667–73.

Rowland Payne, C.M.E., 'Psoriatic science', *British Medical Journal*, 1987; 295: 1158–9.

Raynaud's Disease and Poor Circulation
Standard References

Rheumatoid Arthritis (see Arthritis)
Standard References
O'Farrelly, C. *et al*, 'Association between villous atrophy in rheumatoid arthritis and rheumatoid factor and gliadin-specific IgG', *The Lancet*, 1988; 2: 819–23.
van der Tempel, H. et al, 'The effects of fish oil supplementation in rheumatoid arthritis', *Annals of the Rheumatic Diseases*, 1990; 224: 208–11.

Stress
Guthrie, E., Creed, F., Dawson, D., Tomensen, B., 'A controlled trial of psychological treatment for the irritable bowel syndrome', *Gastroenterology*, 1991; 100: 450–7.
Harvey, R.F., Hinton, R.A., Gunary, R.M., Barry, R.E., 'Individual and group hypnotherapy in the treatment of refractory irritable bowel syndrome', *The Lancet*, 1989; 1: 424–5.
Swedlund, J., Sjoden, L., Ottosson, J.O., Doteval, G., 'Controlled study of psychological treatment for the irritable bowel syndrome', *The Lancet*, 1983; 2: 589–91.
Whorwell, P.J., Prior, A., Colgan, S.M., 'Hypnotherapy in severe irritable bowel syndrome: further experience', *Gut*, 1987; 28: 423–5.

Thyroid Disease
Standard References

Tonsillitis
Standard References

Ulcerative Colitis
Standard References

Urticaria
Standard References
Greaves, M., 'Allergy and the skin – urticaria', *BMJ*, 1998; 316: 1147.

Vaginal Problems
Standard References
Witkins, S.S., Jeremias, J., Ledger, W.J., 'Recurrent vaginitis as a result of sexual transmission of IgE antibodies', *American Journal of Obstetrics and Gynaecology*, 1988; 159: 32–6.

Varicose Veins
Standard References

Further Help and Telephone Advice Lines

If you would like to attend one of the WNAS clinics or need further details about our telephone and postal courses of treatment, you can write to the WNAS at the address below with a large self-addressed envelope and four separate first-class stamps. Please state clearly what you require information about as we receive requests for so many different conditions. The address to write to is:

Women's Nutritional Advisory Service
PO Box 268
Lewes
East Sussex BN7 2QN
Telephone: 01273 487366   Fax: 01273 487576
email: wnas@wnas.org.uk   http://www.wnas.org.uk

We also have a number of advice lines you may be interested in listening to:

THE WNAS ADVICE LINE DIRECTORY	**09062 556615**
Overcome PMS naturally	09062 556600
The PMS diet line	09062 556601
Overcome menopause symptoms naturally	09062 556602
The menopause diet line	09062 556603
Beat sugar craving	09062 556604
Rediscover your zest for life	09062 556605
Overcoming breast tenderness	09062 556606
Overcoming period pain naturally	09062 556607
Get fit for pregnancy & breastfeeding	09062 556608
Skin, nail & hair signs of deficiency	09062 556609
Improve libido naturally	09062 556610
Beat irritable bowel syndrome	09062 556611
Overcome fatigue	09062 556612
Beat migraine naturally	09062 556613
Overcome ovulation pain	09062 556614
Preventing osteoporosis	09062 556644
Self-help for preventing arthritis	09062 556645
Addressing heart diease naturally	09062 556646
Overcoming constipation naturally	09062 556647
Detecting and dealing with allergies	09062 556648

Appendix V
Useful Addresses (UK)

AAA (Action Against Allergy)
PO Box 278
Twickenham TW1 4QQ
020 8892 2711

ACCEPT Clinic
724 Fulham Road
London SW6 5SE
020 7371 7477

Action for ME
PO Box 1302
Wells
Somerset BA5 1YE
01749 670799
Helpline: 0891 122976

Age Concern
Astral House
1268 London Road
London SW16 4ER
020 8679 8000

Al-Anon Family Groups
61 Great Dover Street
London SE1 4YF
020 7403 0888

Albany Trust Counselling
St Paul's Centre
Rossmore Road
London NW1 6NJ
020 8767 1827

Alcohol Concern
Waterbridge House
32–36 Loman Street
London SE1 0EE
020 7928 7377

Alcohol Counselling Prevention Services
34 Electric Lane
London SW9 8JT
020 7737 3579

Alcoholics Anonymous (AA)
General Services Office
PO Box 1
Stonebow House
York YO1 7NJ
0845 769 7555

Allan Sweeney International Reiki and Healing Training Centre
10 Beech Houses
Royal Crescent
Margate
Kent CT9 5AL
01843 230377
www.reiki-healing.com

Allergycare
Health Screening Ltd
1 Church Square
Taunton
Somerset TA1 1SA
01823 325023

Amarant Trust
Gainsborough Clinic
80 Lambeth Road
London SE1 7PW
01293 413000

Anorexia and Bulimia Care
PO Box 30
Ormskirk
Lancashire L39 5JR
01695 422479

Anti-natal Results and Choices
73–75 Charlotte Street
London W1P 4DE
020 7631 0285

Arthritic Association
1st Floor Suite
2 Hyde Gardens
Eastbourne
East Sussex BN21 4PW
020 7491 0233

Arthritis and Rheumatism Council for Research (ARC)
Copeman House
St Mary's Court
St Mary's Gate
Chesterfield
Derbyshire S41 7TD
01246 558033

Arthritis Care
18 Stephenson Way
London NW1 2HD
020 7916 1500

Action on Smoking and Health (ASH)
102 Clifton Street
London EC2A 4HW
020 7840 8300

Association for Post-Natal Illness
25 Jerdan Place
London SW6 1BE
020 7386 0868

**Association for Spina Bifida and
Hydrocephalus**
ASBAH House
42 Park Road
Peterborough
Cambs PE1 2UQ
01733 555988

Association of Breast-feeding Mothers
PO Box 271
Bridgewater TA67 7YT
020 7813 1481

Association of Radical Midwives
62 Greetby Hill
Ormskirk
Lancashire L39 2DT
01695 572776

BACUP
3 Bath Place
Rivington Street
London EC2A 3JR
020 7696 9003
Info.Service: 020 7696 9003

**Bedford and Northampton MS Therapy
Centre**
Bradbury House
155 Barkers Lane
Bedford MK41 9RX
01234 325781

Bliss Baby Life-support Systems
2nd Floor
Camelsord House
89 Albert Embankment
London SE1 72P
020 7820 9471

Breast Cancer Care
Kiln House
210 New Kings Road
London SW6 4NZ
020 7384 2984
Helpline: 080 8800 6000

Bristol Cancer Help Centre
Grove House
Cornwallis Grove
Clifton
Bristol BS8 4PG
0117 980 9500

British Acupuncture Council
63 Jedda Road
London W12 9HQ
020 8735 0400

British Association for Counselling
1 Regent Place
Rugby
Warwickshire CV21 2PJ
01788 550899

**British College of Naturopathy and
Osteopathy**
Lief House
Fumpter Close
120–122 Finchley Road
London NW3 5HR
020 7435 6464

British Diabetic Association
10 Queen Anne Street
London
W1G 9LH
020 7323 1531

British Dyslexia Association
98 London Road
Reading
Berks RG1 5AU
0118 966 2677

British Epilepsy Association
New Anstey House
Gateway Drive
Yeadon
Leeds LS19 7XY
0113 210 8800

British Heart Foundation
14 Fitzhardinge Street
London W1H 6DH
020 7935 0185

British Homeopathic Association
27A Devonshire Street
London W1N 1RJ
020 7935 2163

British Hypnotherapy Association
9 Upper Berkeley Street
London W1H 7DH
020 7723 4443

British Kidney Patient Association (BKPA)
Bordon
Hants GU35 9JZ
01420 472021

British League Against Rheumatism
41 Eagle Street
London WC1R 4TL
020 7242 3313

British Migraine Association
178A High Road
West Byfleet
Surrey KT14 7ED
01932 352468

British Osteopathic Association
8–10 Boston Place
London NW1 6QH
020 7262 1128

British Pregnancy Advisory Service
Austy Manor
Wootton Wawen
Solihull
West Midlands B95 6BX
01564 793225

British School of Osteopathy
Administration and Clinics
275 Borough High Street
London SE1 1JE
020 7930 9254

British Society for Allergy and Clinical
Immunology
66 Western Park
Thames Ditton
Surrey KT7 0HL
020 8398 9240

British Society for Haematology
2 Carlton House Terrace
London SW1Y 5AF
020 8643 7305

British Society of Allergy and
Environmental Medicine
PO Box 7
Knighton RD7 1WT
01703 812124

British Wheel of Yoga
1 Hamilton Place
Boston Road
Sleaford
Lincolnshire NG34 7ES
01529 306851

Brook Advisory Centre
165 Grays Inn Road
London WC1X 8UD
0800 018 5023

Cancer Care Society
Jane Scarth House
39 The hundred
Romsey SO51 8GE
01179 427419

Cancer Link
11–21 Northdown Street
London N1 9BN
080 8808 0000

Cancer Relief Macmillan Fund
89 Albert Embankment
London SE17 EQ
020 7840 7840

Chest, Heart and Stroke Association
123–127 Whitecross Street
London EC1Y 8JJ
020 7490 7999

Coeliac Society
PO Box 220
High Wycombe
Bucks HP11 2HY
01494 437278

College of Health
St Margaret's House
21 Old Ford Road
London E2 9PL
020 8983 1225

College of Traditional Chinese
Acupuncture
Tao House
Queensway
Leamington Spa
Warwickshire CV31 3LZ
01926 422121

Coronary Prevention Group
2 Faviton Street
London WC1H 0BT
020 7935 2889

Cranial Osteopathic Association
478 Baker Street
Enfield
Middlesex EN1 3QS
020 8367 5561

Cruse Bereavment Care
Cruse House
126 Sheen Road
Richmond
Surrey TW9 1UR
020 8940 4818

Cystic Fibrosis Research Trust
11 London Road
Bromley
Kent BR1 1BY
020 8464 7211

Daisy Chain Network
PO Box 392
High Wycombe
Buckinghamshire HP27 0AE
www.daisychain.org.uk

Depression Alliance
35 Westminster Bridge Road
London SE1 7JP
020 7633 0557

Down's Syndrome Association
155 Mitcham Road
London SW17 9PG
020 8682 4001

Drugaid
16 Clive Street
Caerphilly CF83 1GE
0292 088 1000

Eating Disorders Association
1st Floor
Wensum House
103 Prince of Wales Road
Norwich
Norfolk NR1 1DW
01603 621414

European School of Osteopathy
Boxley House
The Street
Boxley
Maidstone ME14 302
01622 671558

Family Planning Association
2–12 Pentonville Road
London N1 9FP
020 7837 4044

Foresight Association for the Promotion of Pre-conceptual Care
28 The Paddock
Godalming
Surrey GU7 1XD
01483 427839

Friends of the Earth Ltd
26–28 Underwood Street
London N1 7JQ
020 7490 1555

General Council and Register of Naturopaths
Goswell House
Street
Somerset BA16 0JG
01458 840072

General Osteopathic Council
176 Tower Bridge Road
London SE1 3LU
020 7357 6655

Gingerbread
16–17 Clerkenwell Close
London EC1R OAP
020 7336 8183

Gullain-Barre Syndrome Support Group
Lincolnshire County Council Offices
Eastgate
Sleaford
Lincs NG34 7EB
01529 304615

Headway – National Head Injuries Association Ltd
4 King Edward Court
King Edward Street
Nottingham NG1 1EW
0115 924 0800

Help for Health Trust
The College of Health
St Margarets House
21 Old Ford Road
London E2 9PL
0115 924 0800

Henry Doubleday Research Association (HDRA)
Ryton Organic Gardens
Ryton on Dunsmore
Coventry CV8 3LG
01203 305517

Herpes Viruses Association
41 North Road
London N7 9DP
020 7609 9061

Homeopathic Development Foundation
19A Cavendish Square
London W1M 9AD
020 7629 3205

Hyperactive Children Support Group
71 Whyke Lane
Chichester
West Sussex PO19 2LD
01903 725182

**Institute for Complementary Medicine
(ICM)**
21 Portland Place
London W1N 3AF
020 7237 5165

International Cerebral Palsy Society
19 St Mary's Grove
London W4 3LL
020 8994 6386

**International Planned Parenthood
Federation**
Regent's College
Inner Circle
Regent's Park
London NW1 4NS
020 7487 7900

La Léche League of Britain
BM 3424
London WC1N 3XX
020 7242 1278

LIFE
Life House
Newbold Terrace
Leamington Spa
Warwickshire CV32 4EA
01926 311511

London Food Commission
3rd Floor
5–11 Worship Street
London EC2A 2BH
020 7837 2250

London Marriage Guidance Council
76A New Cavendish Street
London W1M 7LB
020 7580 1087

Lupus UK
St James House
Romford
Essex RM1 3NH
01708 731251

Margaret Pyke Centre
73 Charlotte Street
London W1P 1LB
020 7530 3600

Marie Curie Cancer Foundation
89 Albert Embankment
London SE1 7TP
020 7599 7777

Marriage Care
Clitherow House
1 Blythe Mews
Blythe Road
London W14 0NW
020 7371 1341

Maternity Alliance
45 Beech Street
London EC2P 1LX
020 7588 8582

Medau Society
8B Robson House
East Street
Epsom
Surrey KT17 1HH
01372 729056

**MENCAP (Royal Society for Mentally
Handicapped Children and Adults)**
MENCAP National Centre
123 Golden Lane
London EC1Y 0RT
020 7454 0454

Migraine Trust
45 Great Ormond Street
London WC1N 3HZ
020 7831 4818

MIND
15–19 Broadway
Stratford
London WC1N 4BO
020 8519 2122

Miscarriage Association
c/o Clayton Hospital
Northgate
Wakefield
West Yorkshire WF1 3JS
01924 200799

Motor Neurone Disease Association
PO Box 246
Northampton NN1 2PR
01604 250505

Multiple Sclerosis Society
25 Effie Road
London SW6 1EE
020 7610 7171

Muscular Dystrophy Group of Great Britain and Northern Ireland
7–11 Prescott Place
Clapham
London SW4 6BS
020 7720 8055

Myalgic Encephalomyelitis Association
Stanhope House
High Street
Stanford–le-Hope
Essex SS17 0HA
01375 642466

National Abortion Campaign
The Print House
18 Ashwin Street
London E8 3DL
020 7923 4976

National Aids Helpline
0800 567123

National Ankylosing Spondylitis Society
PO Box 179
Mayfield
East Sussex TN20 6ZL
01435 873527

National Association for Colitis and Crohn's Disease
PO Box 205
St Albans
Herts AL1 1AB
01727 844296

National Association for the Relief of Paget's Disease
323 Manchester Road
Walkden
Worsley
Manchester M28 3HH
0161 799 4646

National Asthma Campaign
Providence House
Providence Place
London N1 0NT
020 7226 2260

National Back Pain Association
16 Elm Tree Road
Teddington
Middlesex TW1 8ST
020 8977 5474/5

National Childbirth Trust
Alexandra House
Oldham Terrace
London W3 6NH
020 8922 8637

National Council for One-Parent Families
255 Kentish Town Road
London NW5 2LX
0800 018 5026

National Eczema Society
163 Eversholt Street
London NW1 1BU
0870 241 3604

National Endometriosis Society
Suite 50
Westminster Palace Gardens
1–7 Artillery Row
London SW1R 1RL
020 7222 2776

National Federation of Spiritual Healers
Old Manor Farm Studio
Church Street
Sunbury-on-Thames
Middlesex TW16 6RG
01932 783164/5

National Institute of Medical Herbalists
56 Longbrook Street
Exeter
Devon EX4 6AH
01392 426022

National Kidney Federation
6 Stanley Street
Worksop
Nottinghamshire S81 7HX
01909 487795

National Society for Research into Allergy
2 Armadale Road
Hollycroft
Leicestershire LE10 0SZ
01455 250715

Natural Family Planning Centre
Birmingham Maternity Hospital
Queen Elizabeth Medical Centre
Edgbaston
Birmingham B15 2TG
0121 627 2698

Nature Cure Clinic
15 Oldbury Place
London W1M 3AL
020 7935 6213

Pain Society
(The British & Irish Chapter of the International Association for the Study of Pain)
9 Bedford Square
London WC1B 3RA
020 7631 1650

Parkinson's Disease Society
215 Vauxhall Bridge Road
London SW1V 1EJ
020 7931 8080

Patients Association
8 Guildford Street
London WC1N 1DT
0845 608 4455

Phobics Society
Xion Centre
Royce Road
Hulme
Manchester M15 5FQ
0161 227 9898

**Positively Women's Nutritional Advisory
Service**
347–349 City Road
London EC1V 1LR
020 7713 0222

Pregnancy Advisory Service
26 Bedford Square
London WC1B 3HH
020 7637 8962

Psoriasis Association
7 Milton Street
Northampton NN2 7JG
01604 711129

QUIT
Victory House
170 Tottenham Court Road
London W1P 0HA
020 7487 3000

Rape Crisis Centre
PO Box 69
London
WC1X 9NJ
Emergency no. 020 7837 1600
(6–10pm and weekends only)

Raynaud's and Scleroderma Association
112 Crewe Road
Alsager
Cheshire ST7 2JA
01270 872776

Relate
Herbert Gray College
Little Church Street
Rugby
Warwickshire CV21 3AP
01788 573241

Release
388 Old Street
London EC1V 9LT
020 7729 9904

**Royal National Institute for the Blind
(RNIB)**
224 Great Portland Street
London EC1Y 8SL
020 7296 8000

Samaritans
10 The Grove
Slough
Berkshire SL1 1QP
01753 532713

Sanity
63 Cole Park Road
Twickenham
Middlesex TW1 1HT
020 8892 3924

Schizophrenia Association of Great Britain
Bryn Hyfryd
The Crescent
Bangor
Gwynedd LL57 2AG
01248 354048

School of Phytotherapy (Herbal Medicine)
Bucksteep Manor
Bodle Street Green
Nr Hailsham
East Sussex BN27 4RJ
01323 833812/4

**Sexual and Personal Relationships of the
Disabled**
286 Camden Road
London N7 0BJ
020 7607 8851

Shiatsu Society
31 Pullman Lane
Godalming
Surrey GU7 1XY
01788 555051
Admin@shiatsu.org.uk

Sir Michael Sobell House
(Study Centre Coordinator)
Churchill Hospital
Headington
Oxford OX3 7LJ
01865 225860

Society of Teachers of the Alexander Technique
20 London House
266 Fulham Road
London SW10 9EL
020 7284 3338
www.stat.org.uk

SCOPE
6 Market Road
London N7 9PW
020 7619 7100

Spinal Injuries Association
76 James's Lane
London N10 3DF
020 84442 121

Sports England
16 Upper Woburn Place
London WC1H 0QP
020 7273 1500

Stillbirth and Neonatal Deaths Society
28 Portland Street
London W1N 4DE
020 7436 5881

Support after Termination of Pregnancy for Abnormality
73–75 Charlotte Street
London W1P 1LB
020 7631 0285

Terence Higgins Trust
52–54 Grays Inn Road
London WC1X 8JU
020 7831 0330
Helpline 020 7242 1010

The Breast Care and Mastectomy Association of Great Britain (BCMA)
26 Harrison Street
London WC1 8JG
080 8800 6000

Tinnitus Support Services
19–23 Featherstone Street
London EC1Y 8SL
020 7296 8000

Toxoplasmosis Trust
Room 26
61–71 Collier Street
London N1 9BE
Helpline: 020 7713 0599

UK Thalassaemia Society
9 The Broadway
London N14 6PH
020 8882 0011

Tranx (UK) Ltd
National Tranquilliser Advice Centre
Registered Office
25a Masons Avenue
Wealdstone
Harrow
Middlesex HA3 5AH
020 8427 2065 (client line)
020 8427 2827 24hr answering service

Vegan Society
Donald Watson House
7 Battle Road
St Leonards on Sea
East Sussex TN3Y 7AA
01424 427393

Vegetarian Society
Parkdale
Dunham Road
Altrincham
Cheshire WA14 4QG
0161 9280793

Verity
52–42 Featherstone Street
London EC1Y 8RT
020 7251 9009
www.verity-pcos.org.uk

WellBeing
27 Sussex Place
Regent's Park
London NW1 4SP
020 7723 9296

Westminster Drug Project
470 Harrow Road
London W9 3RU
020 7286 3339

Women's Health
52 Featherstone Street
London EC1Y 8RT
020 7251 6580

Women's National Cancer Control Campaign
Souna House
128–130 Curtain Road
London EC2A 3AR
020 7729 1735

Women's Nutritional Advisory Service (WNAS)
PO Box 268
Lewes
East Sussex BN7 1QN
01273 487366
e-mail wnas@wnas.org.uk
www.wnas.org.uk

Women's Therapy Centre
6–9 Manor Gardens
London N7 6LA
020 7263 6200

YMCA
112 Great Russell Street
London WC1B 3NQ
020 7637 8131

Yoga for Health Foundation
Ickwell Bury
Biggleswade
Bedfordshire SG18 9EF
01767 627271

Index

Main references are indicated in **bold**.